CORONARY BLOOD FLOW
Mechanics, Distribution, and Control

Developments in Cardiovascular Medicine

VOLUME 124

The titles published in this series are listed at the end of this volume.

CORONARY BLOOD FLOW
Mechanics, Distribution, and Control

by

JOS A. E. SPAAN
*Professor of Medical Physics,
Cardiovascular Research Institute Amsterdam (CRIA),
Amsterdam, The Netherlands*

KLUWER ACADEMIC PUBLISHERS
DORDRECHT / BOSTON / LONDON

Library of Congress Cataloging-in-Publication Data

```
Spaan, Jos A. E.
    Coronary blood flow : mechanics, distribution, and control / Jos
A.E. Spaan.
    p.   cm. -- (Developments in cardiovascular medicine ; v. 124)
    Includes bibliographical references and indexes.
    ISBN 0-7923-1210-4 (HB : alk. paper)
    1. Coronary circulation.    I. Title.   II. Series.
    [DNLM: 1. Blood Flow Velocity.  2. Coronary Circulation.    W1
DE997VME v. 124 / WG 300 S7337c]
QP108.S62    1991
612.1'7--dc20
DNLM/DLC
for Library of Congress                                         91-7047
```

ISBN 0-7923-1210-4

Published by Kluwer Academic Publishers,
P.O. Box 17, 3300 AA Dordrecht, The Netherlands.

Kluwer Academic Publishers incorporates
the publishing programmes of
D. Reidel, Martinus Nijhoff, Dr W. Junk and MTP Press.

Sold and distributed in the U.S.A. and Canada
by Kluwer Academic Publishers,
101 Philip Drive, Norwell, MA 02061, U.S.A.

In all other countries, sold and distributed
by Kluwer Academic Publishers Group,
P.O. Box 322, 3300 AH Dordrecht, The Netherlands.

Printed on acid-free paper

All Rights Reserved
© 1991 Kluwer Academic Publishers
No part of the material protected by this copyright notice may be reproduced or
utilized in any form or by any means, electronic or mechanical,
including photocopying, recording or by any information storage and
retrieval system, without written permission from the copyright owner.

Printed in the Netherlands

Layout and typesetting: BOB VAN DER LINDEN

Cover picture: Vessels sprouting from subepicardial capillary network
    feeding epicardial fat.
    Made by: drs. M.M. Stork at CVRI, San Francisco

With contributions by:

Jenny Dankelman, Maurice J.M.M. Giezeman, Yves Han,
Ed van Bavel, Jan Verburg, Isabelle Vergroesen,
and Peter A, Wieringa

To my lovely daugthers

Tjitske
and
Nienke

With respect to my Teachers in Science

Pieter C. Veenstra
Ferdinand Kreuzer
John D. Laird

Contents

Foreword by JIE Hoffman   XVII

Author's preface   XIX

Acknowledgements   XXIII

1 **Basic coronary physiology**   1
  1.1 Introduction 1
      1.1.1 Heart function and coronary flow 1
      1.1.2 Control and extravascular resistance 2
      1.1.3 Distribution of supply and demand 3
      1.1.4 Mechanics, control and distribution in the coronary circulation 4
  1.2 Coronary flow mechanics 5
      1.2.1 Inhibition of coronary arterial flow during systole 6
      1.2.2 Retrograde coronary arterial flow, venous flow and intramyocardial compliance 8
  1.3 Regulation of coronary flow 12
      1.3.1 Steady local control of coronary flow 12
      1.3.2 How to define coronary tone? 14
      1.3.3 Rate of adaptation of the coronary circulation to step changes in heart rate 17
      1.3.4 Effect of perfusion pressure step 19
      1.3.5 Reactive hyperemia 20
      1.3.6 Mechanisms of coronary flow control 21
  1.4 Heterogeneity in myocardial perfusion and oxygen supply 24
      1.4.1 Distribution of flow from endocardium to epicardium 24
      1.4.2 Heterogeneity induced by the arterial tree 26
      1.4.3 Heterogeneity of oxygen supply/demand ratio 28
  1.5 Relation between mechanics, control and distribution of coronary flow 28

	1.6	Summary	30
	References		30
2	**Structure and function of the coronary arterial tree**		**37**
	2.1	Basic anatomy	38
	2.2	Collaterals	40
	2.3	Structure of the coronary arterial tree	40
		2.3.1 Ratios between diameters of mother and daughter branches	41
		2.3.2 Growth of arterial cross-sectional area	43
		2.3.3 Length distribution in the arterial tree	44
		2.3.4 Arterial density applying symmetrical branching networks	46
	2.4	Data on filling volume of the coronary arterial tree	49
	2.5	Pressure distribution in the coronary arterial tree	49
	2.6	Symmetrical, dichotomous branching network model	51
		2.6.1 Definition of model structure	52
		2.6.2 Prediction of volume	53
		2.6.3 Prediction of pressure	54
	2.7	Nonsymmetrical dichotomous branching network analysis	58
		2.7.1 Strahler ordering	58
		2.7.2 Fractal models	60
	2.8	Discussion on structure and function of the arterial tree	62
	2.9	Summary	63
	References		64
3	**Structure and perfusion of the capillary bed**		**69**
	3.1	Structure of capillary bed	69
	3.2	Capillary density and volume	70
	3.3	Mechanical properties	72
	3.4	Red cells in the capillary bed	74
		3.4.1 Velocities	74
		3.4.2 Red cell distribution at bifurcations	74
		3.4.3 Hematocrit	76
	3.5	Model of parallel and homogeneous perfused capillary bed	77
	3.6	A model for the heterogeneous perfusion of the capillary bed	79
	3.7	Capillary recruitment in the heart	82
	3.8	Summary	83
	References		84
4	**Structure and function of coronary venous system**		**87**
	4.1	Basic anatomy	87
	4.2	Distribution of coronary venous flow	89
	4.3	Flow and pressure waves in the epicardial veins	92
	4.4	Waterfall behavior of coronary epicardial veins	95

	4.5 Coronary venous compliance	95
	4.6 Summary	96
	References	96

5 Linear system analysis applied to the coronary circulation — 99
5.1 Definitions 100
    5.1.1 System 100
    5.1.2 Linearity 101
    5.1.3 Time and frequency domains 103
    5.1.4 Models 103
    5.1.5 Load line analysis 104
5.2 Linear intramyocardial pump model 106
    5.2.1 Interpretation of the coronary load lines 107
    5.2.2 Intramyocardial pump and the right coronary artery . . . 111
    5.2.3 Shortcomings of the linear intramyocardial pump model . . 111
5.3 Load line analysis of collateral flow 111
5.4 Input impedance 115
    5.4.1 Input impedance during long diastoles 115
    5.4.2 Coronary impulse response in diastole and systole 117
    5.4.3 Model interpretation of coronary input impedance 118
5.5 Nonlinear physical elements and linear
    system analysis 122
5.6 Discussions of the linear models of coronary circulation 125
5.7 Summary 126
References 127

6 Interaction between contraction and coronary flow: Theory — 131
6.1 Systolic extravascular resistance model 132
    6.1.1 Basic behavior of extravascular resistance model 134
    6.1.2 Discussion of extravascular resistance model 134
6.2 The waterfall model 135
    6.2.1 Basic model behavior of the waterfall model 137
6.3 Nonlinear intramyocardial pump model 140
    6.3.1 Pressure dependency of compartmental resistance 142
    6.3.2 Steady state arterial pressure–flow relations during arrest . 144
    6.3.3 Solutions for the subendocardial model layer of the contracting myocardium 146
    6.3.4 Compartmental volume variations 147
    6.3.5 Flow simulations 149
6.4 Variable elastance model 151
    6.4.1 Experimental support 151
    6.4.2 Variable elastance concept 151

　　　　6.4.3　A mathematical intramyocardial pump model with time varying elastance as pump generator 155
　　6.5　Discussion 159
　　6.6　Summary 160
　　References 161

7　Interaction between contraction and coronary flow: Experiment 163
　　7.1　Parallel shift of pressure–flow relations 164
　　7.2　Pressure dependency of coronary resistance 166
　　7.3　Effect of heart rate on microsphere distribution 168
　　7.4　Contractility and microsphere distribution 172
　　7.5　Intramyocardial compliance 174
　　7.6　Pulsations in coronary pressure at constant flow perfusion 178
　　7.7　Diastolic pressure–flow lines 180
　　7.8　Discussion 186
　　7.9　Summary 187
　　References 188

8　Arteriolar mechanics and control of flow　　193
　　8.1　Morphology of the arteriolar wall 194
　　8.2　Myogenic response 195
　　8.3　Arteriolar vasomotion 198
　　8.4　Strain and stress in the arteriolar wall 200
　　8.5　Myogenic responses in relation to autoregulation of flow 205
　　　　8.5.1　Relation between pressure and resistance with and without myogenic tone 206
　　　　8.5.2　Width of the autoregulatory plateau 206
　　　　8.5.3　The optimal strength of myogenic tone 208
　　8.6　Compliance of arterioles 210
　　　　8.6.1　Effect of tone on static compliance 210
　　　　8.6.2　Quasi–static distensibility of dilated coronary arteries . . . 212
　　　　8.6.3　Frequency dependency of distensibility of active and passive small coronary arteries 212
　　8.7　Discussion 214
　　　　8.7.1　Vasodilation 214
　　　　8.7.2　Arterioles and regulation of flow 215
　　8.8　Summary 216
　　References 217

9 Static and dynamic analysis of local control of coronary flow — 219
- 9.1 Introduction — 219
- 9.2 Steady state behavior of flow control — 221
- 9.3 Characteristics of dynamic coronary flow control — 222
  - 9.3.1 Rate of change in flow adaptation — 224
  - 9.3.2 Rate of change of autoregulation — 225
  - 9.3.3 Summary of t_{50} values — 226
- 9.4 Rate of change in myocardial oxygen consumption — 228
  - 9.4.1 Model for the correction of changing oxygen buffers — 228
  - 9.4.2 Transients in oxygen consumption — 230
- 9.5 Oxygen model of coronary flow control — 232
  - 9.5.1 Model definition and equations — 232
  - 9.5.2 Steady state solutions — 233
  - 9.5.3 Dynamic solutions of the oxygen model — 234
  - 9.5.4 Oxygen dose–response curves — 236
- 9.6 Myocardial contraction and dynamics of coronary flow control — 238
- 9.7 The directional effect in dynamic responses of autoregulation — 241
- 9.8 Myogenic response in the coronary circulation — 242
- 9.9 Adenosine model — 243
  - 9.9.1 Adenosine dose–response curves — 245
  - 9.9.2 Experimental evidence for and against the adenosine hypothesis — 247
- 9.10 Discussion — 247
  - 9.10.1 Adaptation of coronary flow in animals and humans — 247
  - 9.10.2 Evaluation of pharmacological coronary vasodilators — 249
  - 9.10.3 Flow adaptation and oxygen extraction — 250
  - 9.10.4 Integration of different possible mechanisms for controlling coronary flow — 251
  - 9.10.5 The use of models on flow control — 253
- 9.11 Summary — 254
- References — 255

10 Water balance within the myocardium — 261
- 10.1 Introduction — 261
- 10.2 Myocardial interstitium and lymph — 263
- 10.3 Transport of water and proteins across the capillary membrane — 266
  - 10.3.1 Routes — 266
  - 10.3.2 Driving forces — 267
  - 10.3.3 Lymph flow and protein concentration — 268
- 10.4 Dynamic changes in interstitial volume and pressure — 270
  - 10.4.1 Heart weight and vascular volume experiments — 271
  - 10.4.2 Lymphatic pressure — 274

10.5 Numbers on permeability, surface area and reflection coefficients . 276
10.6 Compliance of the interstitial space 276
10.7 Transcapillary water transport and cardiac contraction 277
     10.7.1 Waterfall model and linear intramyocardial pump model:
           effect of coronary arterial pressure 279
     10.7.2 Nonlinear intramyocardial pump model: the effect of arterial pressure 281
     10.7.3 Simulated transmural pressure as function of heart rate at constant arterial pressure 282
10.8 Discussion 284
     10.8.1 Transmural differences in water balance 284
     10.8.2 Stabilizing mechanisms in transmural capillary pressure . . 285
     10.8.3 Tissue pressure versus time varying elastance and water balance 286
10.9 Summary 286
References 287

11 Oxygen exchange between blood and tissue in the myocardium 291
11.1 Introduction 291
11.2 Experimental data on oxygen distribution in the myocardium . . . 293
11.3 Oxygen transfer from a single capillary without intercapillary exchange 296
     11.3.1 Krogh solution 298
     11.3.2 Maximal radius of the Krogh cylinder 300
     11.3.3 General solution to the Krogh problem 302
     11.3.4 Decrease of oxygen partial pressure in a perfused capillary applying the Krogh model 303
11.4 Capillary interaction with blood–tissue oxygen exchange 304
     11.4.1 Oxygen pressure distribution 305
     11.4.2 Average oxygen pressures in tissue units and oxygen flow through these 308
     11.4.3 Tissue oxygen distribution in a network model inducing heterogeneous capillary flow 309
     11.4.4 Oxygen histograms 310
     11.4.5 Oxygen pressure history of a red cell travelling through the capillary network 313
11.5 Oxygen diffusion from the ventricular cavity and thoracic space . . 315
11.6 Effect of oxygen consumption localized in the mitochondria 317
     11.6.1 Equations 318
     11.6.2 Effect of mitochondrial oxygen consumption on oxygen pressure distribution 320
     11.6.3 Oxygen pressure near mitochondria 322

Contents

    11.7 Intracellular oxygen transfer and resistance of the capillary wall to oxygen 323
        11.7.1 Diffusion coefficient of oxygen in tissue 323
        11.7.2 Facilitation of oxygen by myoglobin 323
        11.7.3 Diffusion resistance of the capillary wall 325
        11.7.4 Myoglobin as an oxygen store 327
    11.8 Summary 328
    References 328

12 Limitation of coronary flow reserve by a stenosis   **333**
    12.1 Introduction 333
    12.2 Coronary flow reserve 334
    12.3 Coronary stenosis and flow reserve 336
    12.4 Prediction of pressure drop over a coronary stenosis 338
        12.4.1 Pressure drop by viscous losses 338
        12.4.2 Pressure loss by convective acceleration 340
        12.4.3 Dependence of pressure drop over stenosis on stenosis diameter 342
    12.5 Absolute versus relative definition of a stenosis 344
    12.6 Effect of stenosis geometry and flow pulsatility on pressure drop . 346
    12.7 Theoretical optimization of coronary reserve 348
        12.7.1 Effect of heart rate 348
        12.7.2 Reserve and flow ratio in the presence of a stenosis 353
        12.7.3 Hemodilution in the presence of a stenosis 353
    12.8 Reflections on the clinical use of coronary flow reserve 354
    12.9 Summary 357
    References 358

A Equivalent schematic for calculation of pressure distribution   **363**

B Nonlinear pump model   **365**
    References 367

C Calculation of oxygen consumption with changing flow   **369**
    References 371

D The Krogh model   **373**
    D.1 Definition of the problem 373
    D.2 Simplified equation for maximal Krogh radius 375
    D.3 Derivations of the Krogh model 375

Author Index   **377**

Subject Index   **381**

Foreword

by JULIEN IE HOFFMAN

One of the earliest coronary physiologists was Scaramucci who, in 1695, postulated that during systole the contracting myocardium inhibited coronary blood flow. Since then, the many contributions that have been made to our knowledge of the coronary circulation can be arbitrarily divided into three phases based on advances in technical methods. The early phase of research into the coronary circulation, done with great difficulty with crude methods, may be regarded as ending in the 1940s, and it included major discoveries made by such well known investigators as Georg von Anrep, Ernest Starling, Carl Wiggers, and Louis Katz, who formulated much of our basic understanding of the field. After 1940, the field of coronary physiology entered a new phase when instruments for high fidelity registration of coronary flow and pressure became available. This era was dominated by Donald Gregg who combined careful attention to the function of these instruments (some of which he helped to develop) with an extraordinary ability to discern mechanisms from apparently minor changes in coronary flow and pressure patterns. His book 'The Coronary Circulation in Health and Disease' set a new standard in the field. After 1960, techniques for measuring regional myocardial blood flow became available, and enabled a large group of eminent investigators to make major advances in understanding the physiology and pathophysiology of myocardial blood flow. In this period, the book 'The Coronary Circulation in Health and Disease' by Melvin Marcus not only summarized the field to date, but related the physiology clearly to the clinical applications in a way that the previous book by Gregg was unable to do.

Now the present book by Dr. Spaan begins a new phase, based not on new measuring techniques but on the introduction of two approaches that will be new to most readers who are interested in the coronary circulation. First, it incorporates a great deal of information about the microcirculation, often based on work from Dr. Spaan's laboratory; this information forms the basis for explaining findings at the macroscopic level. Second, Dr. Spaan's background in bioengineering has allowed him to evaluate transient responses and nonlinearities, and, based on these, to discuss the advantages and disadvantages of various models of the coronary circulation. Most physiologists in this field are restricted to simple linear models by their unfamiliarity with nonlinear concepts, but Dr. Spaan has been able to incorporate these nonlinear concepts in a way that most readers will understand. By patiently dissecting out the logical outcome of the major theories in the field of coronary blood flow, Dr. Spaan has demonstrated for each where predictions based on existing knowledge break down to reveal their weaknesses. What is particularly revealing is that a given set of experimental data can be fitted equally well by several different models, all of which give similar results over the range of pressures and flows examined. Not only does Dr. Spaan explain why this happens, but he indicates where new experiments might usefully discriminate among the different theories. The amount of information provided is prodigious, and one of the great contributions of this book is to point out where new investigative efforts should go. The stimulation given to coronary investigation by this book will alter the field for years to come.

Author's preface

The approaching possibility of clinically assessing the magnitude and distribution of coronary blood flow in humans creates a challenge; a meaningful interpretation of these measurements requires a profound knowledge of the determinants of coronary flow. This book has been written to help those working in the field of coronary circulation, either as clinicians, research workers, or both together. Moreover, it surveys concepts in modern coronary physiology for all interested in this area, an area in which insights are developing at a rapid rate. Elementary concepts in coronary physiology have been emphasized so that even those without much prior knowledge of the subject can understand what has been achieved and what still remains to be done.

Coronary blood flow makes it possible for the heart to beat. Unfortunately, by beating to generate the driving pressure for blood flow, the heart adds an extra resistance to the coronary circulation. In the healthy heart this burden is easily handled. However, in diseases of the coronary arteries or the heart muscle, this burden may restrict the ability of the coronary circulation to allow for an increased work load or even to sustain a basic level of performance. Medicine has developed to the stage where interventions that prolong life and improve its quality have become daily routines. In achieving this goal, the function of the coronary circulation at all levels from the larger extramural arteries to the smaller parts of the microcirculation needs to be understood in all its ramifications.

The coronary circulation is a system that cannot be understood from a single discipline alone. A limited list of essential disciplines includes cardiology, physiology, biochemistry, and engineering. The professional attitudes of practitioners of these disciplines is quite diverse, and interaction between them is a prerequisite for progress in the physiology, pathophysiology, and management of the diseases of this crucial part of the circulation. For example, the role of fluid mechanics in understanding the coronary circulation is obvious from history. Important scientist like Poiseuille, Bernoulli, Young, and many others had a primary interest in the circulation. However, an understanding of fluid mechanics is not enough to understand coronary blood flow. At a very local level, the flow magnitude is tuned to the metabolic needs of the heart by a control system based on feedback. In this information circle, molecular and mechanical signals interact. The resulting behavior of coronary flow control can be analyzed by the laws applied in control engineering which dictate the behavior of man-made systems.

The field of coronary research is directed at old problems but is continuously renewing its concepts as new information and techniques become available. This book attempts to elucidate those concepts in so far as they concern the mechanics, distribution and control of coronary blood flow at the levels of the major coronary arteries and veins, and also in the coronary microcirculation. There is no intent to provide a complete review of the literature on coronary research, nor to cover clinical diagnostics or interventions.

My background is in Engineering. My graduation work concerned the field of artificial organs. After graduation in 1971 I moved more and more towards the application of physical and engineering principles to biological systems, and in particular to the coronary circulation. In these past twenty years I have, in varying degrees of intensity, worked in close cooperation with clinicians and physiologists. I have learned from their ability to understand physical principles even when their background for appreciating mathematical methods was not strong. In this book I have attempted to convey the physical and engineering principles with a minimum of mathematical formalisms. The subsections are organized in such a way that the basics of the analyses and their outcome can be understood with only a basic appreciation of mathematical methods. If, however, readers have suggestions about ways to improve the presentation or content of this book, their comments will be appreciated.

Writing a monograph on my own was done mainly to preserve a unity of presentation in all the chapters. This does not mean that the book is the exclusive result of my thinking and work, as acknowledged by the authorship of my co-workers in the last chapters. The book reflects the work that I have done with many others. The diffusion of oxygen was the subject of my PhD thesis that I performed under the stimulating supervision of Pieter Veenstra, Professor of Mechanical Engineering, and Ferdinand Kreuzer, Professor of Physiology. My interest in the coronary circulation was aroused by John Laird, Aeronautical Engineer and for nine years Professor of Physiological Physics. He brought me from a University of Technology into a Medical Faculty. In fact, the directions outlined in this book were born during our years of collaboration. Furthermore, without the ideas and experimental work of the other scientists and technical staff who worked with me for various periods, I would not have been able to write this book. The steady development of my concepts of the coronary circulation is certainly due to the stimulating interaction with colleagues all over the world. I am grateful to be part of this interaction and for the stimulation and the many friends that it brought me.

I would like to express my profound gratitude for the editorial work and stimulation that I received from my colleagues, Julien Hoffman and Bill Chilian.

Author's preface

Professor Hoffman, in particular, contributed a great deal to my thinking in the months that I worked in his laboratory and by many subsequent discussions. He taught me the importance of understanding problems of the distribution of myocardial blood flow. The contributions of Julien Hoffman and Bill Chilian in style and content of this book are numerous. In addition, their patience with this slowly maturing author have made this book finally possible. Patience also was shown by the publisher, Heleen Liepman, who stimulated my ambition to undertake the enterprise of writing a monograph.

A key person in the creation of this monograph was Bob van der Linden. As a self-confident student he offered his ingenuity and in particular his enthusiasm to typeset the manuscript in Latex. His collaboration was a deed of friendship. His moral support and willingness to alter the text repeatedly were admirable. We sometimes spoke about "our book", which it probably is. I would also like to thank many more people than I can list for their support and assistance on numerous occasions, as, for example, with Mirage (Jenny Dankelman), Unix and Kermit (Peter Lucas), and Latex (Erwin Furth, Yves Han). Masami Goto was always helpful in pointing out specific topics of scientific interest and in reading chapters. Karin Griblin-Laird helped me with grammar. Without here support I would not have been able to express my thoughts in English. Annelies Strackee helped me by reading the proofs of the manuscript. Secretarial support was professional and provided by Lois Nelissen and Marijke Lensing.

For at least the last year I have been very preoccupied by the monograph. I exhausted the patience of my children, friends and colleagues. I am, however, very grateful for their forbearance, stimulus, and at times their protective intolerance when spending all my time with the book. In particular, Mar was a true friend during a difficult time. She encouraged me when I doubted if my efforts would ever come to fruition.

Finally, I learned a lot by writing this book, and hope that I have been of service to others in contributing to a better understanding of Coronary Blood Flow.

JOS AE SPAAN

Acknowledgements

Much new material in this book is the result of support from different sources, for which I'm grateful:

- Dept. of Physiology and Physiological Physics University of Leiden (1976 - 1986)

- Dept. of Medical Physics and Informatics University of Amsterdam (1986 - present)

- Dept. of Measurements and control Delft University of Technology

- Netherlands Foundation for Research (NWO)
    Medical Sciences
    Foundation for BioPhysics

- Dutch Heart Foundation

Chapter 1

Basic coronary physiology

1.1 Introduction

1.1.1 Heart function and coronary flow

THE HEART PROPELS BLOOD through the vascular system. It thereby maintains the delicate balance between the functions of different organs in our body by transporting fuel and waste products. Strategic stocks and waste storage capabilities differ from substance to substance and from organ to organ and are meant to compensate for transient shortcomings in the transport of substances. Supply of oxygen to the brain determines the lower boundary of time in which the process may fail. The heart is the key organ in the overall process of supply. When the heart fails completely, awareness is gone within seconds and brain death occurs within minutes. Apart from these elementary functions, blood flow is essential for carrying away heat produced by metabolism in the organs, for transporting signal substances like hormones, and for circulating cells for the defence against alien organisms and structures.

The mechanical work needed for pumping blood is performed by the heart muscle or myocardium. The amount of mechanical work under resting conditions can easily be calculated from the product of cardiac output and aortic pressure. In units usually used in physiology, cardiac output is 5 liters per minute and mean aortic pressure is 100 mm Hg. After conversion of units these numbers result in a mechanical work of only 4 Watts. This can be compared with the power of the back light of an average Dutch bicycle, which is a reason not to be impressed by this number. It is the continuity of functioning and the range of adaptation to increased demand that enforces admiration for this organ. Within a duration of life of 70 years and an average heart rate of 70 beats per minute one arrives at an estimate of 2.6×10^9 contractions. The total blood volume pumped is 200×10^9 liters which can fill a mammoth oil tanker. During severe exercise, cardiac output may increase by a factor of four to six, showing that the heart is well designed to adapt to a variety of conditions.

As for every other organ, the heart depends for its functioning on the blood flowing through its vessels, the coronary circulation. As a tax on the whole circulation about 5 to 10% of the cardiac output is shunted through these coronary vessels to make cardiac functioning possible. The inlet for the coronary system is within the region of the aortic valve structure and consists basically of two major vessels which are the first to branch from the aorta. These vessels, discussed in Chapter 2, run over the surface of the heart, giving rise to branches which penetrate the heart muscle and in turn branch into smaller vessels in order to supply the capillary network of the heart with blood. This capillary network is another technical miracle. The capillaries are vessels with a diameter of only 5 μm through which the red cells flow in a single line. The network, discussed in Chapter 3, is very dense with an average intercapillary distance of 20 μm. This network is interwoven with the muscle fibers whose periodic shortening and relaxation cause the heart to beat. Oxygen and other substrates are exchanged between blood and muscle cells at the capillary level. Capillary blood velocity is in the order of $1 \text{ mm} \cdot \text{s}^{-1}$. An estimate of capillary volume flow comes from the product of velocity and capillary cross-sectional area and amounts to 0.02 μl per second. A liquid drop is typically about 20 μl and consequently a capillary in the heart transports under control conditions only 4 drops of blood each hour. The small amount of blood flow per capillary is compensated for by the large amount of capillaries, about 3200 per mm^2 in a cross section perpendicular to the capillary direction.

1.1.2 Control and extravascular resistance

Coronary blood flow is not a constant quantity but is adapted to the metabolic needs of the heart. The heart has a control system to regulate the coronary blood flow to a level close to the minimum required for the supply of oxygen. Under normal conditions the heart extracts about 70% of all the oxygen from the blood flowing through its arteries. During exercise, oxygen consumption of the heart may increase by a factor of five which has to be accommodated by an increase of coronary blood flow. This increase is made possible by dilation of the small arteries with diameters between 20 and 400 μm. The dilation is controlled by a local regulatory process which tunes the supply of oxygen to the heart to the metabolic demands and compensates for mechanisms that could disturb the balance between supply of and demand for oxygen.

Mechanisms disturbing the supply and demand ratio may be physiological or pathophysiological. An important physiological disturbance of coronary flow is the contraction of the heart itself. The same factors that generate the pressure in the left ventricle in order to propel blood through the cardiac system compress the vessels, small and large, within the heart muscle. These compressing forces impede coronary blood flow and their effects are often referred to as extravascular resistance. A simple increase in heart rate increases not only the demand for blood flow but also increases the extravascular resistance. Hence, by increasing heart rate, arteriolar dilation must compensate for both increase in demand and increase of extravascular resistance. A different physiological factor that may disturb the balance between demand and supply is arterial blood pressure. Arterial blood pressure may vary with work, sleep or for other reasons. The local coronary flow control mechanism compensates for these disturbances in inlet pressure of the coronary system.

A well recognized pathophysiological mechanism affecting the supply of blood in a negative way is atherosclerosis. This disease process may result in either local or more distributed narrowing of the larger coronary arteries. Such a narrowing adds to the resistance of the coronary system. The local flow control process will recognize such an obstruction as a reduction in pressure and respond by vasodilation. That is the reason why the disease of coronary atherosclerosis may progress unnoticed for such a long time. However, the additional resistance to flow reduces the range of oxygen demand over which the coronary circulation is able to respond by increasing supply. That is why angina pectoris, a chest pain that is related to a shortage of blood supply to the myocardium, may be induced by exercise. The need to compensate for the arterial narrowing will exhaust the dilatory capabilities of the coronary resistance vessels and bring the control system to the limit of its working range. Exercise increases demand and the extravascular resistance to such an extent that supply will fail to compensate for the increased demand.

1.1.3 Distribution of supply and demand

The heart muscle is not a very homogeneous organ. It is organized in fibers and bundles which are wound around the cavities at angles with the equator between -60^0 and $+60^0$, depending on the depth within the muscle. Within the cavities papillary muscles, which can be considered as folds from the subendocardium, make the inner surface irregular. This all causes the required mechanical behavior of heart muscle to vary over the wall even under normal physiological conditions. In terms of flow, too, distribution inhomogeneities need to be considered. In part these inhomogeneities are induced by the spatial variation in heart muscle mechanics causing inhomogeneities in demand and extravascular resistance. However, inhomogeneities are also the result of the vascular bed itself. The arterial tree does, as a rule, not branch symmetrically.

The stochastic nature of the arterial branching pattern induces a heterogeneous distribution of flow over the arterioles. Local control may smooth out some of these differences. When flow through an artery is expressed per unit weight of tissue perfused by it one would expect a local match of demand and supply. However, the site of action of control is over a range of arterial diameters from 400 μm down. Hence, 'local' is also a notion with a limited validity. Because of the vague boundaries of areas of influence of tissue on smooth muscle in control vessels at different levels in the tree, an inhomogeneous distribution of flow is to be expected. It is obvious that local disturbances, as for example a small artery narrowing, will further increase the heterogeneity in cardiac function and in flow distribution.

It seems very important to understand the heterogeneous nature of distribution of mechanical, biochemical and flow distribution and their relations with quantities that can be measured on a macroscopic scale such as pressure–volume relations of the ventricles, arterial venous differences in substrate concentrations, and flow in large coronary arteries. This understanding is not only an intellectual challenge. Myocardial disfunction often starts locally and is compensated for by the remaining muscle. Insight into the coherence between events at the micro and macro level may further our understanding of the beginning and progression of disease processes.

1.1.4 Mechanics, control and distribution in the coronary circulation

This introductory section underlines three important topics of coronary research: mechanics, control and distribution. The mechanics of coronary circulation covers all the relations between mechanical quantities such as pressure, flow, contraction, tension and so on. Control of the coronary circulation consists of all the mechanisms that play a role in feedback between cardiac function and coronary flow. Arteriolar smooth muscle mechanics plays a central role in this field of study. Distribution is a key word that relates to all properties of the coronary circulation and its determinants. In this book we will focus on the distribution of blood and oxygen over the wall, the control of blood flow and the mechanical interactions between heart contraction and the coronary circulation. It will be clear that all three fields of research are interrelated and these connections will be discussed in the succeeding chapters.

The remainder of Chapter 1 is meant to provide a brief review of coronary physiology organized into three sections. In these sections typical observations are highlighted and are discussed in detail in Chapters 2–12. The material is restricted merely to observations and forms an indication of concepts that are presently under discussion in the literature. It is meant to raise curiosity about the fundamental properties of the coronary circulation[1].

---

[1]Some older and more recent reviews are [39, 32, 46, 51, 63, 68, 80]

1.2 Coronary flow mechanics

For a long time, there have been discussion about whether contraction would impede or facilitate coronary blood flow. The pulsatility of coronary arterial and venous flow was already noticed in the seventeenth century by Scaramucci [75] who nowadays is considered as the founder of coronary physiology. As demonstrated in Figures 1.1 and 1.4, coronary arterial flow is low or even retrograde in systole while at the same time coronary venous outflow is high. In diastole, the reverse occurs: arterial flow is high but venous flow is low. Hence, the isolated observation of coronary arterial flow may lead to the conclusion that contraction impedes coronary flow whereas the isolated observation of venous flow can be interpreted that contraction augments coronary flow. Porter [69], at the end of the nineteenth century, observed that time averaged flow increased with heart contraction and hence augmented coronary flow. However, he did not appreciate at that time that flow was under the influence of metabolic control. Most likely, coronary flow increased in his experiments because of an increased demand. The definitive conclusion that contraction is an impeding factor for coronary flow came with a study of Sabiston and Gregg [74], who applied a rotameter in a perfusion line connecting a carotid artery with the left main coronary artery. The time resolution of the instrument was good enough to demonstrate a sudden sustained rise in coronary flow when the heart was arrested by vagal stimulation. The crux of their conclusions has been confirmed by many. However, the experiments of Sabiston and Gregg were repeated recently in a systematic fashion by Katz and Feigl [52] and it appeared that the magnitude of the effect was overestimated in the earlier study, probably because of the errors introduced by the rotameter.

Although nowadays we accept that time averaged coronary flow as measured in large coronary arteries and veins is impeded by heart contraction, the mechanism of this impeding effect is still uncertain. For a long time compression of blood vessels within the myocardium was thought to be caused by tissue pressure related to pressure in the pumping chambers of the heart. However, at present the notion is developing that the impeding effect might be caused by changing stiffness of the heart muscle [56, 58, 89]. The final study on this subject has not been performed yet. The fact that arterial and venous flows are out of phase must mean that intramyocardial blood volume varies during the heart cycle. This volume must increase during diastole and decrease during systole. Because of mass balance the rate of volume change is proportional to the difference between arterial inflow and venous outflow. The contribution of rate of volume change to coronary flow is referred to as capacitive flow. Volume changes throughout the cardiac cycle are brought about by squeezing of intramyocardial blood vessels, either by tissue pressure or by varying wall stiffness. This effect has been named intramyocardial pump action [83]. If a vessel varies in volume its resistance will vary as well. The effects on coronary arterial and venous flow to be expected from these volume variations, apart from capacitive flow components, are hard to predict. Much depends on where these volume variations occur. If they are concentrated in a certain type of vessel, the relative volume changes there will be large and large resistance variations are to be expected. If, however, the volume variations are well distributed the resistance variations will be small. Hence, in describing the flow variations in arteries and veins one has to consider the interaction between capacitive flow and resistance variations (Chapters 5, 6 and 7).

1.2.1 Inhibition of coronary arterial flow during systole

The interaction between heart contraction and coronary arterial flow has received much attention in this century. The difference between flow in the left and right coronary arteries, as well as some peculiarities of the left coronary flow wave form, have been the basis of the hypothesis that the effect of contraction was mediated by tissue pressure related to ventricular cavity pressure.

The coronary flow measured in a major coronary branch of a conscious dog is shown in Figure 1.1. The aortic and coronary arterial pressures are also given. The flow tracing exhibits the following characteristics. In diastole, flow decreases, as does arterial pressure. A little flow wave (a) coincides with atrial contraction; however, a sudden drop in flow is seen at the first sign of the q wave in the electrocardiogram when pressure in the left ventricle starts to rise (b). The sudden rise in aortic pressure causes flow to exhibit a spike (c). The contraction of the heart impedes coronary inflow and, despite the higher coronary arterial pressure, the coronary flow drops in mid systole (d). After closure of the aortic valve and fall of left ventricular pressure, coronary flow rises rapidly (e) and diastolic decay of flow starts again.

The flow in the right coronary artery exhibits a different pattern, as illustrated in Figure 1.2. It should be noted that the right coronary flow signal follows the aortic pressure signal during systole, in contrast to the left coronary arterial flow, which was inhibited. This difference has long been considered evidence that the mechanism of systolic inhibition was related to the pressure in the ventricles. This point of view was lent additional support by the observation that the right coronary arterial flow wave also showed systolic inhibition of flow when right ventricular pressure was increased by pulmonary stenosis. The flow waves in the right and left coronary artery were then quite similar [62]. Recently, observations have been published suggesting that flow wave forms in small side branches of the right coronary artery are more pulsatile than in its most proximal part [45].

There were also other experimental observations supporting the concept of cavity pressure as the cause of systolic arterial flow inhibition. Microsphere distribution over the free left ventricular wall after abolishing tone in the arterioles revealed that the inhibition of time averaged flow was largest in the subendocardial layer, or the layer closest to the left ventricular cavity (e.g., Figure 1.10).

1.2 Coronary flow mechanics

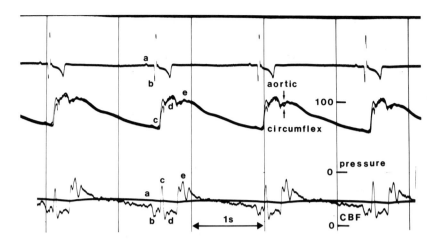

Figure 1.1: *Tracing of left coronary arterial flow measured with an electromagnetic flow probe in a conscious dog. Top signal is the electrocardiogram. Aortic and coronary pressure signals are in the middle. Mean and phasic coronary flow signals are at the bottom. a = atrial contraction, b = onset of left ventricular contraction, c = rise in aortic pressure due to opening of the aortic valve. For further explanation, see text. (Courtesy of Dr. R.A. Olsson.)*

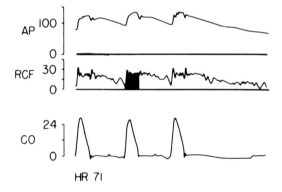

Figure 1.2: *Tracing of right coronary arterial flow measured with an electromagnetic flow probe in a conscious dog. Top signal: aortic pressure, middle signal: right coronary flow, and bottom panel: cardiac output. The time scale is estimated from the heart rate specified by the authors. Note that right coronary arterial flow is not decreased in systole when measured in the proximal part of the artery. (From Lowensohn et al. [62], by permission of authors and American Heart Association, Inc.)*

Experimental [43] and theoretical [3] evidence indicates that tissue pressure is about equal to left ventricular pressure in the subendocardium and gradually decreases to atmospheric in the subepicardium. This concept of tissue pressure as the intermediate between cavity pressure and intramyocardial vascular compression is compatible with the selective subendocardial flow reduction. Incidental observations that left coronary flow was also pulsatile when the heart was beating and empty as occurs during graft surgery [70] were ascribed to tissue pressures generated by the large deformations of the ventricle in this condition. It is only recently that convincing evidence has been presented that the pulsatility of coronary arterial flow is related more to the contractility of the ventricular wall than to the left ventricular pressure generated by it [56, 57, 58]. The concept of time varying elastance was postulated as a mechanism to explain the pulsatility of coronary arterial flow. The impediment of systolic arterial flow was thought to be caused by direct interaction between myocyte contraction and myocardial microvessels, analogous to the compression of the left ventricular cavity by the left ventricular wall. This concept is in agreement with other recent measurements on blood velocity in small arteries on the left and right atrium. Flow in these vessels is also completely inhibited in systole, and this inhibition is unlikely to be caused by the small pressure waves within the atria [50]. Moreover, it should be noted that earlier studies also pointed to a dominant role of the inotropic state of the heart [65, 66]. The different concepts of systolic inhibition of flow will be analyzed in depth in Chapters 5, 6 and 7. At this point it should be noted that there is a controversy which urgently requires a solution. The theory based on direct interaction between myocyte contraction and microvessels does not explain why the right coronary arterial flow wave resembles the aortic pressure wave and, moreover, seems not to be in agreement with the observations that myocardial perfusion is inhibited by cardiac contraction in the subendocardium in contrast to the perfusion of the subepicardium.

1.2.2 Retrograde coronary arterial flow, venous flow and intramyocardial compliance

For a long time the concepts to explain the systolic inhibition of coronary arterial flow ran along lines which only served to explain a reduction of flow in systole since these explanations included, for example, an increase in resistance during systole [41] or an increase in so-called back pressure thought to be related to a collapse of coronary microvessels [29]. However, flow in a coronary artery may be retrograde a phenomenon already noticed by Porter in 1898 [69]. Zero flow seems not to be a natural threshold for coronary flow. An example of retrograde flow is provided in Figure 1.3. This figure illustrates tracings obtained from an experiment on an anesthetized open chest dog in which the left main coronary artery was cannulated and perfused at approximately constant pressure. Paired

1.2 Coronary flow mechanics

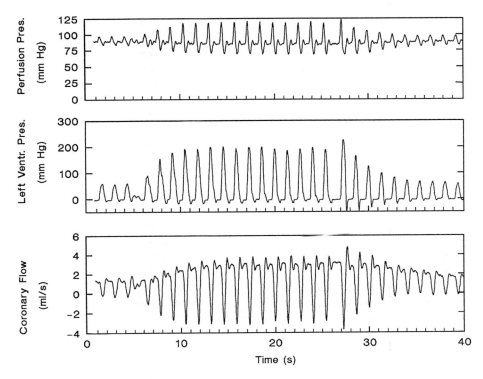

Figure 1.3: *Retrograde systolic flow in cannulated left main stem preparation in the anesthetized dog caused by paired pacing. Top panel: perfusion pressure, middle panel: left ventricular pressure, bottom panel: coronary flow in the left main stem. Note the negative left ventricular pressure and concomitant overshoot of initial diastolic coronary flow.*

pacing of the left ventricle resulted in both an increase in left ventricular pressure due to an increased contractility and a significant backflow into the cannula while coronary arterial pressure was maintained. Retrograde flow can also be observed at normal contractility and constant perfusion pressure if this pressure is reduced below 70 mm Hg [79].

Backflow is only possible when volume is displaced from the coronary artery back into the cannula. It cannot be explained by any such mechanism as change in resistance since at most this would only cause flow to cease. Hence, retrograde flow is direct evidence that blood is pumped back from the intramyocardial vessels. This must be accompanied by a reduction of intramyocardial blood volume [83]. This pump action can be explained on the basis of tissue pressure related to ventricular pressure as well as on the basis of the varying elastance concept. Both predict compression of the intramyocardial blood vessels. It should be noted that with the intervention shown in Figure 1.3, it is impossible to distinguish whether contractility or cavity pressure was the cause of the increase in pulsatility of the coronary arterial flow. Since contractility and left ventricular pressure will normally alter concomitantly, special experimental conditions have to be created to distinguish the two (see Chapters 6 and 7).

Intramyocardial pump action is also clear from the waves in the coronary venous flow. Coronary venous flow is high in systole and low in diastole. This holds for the flow in veins of the left ventricle [69, 81, 90], right ventricle [45] and the atria [50].

An illustration of the pulsatility of the flow in the great cardiac vein is illustrated in Figure 1.4. The results are from a preparation similar to the one in Figure 1.3 but with the additional cannulation of the great cardiac vein. Blood from this cannula was drained into a pressure reservoir, while maintaining mean venous pressure at a reasonably constant level. Venous flow was measured with a cannulating flow probe directly attached to the venous cannula. Venous flow is out of phase with arterial flow. This indicates a periodically changing blood volume between the two cannulas during the heart beat.

Intramyocardial blood volume is, indeed, not constant as is clear from the continuation of coronary venous flow after coronary arterial occlusion as is shown in Figure 1.4. The decay of coronary venous outflow is evidence for the decrease of intramyocardial blood volume after the arterial inflow ceases. The coronary venous outflow decay should be interpreted in conjunction with the decay of coronary peripheral pressure, the pressure distal to the occlusion of the perfusion line. This pressure is maintained in the first systole after occlusion due to compression of the intramyocardial vessels. It then gradually drops. In the coronary peripheral pressure decay curve, a dotted line has been drawn by eye to indicate the beat averaged peripheral pressure. The concomitant decay of coronary peripheral pressure and venous outflow is characteristic of the presence of compliance of the intramyocardial vessels. The beat averaged peripheral pressure was extrapolated back to the time of arterial occlusion. The value $P_{ib,0}$ thus obtained might be considered as the average intramyocardial blood pressure before the occlusion and equal to the averaged intramyocardial blood pressure during perfusion.

Both peripheral coronary pressure and coronary venous outflow decay are characterized by a time constant longer than a heart beat. Hence, one has to conclude that at the microvascular level there is no equilibration in vascular volume, and hence pressures, within a heartbeat.

Chapter 7 will demonstrate that if the heart is arrested, intramyocardial blood volume increases due to the reduced compression of the intramyocardial microvessels. Hence, the volume of the intramyocardial microvessels, and consequently their diameter, depends on both perfusion and heart contraction. At least two mechanisms affecting both arterial and venous pressure and flow can be inferred

1.3 Coronary flow mechanics

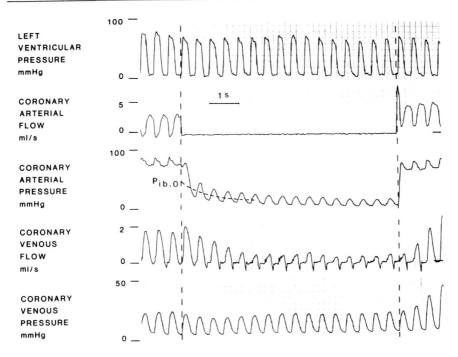

Figure 1.4: *Coronary venous flow before and during a coronary arterial occlusion. Left main coronary artery was cannulated and perfused artificially. The great cardiac vein was also cannulated and drained into a pressure controlled reservoir. The dotted curve in the middle panel was drawn by eye to indicate the course of the time averaged coronary arterial pressure after occlusion, except for the first 0.5 s. Extrapolation back to time of occlusion yields $P_{ib,0}$, which may reflect time averaged intramyocardial blood pressure during perfusion prior to occlusion. (Redrawn from [81].)*

from the change of microvascular volume. The first is capacitive flow which is due to the rate of change of volume of the blood vessels. It affects only the flow transients. The second mechanism is the resistance of the microvessels that increases with decreasing vessel diameters. An increase of resistance will decrease time averaged flow. However, during the time that resistance is actually changing the rate of change of resistance also affects the transients in flow. Hence, transients in arterial or venous flow may not solely be interpreted in terms of capacitive flow.

Because of all these interactions, the interpretation of coronary arterial and venous flow signals is complicated. Interaction between systole and diastole should be taken into account [2, 15, 46, 47, 90]. Models which may be very helpful in unravelling these interactions are examined in Chapters 6 and 7.

1.3 Regulation of coronary flow

The tight relation between coronary flow and oxygen consumption of the heart was not well appreciated until the work of Barcroft and Dixon [8] at the beginning of this century. Tuning of flow to oxygen consumption is effectuated by the smooth muscle within the walls of the resistance vessels. From studies on epicardial small arteries in situ, isolated coronary resistance vessels, and other whole organ studies one may presently conclude that at least three mechanisms must be involved in the control of coronary flow:

1. a mediator between myocyte metabolism and coronary resistance vessels,

2. myogenic tone (the tone induced by stretch), and

3. flow dependent dilation.

These mechanisms must be tuned in order to let the control system behave as it does. However, the interactions between these mechanisms are just beginning to receive attention in coronary research. The study of flow control in the coronary circulation at the level of resistance vessels is limited because intramyocardial resistance vessels cannot be studied in situ with the present techniques available. Hence, the relations between pressure and flow in the major coronary arteries are still the major source of information of the control function of the coronary circulation. In this section we will briefly define the steady state and dynamic behavior of the coronary control system and the working range of flow control as evidenced by reactive hyperemia. A short review of candidate mechanisms for flow control is presented as well. Flow control as studied from isolated resistance vessels will be discussed in Chapter 8. An extensive analysis of local coronary flow control is provided in Chapter 9.

1.3.1 Steady local control of coronary flow

The control of coronary flow is demonstrated in Figure 1.5. These results from our laboratory [87, 88] were obtained in anesthetized open chest goats in which the left main coronary artery was cannulated. Such a cannulation facilitates the proper study of the control of coronary flow by maintaining coronary arterial pressure independent of the aortic pressure [40]; in an intact preparation the generation of perfusion pressure, being the aortic pressure, requires cardiac work and hence is related to oxygen consumption [1, 39]. The top panel of Figure 1.5 illustrates the coupling between coronary flow and oxygen consumption at two different values of perfusion pressure. Oxygen consumption was varied by volume loading of the animal's vascular system. It is important to note that the relationship between flow and oxygen consumption is not unique but coronary arterial pressure dependent. Often, a unique relation is suggested in the literature with

1.3 Regulation of coronary flow

reference to the data of Eckenhoff *et al.* [31] who compiled the early data on the relation between coronary flow and oxygen consumption. In these experiments, however, coronary arterial pressure was not controlled and had probably changed with oxygen consumption.

The coupling between coronary flow and oxygen consumption is often referred to as exercise or functional hyperemia although I prefer the term metabolic adjustment of coronary flow since, basically, this is what happens.

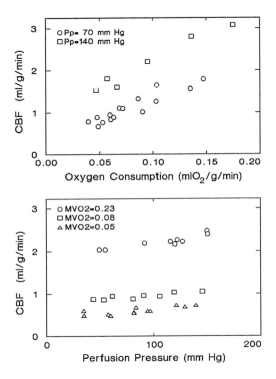

Figure 1.5: *Local control of coronary flow. Top panel: Illustration of metabolic flow adjustment, i.e., the relation between coronary blood flow and myocardial oxygen consumption at constant perfusion pressure. Oxygen consumption, MVO_2, was altered by volume loading of the animal. Bottom panel: Illustration of autoregulation, i.e., the relation between coronary blood flow and coronary perfusion pressure at constant MVO_2. The low MVO_2 value was obtained by the administration of hexamethonium, the high value by the administration of norepinephrine. Top and bottom panels were obtained from different animals. (Redrawn from Vergroesen et al. [87].)*

The bottom panel of Figure 1.5 illustrates what is generally denoted as autoregulation. Coronary flow is only slightly dependent on perfusion pressure when oxygen consumption is kept constant. If mechanical conditions such as heart rate and left ventricular systolic pressure are kept constant, oxygen consumption of the heart will continue to rise with increasing coronary perfusion pressure. This is probably due to the stiffening of the framework of the heart by the higher intraluminal pressures, reducing the efficiency of the heart to pump blood [28]. The phenomenon of oxygen consumption increased by perfusion pressure is generally referred to as Gregg's phenomenon. The results in the bottom panel of Figure 1.5 are therefore corrected for changes in myocardial oxygen consumption induced by the changes in perfusion pressure. This was made possible by the fact that the sensitivity of flow to oxygen consumption was measured at constant perfusion pressure and oxygen consumption was altered by changing the mechanical work of the heart.

The relationships between flow, CBF, oxygen consumption, MVO_2, and perfusion pressure, P, are essentially described by a linear equation:

$$CBF = aMVO_2 + bP + c \qquad [1.1]$$

The constants a and b represent the sensitivities of flow for MVO_2 and perfusion pressure respectively. The former may be influenced by alpha-adrenergic blockade [67] and there is some evidence that the latter may be effected by alpha-adrenergic blockade as well. The constant c is an empirical constant. The importance of this equation will be analyzed in Chapter 9.

1.3.2 How to define coronary tone?

Since coronary flow is controlled at the arteriolar level it is desirable to be able to define the state of these vessels and how their state is changed by interventions. For this the notion 'tone' is often applied. However, tone is not a very precisely defined concept in coronary physiology. It is a loosely used term related to the wall tension in the small arteries and arterioles, the wall tension of these vessels being modulated by the smooth muscle in their walls and also by transmural pressure. Coronary flow is undoubtedly controlled by adjustment of smooth muscle activity. Since wall tension is impossible to measure, an index is needed to reflect its effect; generally this index is the concept of resistance and is regarded as equivalent to tone. The definition of a sensible resistance index which can be estimated from measurable quantities, however, is not simple. In general, flow and pressure in the coronary arteries are the quantities available from which resistance can be estimated. At least one of these signals varies in time and, without a perfusion system, both these signals do. It has long been thought [41] that at the end of diastole, the ratio between pressure and flow, or the so called end-diastolic resistance, reflected the resistance of the coronary bed free of the compression effect of systole. However, as shown by Figure 1.4, there is no coronary venous flow at the end of diastole but coronary inflow is still high. Hence, the coronary system at the end of a normal diastole can not be considered as a simple series of tubes with resistance. The flow characteristic of rigid tubes with constant resistance in series is that flows in the various compartments are equal. Since blood is stored in between the coronary artery and vein during diastole, the effect of a compliance of the intramyocardial vessels should be incorporated in the quantification of tone from coronary pressure and flow signals. This poses little difficulty in the theory of linear systems analysis. A periodically changing signal such as coronary arterial flow and pressure might be treated as a superposition of a time varying component, with time averaged value of zero, and a steady component equal to the time averaged value of the signal. If the coronary system were linear, the relation between time averaged pressure and flow would be determined solely by the resistance of the vascular bed and the vascular compliance would be irrelevant; the ratio between time averaged pressure and flow would then be a correct measure of resistance. However, the coronary system is nonlinear and per definition the superposition principle is not applicable to nonlinear systems, as will be discussed in Chapter 5 (e.g., Figure 5.2). The complication of nonlinearities in defining resistance will be further illustrated by means of the concept of end-diastolic resistance.

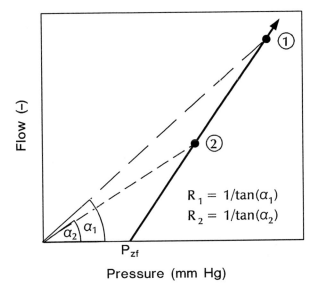

Figure 1.6: Schematic illustration of the diastolic coronary pressure–flow relation. This relation has an intercept with the pressure axis at a pressure value far higher than venous pressure (e.g., Chapter 7). The dotted lines are the pressure–flow relations which are implicitly assumed when end-diastolic resistance index is used to define coronary resistance. α_1 and α_2 are slopes of pressure flow relations defining resistances R_1 and R_2 respectively. A decrease in coronary arterial pressure would be interpreted as inducing vasoconstriction. Both axes have arbitrary units. Relative values of end-diastolic and zero flow pressure, P_{zf}, are realistic with respect to the initial diastolic pressure value.

The problems involved with the interpretation of the end-diastolic resistance index are illustrated in Figure 1.6. This figure gives a schematic illustration of the relation between pressure and flow during diastole. As is clear from this figure the coronary diastolic pressure–flow relation does not pass through the pressure axis at a pressure equal or close to venous pressure [12] but much higher.

The interpretation of the diastolic pressure–flow line is still a subject of discussion [54, 55, 77, 78] (see Chapter 7). The application of the end-diastolic resistance index as an index of resistance implies the assumption of a pressure–flow relation passing through the origin. The inverse of the slope of the line equals the assumed end-diastolic resistance. Now, when coronary arterial pressure is changed rapidly, flow will alter according to the diastolic pressure–flow relation. The figure illustrates what happens when pressure is decreased. There will be an increase in the diastolic resistance index which will be interpreted as a rapid increase in coronary tone. This is completely opposite to the result expected from such a decrease in perfusion pressure, since autoregulation, provided that there is time to react, is supposed to induce a vasodilation after a decrease in arterial pressure. Moreover, since normally diastolic coronary pressure will follow the aortic pressure decay, the end-diastolic resistance index could lead to the conclusion that arterioles would adapt their tone continuously during diastole and systole would induce a rapid vasodilation.

Also, the ratio between mean pressure and mean flow bears no unique relationship to the arteriolar resistance as can be illustrated by the events related to an increase in heart rate. When heart rate increases there is an extra impediment of time averaged coronary flow, referred to as extravascular resistance. This becomes particularly clear when vasomotor tone is pharmacologically abolished and coronary arterial pressure maintained. Coronary flow will decrease as heart rate increases. When heart rate is increased with intact response of the resistance vessels, the arterioles will dilate. However, part of the dilation has to compensate for the increased compression of the coronary microvessels. Hence, the ultimate reduction in ratio between pressure and flow will be an underestimate of the decrease of the resistance in the coronary resistance vessels.

The conclusion at this time must be that a proper estimation of arteriolar resistance under normal beating conditions of the heart and especially during transients in one of its determinants is at present not possible. Hence, in each study directed at coronary control and based on coronary arterial or venous pressure–flow relations, the consequences of the choice of index need careful evaluation. In general, the ratio between beat averaged pressure and flow should be preferred to a diastolic index, since in the beat averaged index the possible compliance effects during systole and diastole will, at least in part, cancel each other out. Moreover, especially at higher heart rates, diastole will be too short for the coronary arterial flow to reach a plateau phase, and to allow a well-defined estimation of flow and pressure.

1.3.3 Rate of adaptation of the coronary circulation to step changes in heart rate

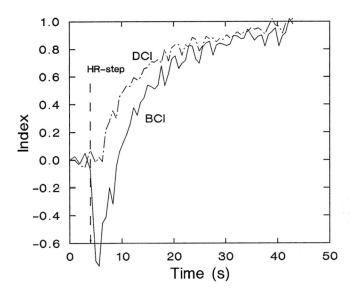

Figure 1.7: Dynamic change in normalized coronary arterial pressure/flow ratio following a sudden change in heart rate. BCI: pressure and flow were averaged per beat. DCI: pressure and flow were averaged over diastole alone. Measurements were performed in the anesthetized goat with cannulated coronary artery perfused at constant pressure. The curves were averaged over 14 interventions. Note the initial reversed response of BCI but delayed response of DCI. (Redrawn from [82].)

The heart is an organ which can rapidly change its performance and it is vital that flow can adapt appropriately to this. This implies that, on the one hand, the resistance vessels are able to dilate rapidly enough to meet the increased oxygen demand. On the other hand, this adaptation should proceed in such a way that no instabilities in supply occur which may lead to a depression of function because of temporary undersupply. Apart from these practical reasons, the study of the dynamics of coronary control might be helpful in identifying specifications of messengers involved in the control loop.

In order to characterize the dynamics of coronary flow adjustment, experiments were performed in anesthetized open chest goats with a cannulated left main coronary artery perfused at constant pressure. The heart was electrically paced and its rate was suddenly altered. The response of coronary flow to this intervention was recorded. Two indices were used to characterize the response of the coronary circulation. The first was based on the mean coronary resistance index discussed above. Pressure and flow were averaged per beat and their ratio calculated. This ratio increases with vasoconstriction and decreases with vasodilation. In order to allow the comparison of the time course of the coronary response during constriction and dilation and at different magnitudes of the response, the index was further normalized. The new index, BCI, is zero before the heart rate change and one after coronary flow has established a new steady state [13]. The second index was based on a diastolic resistance index, DCI. Pressure and flow were both averaged over the duration of diastole and their ratio taken. This ratio was subsequently also set to zero before and one after the change in heart rate. The indices are both defined by (see also Equation [9.2])

$$\text{Index} = \frac{\overline{P(t)/Q(t)} - \overline{P_i/Q_i}}{\overline{P_e/Q_e} - \overline{P_i/Q_i}} \qquad [1.2]$$

where

Index is either BCI or DCI,
BCI is Index where $P(t)$ and $Q(t)$ are averaged per beat,
DCI is Index where $P(t)$ and $Q(t)$ are averaged per diastole,
$P(t)$ is pressure as function of time,
$Q(t)$ is flow as function of time,
$\overline{P_i}$ is average pressure prior to intervention,
$\overline{Q_i}$ is average flow prior to intervention,
$\overline{P_e}$ is average pressure after intervention,
$\overline{Q_e}$ is average flow after intervention.

The response of the coronary system to a sudden increase in heart rate as defined by the course of these two indices is shown in Figure 1.7. The heart rate step was from 60 to 90 beats per minute. Higher heart rates did not permit a good estimation of diastolic flow. The results in Figure 1.7 are the averaged results of 9 goats and in total 14 interventions. The responses to the increase and decrease of heart rate were all averaged. However, understanding the responses may be facilitated by assuming that they were the result of an increase in heart rate alone. Because pressure was maintained at a constant level, the responses reflect the relative changes in beat averaged and diastolic averaged flow respectively. Hence, the course of the indices indicates that both mean flow and diastolic flow increase with an increase in heart rate due to metabolic flow adjustment.

The diastolic index remained constant for a few seconds and then started to increase. The half time for the response is in the order of 7.5 s. The beat index first has a phase in which the response goes in the opposite direction. The time needed to reach half the final response was in the order of 15 s.

The difference in time constants between the two responses illustrates again the problems in the definition of an index. If the diastolic index reflected arteriolar resistance, this resistance would change with a t_{50} of 7.5 s. If the beat index is the correct one, arteriolar resistance would change with a t_{50} of 15 s. Hence, because of the uncertainty in the way smooth muscle tone is linked to a coronary index, there is an uncertainty by a factor of two in the rate of responses of arteriolar resistance.

The initial reversal of response of the beat index must be due to a sudden change in compression of the myocardial microcirculation. Such a change induces both a compliance effect and a change in impediment of coronary flow. The responses of the coronary indices to a change in heart rate will be discussed in more detail in Chapter 9.

1.3.4 Effect of perfusion pressure step

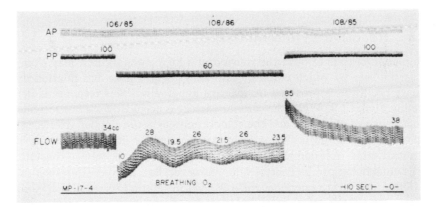

Figure 1.8: *Response of coronary arterial flow to a step change in perfusion pressure under normoxic conditions. Measurements are from an anesthetized dog with cannulated left main coronary artery being perfused at constant pressure. The flow pulsations are rather small which probably is due to the perfusion system applied. (From Driscol et al. [30], by permission of the authors and of the American Heart Association, Inc.)*

The steady state of coronary flow control could be defined by flow adjustment to metabolism and autoregulation. An autoregulatory response is induced by a change in coronary arterial pressure. Hence, a complete characterization of the dynamics of coronary flow control requires, next to the adaptation of coronary flow to a heart rate change, also the adaptation to a change in coronary arterial pressure. Such responses were published by Driscol et al. [30], and are illustrated in Figure 1.8. Their results were also obtained in a preparation with a cannulated main coronary artery, but in the anesthetized dog. Perfusion pressure was dropped suddenly from 100 to 60 mm Hg and returned to 100 mm Hg after approximately one minute of stabilization at 60 mm Hg. Flow was first seen to vary with pressure but was then directed towards its control value by vasoconstriction in the positive pressure step and by vasodilation when the pressure step was reversed. The type of flow response provoked depends on the direction of pressure change. The response to a downward pressure step exhibits oscillations which are absent in the response to an upward pressure step. Oscillations in flow in response to a decrease in pressure have been confirmed by others [23] and also in our laboratory [19]. Driscol et al. [30] reported that oscillations disappeared with anoxia. Such oscillations are absent when perfusion alterations are induced with coronary constrictions in conscious animals [16]. A further experimental characterization of the dynamics of coronary tone is discussed in Chapter 9. However, as a preliminary conclusion we may state that the t_{50} for the change of flow, either due to a change in metabolism or to a change in perfusion pressure, is about 5–15 seconds.

1.3.5 Reactive hyperemia

A simple illustration of both the range over which coronary flow may change as well as the rate by which coronary flow may recover after full dilation due to coronary occlusion is provided by reactive hyperemia. This response is demonstrated in Figure 1.9. When the coronary artery is occluded for a few seconds, the heart is deprived of oxygen and the smooth muscle in the smaller arteries relaxes completely. When the occlusion is released, coronary flow increases far above the control value. As soon as the oxygen supply is restored, oxygen consumption returns quickly back to its control value; however, flow is slower to return to control. Often the term repayment ratio is used in relation to reactive hyperemia. For flow, it is the ratio between volume above control that flows through the coronary artery after occlusion and the volume that would have passed during the time of occlusion if flow had not been disrupted. For occlusion of durations between 10 and 15 seconds this ratio is about four [17]. A similar definition holds for oxygen consumption; this latter ratio is about one [73]. Earlier numbers on oxygen repayment ratio were higher [18] but were due to an inappropriate application of the steady state Fick equation to a transient phenomenon like reactive hyperemia.

The peak value of flow following an occlusion of about 15 s is the maximal flow that can be obtained for an ischemic stimulus and varies linearly with coronary arterial pressure [21]. It is, however, not the maximal flow that can be obtained at the same conditions of perfusion pressure, heart rate and left ventricular pressure; some vasodilators can increase flow considerably further [38]. This difference can be explained in part by the different conditions: dynamic versus static. Moreover, heterogeneity in reperfusion may also cause disparity between the occurrences of peak flow in certain layers. It has been shown that peak reactive hyperemic flow occurs later in the subendocardium than in the subepicardium [27]. Hence, the spread in time of occurrence of peak reactive hyperemic flow in segments of

1.3 Regulation of coronary flow

the heart muscle may result in a lower value of peak reactive hyperemic flow, measured in a large coronary artery, than if all segments have a synchronous peak flow.

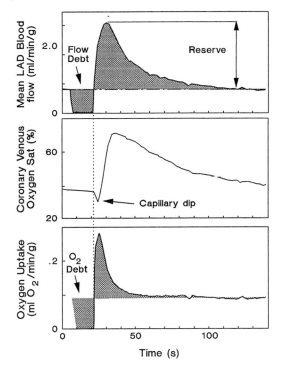

Figure 1.9: Reactive hyperemic response after a 15 s occlusion. Flow increases to a multiple of its control (top panel). Oxygen consumption is back to control in a few seconds (bottom panel) while venous oxygen saturation is still above its control (middle panel). The ratios between the marked areas after restoration of flow and during occlusion are referred to as repayment ratio of flow (top panel) and oxygen (bottom panel) respectively. (Redrawn from Ruiter et al. [73].)

The difference between the control flow and the peak reactive hyperemic flow is often used as approximation of coronary reserve. At present, the usefulness of this quantity is evaluated for application in clinical evaluation of patency of coronary arteries and many other items, e.g., transplant rejection. The peak of the response is reduced by coronary stenosis, which increases the uncontrolled resistance in the coronary bed. There are, however, several other factors that affect the magnitude of this reserve. In the first place, the level of the initial flow is of importance. The peak of reactive hyperemic flow can furthermore be reduced by the level of compression of the coronary microvessels. The clinical application of coronary reserve will be discussed in more detail in Chapter 12.

1.3.6 Mechanisms of coronary flow control

The static and dynamic behavior of coronary flow control is consistent with that of a control system based on feedback. From control engineering theory it is known that the existence of an error signal is essential for a feedback system.

Hence, in order to understand completely the control loop regulating coronary flow we have to identify an endogenous factor that fulfills the role of an error signal. The requirement for such an error signal is that it has to increase coronary resistance when flow is above its working point and to decrease coronary resistance when flow is too low. Moreover, the substance or mechanism which fulfills the role of an error signal must be able to adjust arteriolar resistance at a rate similar to the rate of change of the coronary indices as defined, for example, by Figure 1.7. At this moment, no definitive identification of this error signal has yet been made.

There are many endogenous factors that are known to affect the level of coronary tone as judged by either the mean coronary or end-diastolic coronary index. However, the simple observation that an endogenous factor has an effect on one of these indices does not make it a candidate for the error signal. The recently discovered substance endothelin [92] is a very potent endogenous vasoconstrictor, but is unlikely to be such a factor since its effect is too long lasting to allow the rapid changes in indices discussed above. Below, we present a short inventory of substances and mechanisms currently being discussed in relation to the regulation of coronary flow. Most of these mechanisms will be discussed more extensively in Chapters 8 and 9.

Adenosine has been a popular candidate for the error signal. Many studies have appeared to link interstitial adenosine to the metabolic level of the heart. An increase in cardiac work results in more endogenous adenosine production and this could be responsible for the coronary flow adjustment to metabolism. The required dependency of interstitial adenosine concentration on flow was formulated with the adenosine hypothesis [14] but was inadequately studied. The adenosine hypothesis met criticism after a series of experiments in which the interstitium was saturated with adenosine deaminase, ADA, at a concentration that should have broken down all interstitial adenosine [6, 22, 42, 59]. Coronary autoregulation and flow adjustment seemed not to be affected by the infusion of ADA. However, isolated coronary arterioles are sensitive to adenosine at concentrations that exist within the interstitium [85].

Tissue oxygen tension is a classical candidate for the control of organ flow. Chapter 9 shows that the coronary flow control system seems to be designed to keep tissue oxygen tension within reasonable limits as may be judged from coronary venous oxygen saturation. Normally, coronary venous oxygen saturation is in the range of 30 to 50%. On the other hand, during extreme exercise coronary venous oxygen saturation may decrease to 9% and still the heart may function perfectly, even at an oxygen consumption rate four times above control [71]. This illustrates that normally the heart does not work on the verge of ischemia and tissue oxygen pressure may vary over a wide enough range to act as an error signal. As illustrated in Figure 1.9 coronary venous oxygen pressure is still far above control during reactive hyperemia when oxygen consumption is already back to control. Hence, a possible relation between coronary resistance and tissue oxygen pressure during steady state, needs not to be present during transients. The problem with the oxygen hypothesis is that no direct effect of tissue oxygen pressure on isolated coronary arterioles is apparent. However, no direct effect is necessary as long as there is a mediator between tissue oxygen tension and coronary resistance vessels.

ATP-sensitive potassium channels have an essential role in anoxic vasodilation as was recently demonstrated by Daut *et al.* [20]. When these channels were blocked in Tyrode perfused rat hearts the vasodilatory response to a coronary occlusion as well as to anoxic perfusion disappeared completely. However, as can be judged from their figure, illustrating a typical result, there was no maximal constriction when these channels were blocked, indicating that normal control of flow is still possible. This would imply that normal regulation of flow is different from anoxic vasodilation. It might still be too early to come to this conclusion. An important experiment to be performed, should be directed at establishing the extent to which these channels play a role in the normal local control of coronary circulation.

Myogenic tone can be altered by a change of pressure alone. In 1902, Bayliss [11] reported that diameters of arterioles could constrict upon an increase in distending pressure and dilate following a decrease in pressure. The dynamic response is known as the myogenic response. It has recently been established [60] that small isolated coronary arteries and arterioles also exhibit spontaneous tone and a myogenic response. Coronary resistance vessels have the intrinsic ability to modulate flow such that an autoregulation curve may result. However, it is not clear how spontaneous myogenic tone is modulated by metabolism. Moreover, it is not a priori clear how a cascade of resistance vessels in series with myogenic tone act as a system. Vasoconstriction of proximal vessels will reduce pressure for distal vessels, thereby diminishing the stimulus for their myogenic response.

Flow induced relaxation is an endothelial mediated response [34, 35, 36, 48, 49, 61]. Arteries, including resistance vessels, dilate when flow through them is increased. It should be noted, however, that this response in itself cannot be the error signal for the control of coronary flow. If the flow mediated response were the only mechanism the resistance vessels would always be maximally dilated. An increase in flow would induce relaxation, which in turn would increase flow and so on. However, the flow induced relaxation may act as an amplification of a tissue oriented error signal which affects the smallest arterioles but not the more upstream resistance vessels. The flow increase induced by dilation of these smallest vessels may then result in flow mediated dilation of the proximal resistance vessels.

Interstitial oncotic pressure has been suggested as factor in the control of coronary autoregulation because of its effect on vascular smooth muscle tone [5]. However, on the basis of system analysis directed to the sensitivities of the different subprocesses involved it was concluded that the gain of this feedback loop is not sufficient to explain coronary autoregulation [44].

1.4 Heterogeneity in myocardial perfusion and oxygen supply

Heart function is the result of concerted action between myocardial fibers. Despite this, there may be variations over the myocardium in mechanical work and compressive effects on microvessels. Apart from these external effects the more or less stochastic nature of the coronary arterial tree will also contribute to an inhomogeneous distribution of blood flow. Such an inhomogeneity is especially to be expected when the arterioles have lost their tone, either by pharmacological intervention or by ischemia. When coronary regulation is intact one would expect that heterogeneity induced by all these effects may be smoothed out because control of flow is realized at the local level. In this instance it is tempting to extrapolate relations between flow and oxygen consumption as determined from large epicardial arteries and veins to the microscopic level, i.e., the smallest arterioles. However, there is plenty of evidence that such an extrapolation is impermissible.

The variation of flow over the wall from endocardium to epicardium has been recognized for a long time (Chapters 6 and 7); in the past ten years, however, emphasis has been placed on heterogeneous distribution of flow over very small tissue units weighing about 0.1 g [4]. At a much smaller level, that of the capillaries, heterogeneity is due to the structure of the capillary bed (Chapter 3). Regional measurements of tissue oxygen pressure and small venous oxygen saturation also revealed a substantial variation (Chapter 11). This section is meant as a brief introduction to the rapid growing area of research on heterogeneity.

A proper understanding of the factors governing the heterogeneity of blood and oxygen distribution is vital not only from a fundamental point of view but also for understanding pathophysiology. The subendocardium is more vulnerable for ischemia than the subepicardium (Chapter 12). Moreover, often patchy necrosis in heart muscle is found pointing into the direction of selective local underperfusion.

1.4.1 Distribution of flow from endocardium to epicardium

When local control of coronary flow is intact, the flow distribution over the myocardial wall as measured by the microsphere technique is quite homogeneous in the plateau range of the autoregulation curve [72]. Obviously, this is due to the regulation of smooth muscle tone at the regional level. However, when local control is obliterated by, e.g. adenosine, the flow distribution is determined

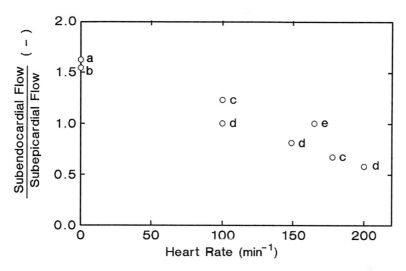

Figure 1.10: Ratio between flow in the subendocardium and subepicardium in the heart of dogs as a function of heart frequency and selected on the following criteria: maximal vasodilation and average coronary arterial pressure equals 100 mm Hg. Data are from the following references: a: [91], b: [24], c: [25], d: [7], e: [26]. (Redrawn from Bruinsma et al. [15].)

by the interplay of mechanical forces related to coronary arterial pressure and stresses in the wall. In Figure 1.10, data on the ratio between subendocardial and subepicardial flow are compiled from several studies selected for the following criteria. Mean coronary arterial pressure had to be close to 100 mm Hg and the coronary vessels had to be dilated maximally by a drug. The result should be read as follows: if the heart is arrested, subendocardial flow exceeds subepicardial flow by as much as 50%. Hence, the conclusion is that the uncompressed vascular structure results in a lower vascular resistance in the subendocardium. The endo/epi ratio decreases with heart rate, becoming about unity at a heart rate of 100 beats $\cdot$ min^{-1} and 0.5 at 200 beats $\cdot$ min^{-1}. From the studies reporting on flow distribution at different heart rates one has to conclude that the decreasing ratio is due to the decrease of subendocardial flow. Subepicardial flow is constant or even increases slightly with heart rate. Hence, compression of the intramyocardial vasculature is almost absent in the outer myocardial layer which is evidence that during normal performance of the heart, the shortening of the muscle fibers themselves has little effect on the perfusion of the tissue. The subendocardial compression may reduce flow through that region by a factor of three.

The difference between subendocardial and subepicardial impediment by contraction has long been attributed to higher tissue pressures at the layers close to the left ventricular cavity. However, subendocardial flow reduction was also found when the heart was beating but empty [86]. The present alternative hypothesis for interaction between heart contraction and coronary flow is based on time varying elastance of the myocardium [56]. This hypothesis is consistent with flow impediment in the empty beating heart but as yet presents no explanation for why this should be pronounced in the subendocardium but absent in the subepicardium. The conclusion must be that at the moment there is no satisfying hypothesis to explain these regional differences.

1.4.2 Heterogeneity induced by the arterial tree

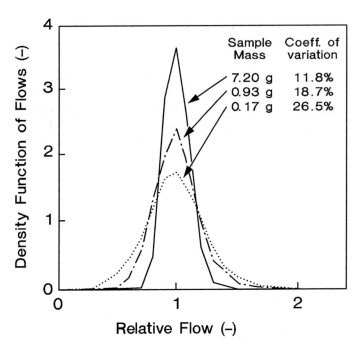

Figure 1.11: Dispersion of flow, expressed as coefficient of variation, in 10 baboons as measured by microspheres. The flows are presented relative to the mean of each distribution. The average piece mass for each distribution is given in the figure. Control of coronary flow was intact. Note the wide range of flow around the mean and that spread is larger with smaller samples. (Redrawn from Figure 4 of Bassingthwaighte et al. [10].)

Despite variabilities in vascular architecture, one would assume that because of the local nature of coronary control and the presumably homogeneous distri-

1.4 Heterogeneity in myocardial perfusion and oxygen supply

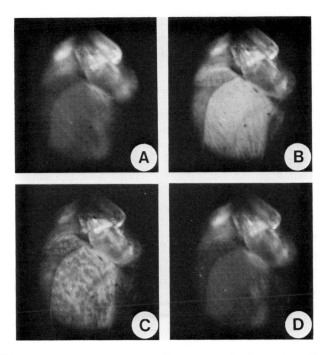

Figure 1.12: *Illustration of the patchy fluorescence by NADH in a Tyrode perfused rat heart. A: control perfusion at high oxygen pressure. B: anoxic perfusion. C: 2 s. after reperfusion with high partial oxygen pressure. D: 5 s. after reperfusion at high partial oxygen pressure. Panels A and D are controls for the measurement in B and C. (Measurements performed by Hans Vink in the Lab. of Medical Physics, University of Amsterdam.)*

bution of oxygen consumption, flow distribution would be quite even. On the contrary, a variation in microsphere density has been found, exceeding that which could be expected from methodological scatter [4, 9, 64, 93] . This is illustrated in Figure 1.11. The spread around the mean is tremendous. There are a significant number of tissue samples with a flow of less than half the mean. This is a striking finding since such a flow level in the main coronary artery, corrected for the weight of tissue perfused, would result in global ischemia of the myocardium. Coronary venous oxygen saturation is about 30%, and hence a reduction of coronary arterial flow by a factor of two cannot be compensated for by a larger oxygen extraction.

The standard deviation relative to the mean of the flow distribution appeared to increase when the myocardium was cut into smaller and smaller pieces. The dependency of the standard deviation on the weight of the sample pieces followed a mathematical description known as fractal [10]. Fractals come about as result of stochastic processes [37] and it has been suggested that for the coronary flow distribution this results from the stochastic distribution of the arterial network.

1.4.3 Heterogeneity of oxygen supply/demand ratio

Heterogeneity in either vascularity or myocardial oxygen consumption was published by Steenbergen et al. [84]. They perfused rat hearts with a saline solution and studied the epicardial fluorescence of NADH. With a lack of oxygen in tissue, NAD is converted into NADH which emits light at 465 nm wavelength when excited by radiation at 355 nm. When perfused with the saline solution at a high oxygen concentration there is practically no NADH fluorescence. Perfusion with solution with a very low oxygen partial pressure results in a homogeneous fluorescence. At an intermediate value of oxygen supply the NADH fluorescence becomes patchy, illustrating that either the distribution of oxygen or oxygen consumption is not homogeneous. Patchy NADH fluorescence can also be observed in the starting phase of the reactive hyperemic response as illustrated in Figure 1.12. Note that the patchy areas of NADH fluorescence vary considerably in area.

Sestier and coworkers [76] analyzed whether or not the heterogeneity in distribution of flow is constant in time. They injected microspheres 20–30 seconds apart and concluded that the distribution changed in time. In this way, a temporal heterogeneity might compensate for a spatial heterogeneity, meaning that an area having low flow at one moment would receive more flow later and vice versa. Temporal fluctuations in microsphere distribution have also been studied by others [53, 64] who concluded that these variations caused only about one third of the variation between regions. A stable spatial heterogeneity of perfusion is in agreement with the observations of Steenbergen et al. [84] that the patchy pattern of NADH fluorescence is always the same whether this was obtained by low oxygen pressure of the perfusion solution or by a reduced flow at high oxygen pressure. This implies that especially when it comes to perfusion conditions critical for oxygen supply the ischemic zones are stationary and do not vary position in time.

1.5 Relation between mechanics, control and distribution of coronary flow

The three themes of this book, mechanics, regulation and distribution, may be considered at different levels in the heart. Contraction of the heart impedes coronary arterial flow in systole. The interaction of fiber contraction and perfusion causing this impediment is at the local level and may exhibit quite a variation in magnitude or even mechanism over the myocardial wall. This variation in interaction may either be the result of a variation in fiber mechanics or in perfusion. Spatial variations exist under normal physiological conditions and will increase in magnitude and nature when pathological conditions arise. From measurements in the large coronary arteries it is possible to conclude that a powerful control mechanism adjusts flow to the metabolic needs of the heart. This control is brought about by feedback at the local level and one would therefore expect that at the level of small tissue units the flow would be matched to the local needs, at least under normal physiological conditions.

The studies on flow distribution have revealed that flow is distributed heterogeneously. On the assumption that flow would be matched to metabolism, as concluded from the observations on the epicardial arteries, one might expect a heterogeneity in metabolic functions spatially correlated with the flow heterogeneity. A large heterogeneity in metabolic parameters has indeed been found but not the spatial correlation [33]. Hence, the question arises to what extent the pathways for control of flow, again in nature or magnitude of signals, are similar in all parts of the heart. An important conceptual step that has to be made in coronary research is that of interaction between distribution and control, at different spatial distances within the myocardium. For example, blood flow is important to the supply of oxygen to the heart. However, in the very last stage of the transfer process diffusion is of importance. Oxygen may diffuse over more than an intercapillary distance. Moreover, the anatomy of the capillary gives rise to stochastic distribution of blood flow. This, in combination with intercapillary diffusion of oxygen, may uncouple the direct relation between blood flow and oxygen supply to small regions of the heart. It seems important that these relations be established.

Another important point that needs more insight and quantification is related to the distribution of the control function of small arteries and arterioles. Under normal physiological conditions pressure starts to fall in epicardial small arteries of 400 μm diameter. The control of flow requires tuning between vascular resistance and metabolism at the local level. Because of the small distances involved, it is not hard to accept that the small arterioles are under the direct influence of metabolic processes. However, this influence will be much weaker at the level of larger vessels. Moreover, an unstable control mechanism would result if the larger resistance vessels were under the control of only the myocytes in their direct environment. If, because of anatomical reasons, the cells surrounding a segment of a resistance vessel were amply supplied by oxygen, the metabolic control signal might lead to local vasoconstriction, thereby reducing the supply to the myocytes depending on blood flow through this segment.

Our lack of understanding of interaction of the different mechanical, regulatory and distribution processes is still enormous. This book attempts to focus on some of these problems, thereby striving to resolve these questions.

1.6 Summary

Coronary arterial and coronary venous pressure and flow signals are time varying and are the result of interaction between perfusion source on the one hand and compression due to muscle contractions on the other hand. Because arterial and venous flows are out of phase, the notion 'perfusion of the heart' can only usefully be applied to the time average of the flow through the heart muscle. Mean coronary flow is controlled by a local mechanism and depends primarily on oxygen consumption of the heart, although it is also dependent on perfusion pressure. The time needed to change flow by the local control mechanism requires many seconds. At normoxic conditions the dynamic response of coronary flow depends on the direction of the pressure changes: oscillatory with a pressure step-down and overdamped with a pressure step-up. Intramyocardial blood-volume is not constant but depends on blood pressure and compression due to heart contraction. Blood volume variation affects coronary arterial and venous flow, capacitive flow and resistance variations. The perfusion of the heart is heterogeneous at different levels. With elimination of local control, flow at the subendocardium can differ strongly from that in the subepicardium. This is due to the compression of vessels in the subendocardium, and this compressive effect in turn depends on heart rate. Flow is also heterogeneous within a layer at constant depth in the myocardium, and at the capillary level. One should therefore be cautious in extrapolating findings from measurements in the larger arteries and veins to small areas of myocardium.

References

[1] ALLELA A, WILLIAMS FL, BOLENE-WILLIAMS FC, KATZ M (1955) Interrelation between cardiac oxygen consumption and coronary blood flow. *Am. J. Physiol.* **183**: 570–576.

[2] ARTS MGJ[2] (1978) *A mathematical model of the dynamics of the left ventricle and the coronary circulation.* PhD Thesis. University of Limburg, Maastricht, The Netherlands.

[3] ARTS T, VEENSTRA PC, RENEMAN RS (1982) Epicardial deformation and left ventricular wall mechanics during ejection in the dog. *Am. J. Physiol.* **243** (*Heart Circ. Physiol.* **12**): 379–390.

[4] AUSTIN RE JR, ALDEA GS, COGGINS DL, FLYNN AE, HOFFMAN JIE (1990) Profound spatial heterogeneity of coronary reserve. Discordance between patterns of resting and maximal myocardial blood flow. *Circ. Res.* **67**: 319–331.

---

[2] Arts MGJ is the same person as Arts T [3].

[5] AVOLIO AP, SPAAN JAE, LAIRD JD (1980) Plasma protein concentration and control of coronary vascular resistance in isolated rat heart. *Am. J. Physiol.* **238** (*Heart Circ. Physiol.* **7**): H471–H480.
[6] BACHE RJ, DAI XZ, SCHWARTZ JS, HOMANS DC (1988) Role of adenosine in coronary vasodilation during exercise. *Circ. Res.* **62**: 846–853.
[7] BACHE RJ, COBB FR (1977) Effect of maximal coronary vasodilation on transmural myocardial perfusion during tachycardia in the awake dog. *Circ. Res.* **41**: 648–653.
[8] BARCROFT J, DIXON WE (1906) The gaseous metabolism of the mammalian heart. Part 1. *J. Physiol. Lond.* **35**: 182–204.
[9] BASSINGTHWAIGHTE JB (1988) Physiological heterogeneity: fractals link determinism and randomness in structure and function. *New Physiol. Sci.* **3**: 5–10.
[10] BASSINGTHWAIGHTE JB, KING RB, ROGER SA (1989) Fractal nature of regional myocardial blood flow heterogeneity. *Circ. Res.* **65**: 578–590.
[11] BAYLISS WM (1902) On the local reactions of the arterial wall to changes in internal pressure. *J. Physiol. Lond.* **28**: 220–231.
[12] BELLAMY RF (1978) Diastolic coronary artery pressure-flow relations in the dog. *Circ. Res.* **43**: 92–101.
[13] BELLONI FL, SPARKS HV JR (1982) Dynamics of myocardial oxygen consumption and coronary artery pressure-flow relationship in the dog. *Circ. Res.* **50**: 377–385.
[14] BERNE RM (1980) The role of adenosine in the regulation of coronary blood flow. *Circ. Res.* **47**: 807–813.
[15] BRUINSMA P, ARTS T, DANKELMAN J, SPAAN JAE (1988) Model of the coronary circulation based on pressure dependence of coronary resistance and compliance. *Basic Res. Cardiol.* **83**: 510–524.
[16] CANTY JM JR (1988) Coronary pressure-function and steady-state pressure-flow relations during autoregulation in the unanesthetized dog. *Circ. Res.* **63**: 821–836.
[17] COFFMAN JD, GREGG DE (1960) Reactive hyperemia characteristics of the myocardium. *Am. J. Physiol.* **199**: 1143–1149.
[18] COFFMAN JD, GREGG DE (1961) Oxygen metabolism and oxygen debt repayment after myocardial ischemia. *Am. J. Physiol.* **201**: 881–887.
[19] DANKELMAN J, SPAAN JAE, STASSEN HG, VERGROESEN I (1989) Dynamics of coronary adjustment to a change in heart rate in the anaesthetized goat. *J. Physiol. Lond.* **408**: 295–312.
[20] DAUT J, MAIER-RUDOLPH W, VON BECKERATH N, MEHRKE G, GÜNTHER K, GOEDEL-MEINEN L (1990) Hypoxic dilation of coronary arteries is mediated by ATP-sensitive potassium channels. *Science* **247**: 1341–1344.
[21] DOLE WP, MONTVILLE WJ, BISHOP VS (1981) Dependency of myocardial

reactive hyperemia on coronary artery pressure in the dog. *Am. J. Physiol.* **240** (*Heart Circ. Physiol.* **9**): H709–H715.

[22] DOLE WP, YAMADA N, BISHOP VS, OLSSON RA (1985) Role of adenosine in coronary blood flow regulation after reductions in perfusing pressure. *Circ. Res.* **56**: 517–524.

[23] DOLE WP, NUNO DW (1986) Myocardial oxygen tension determines the degree and pressure range of coronary autoregulation. *Circ. Res.* **59**: 202–215.

[24] DOMENECH RJ (1978) Regional diastolic coronary blood flow during diastolic ventricular hypertension. *Cardiovasc. Res.* **12**: 639–645.

[25] DOMENECH RJ, GOICH J (1976) Effect of heart rate on regional coronary blood flow. *Cardiovasc. Res.* **10**: 224–231.

[26] DOWNEY HF, BASHOUR FA, STEPHENS AJ, KECHEJIAN SJ, UNDERWOOD RH (1975) Uniformity of transmural perfusion in anesthetized dogs with maximally dilated coronary circulations. *Circ. Res.* **37**: 111–117.

[27] DOWNEY HF, CRYSTAL GJ, BASHOUR FA (1983) Asynchronous transmural perfusion during coronary reactive hyperemia. *Cardiovasc. Res.* **17**: 200–206.

[28] DOWNEY HF, MURAKAMI H, KIM SJ, WILLIAMS AG JR (1990) Mechanism of Gregg's phenomenon: alteration of ventricular end-diastolic segment length. *FASEB J.* **4**(3): A403.

[29] DOWNEY JM, KIRK ES (1975) Inhibition of coronary blood flow by a vascular waterfall mechanism. *Circ. Res.* **36**: 753–760.

[30] DRISCOL DE, MOIR TW, ECKSTEIN RW (1963) Vascular effect of changes in perfusion pressure in the non-ischemic and ischemic heart. *Circ. Res.* **15** *Suppl.* I: 94–102.

[31] ECKENHOFF JE, HAFKENSCHIEL JH, LANDMESSER CM, HARMEL M (1947) Cardiac oxygen metabolism and control of the coronary circulation. *Am. J. Physiol.* **149**: 634–649.

[32] FEIGL EO (1983) Coronary physiology. *Physiol. Rev.* **63**: 1–205.

[33] FRANZEN D, CONWAY RS ZHANG H, SONNENBLICK EH, ENG C (1988) Spatial heterogeneity of local blood flow and metabolite content in dog hearts. *Am. J. Physiol.* **254** (*Heart Circ. Physiol.* **13**): 344–353.

[34] FLEISCH A (1935) Les réflexes nutritifs ascendants producteurs de dilatation artérielle. *Arch. Int. Physiol.* **XLI**: 141–167.

[35] FURCHOTT RF (1983) Role of endothelium in responses of vascular smooth muscle. *Circ. Res.* **53**: 557–573.

[36] FURCHOTT RF, ZAWADZKI JV (1980) The obligatory role of endothelial cells in the relaxation of arterial smooth muscle by acetylcholine. *Nature* **288**: 373–376.

[37] GOLDBERGER AL, RIGNEY DR, WEST BJ (1990) Chaos and fractals in human physiology. *Scientific American* **262**: 34–41.

[38] GRATTAN MT, HANLEY FL, STEVENS MB, HOFFMAN JIE (1986) Transmural coronary flow reserve patterns in dogs. *Am. J. Physiol.* **250** (*Heart Circ. Physiol.* **19**): H276–H283.
[39] GREGG DE (1950) *The coronary circulation in health and disease.* LEA AND FEBIGER, Philadelphia.
[40] GREGG DE (1963) Effect of coronary perfusion pressure or coronary flow on oxygen usage of the myocardium. *Circ. Res.* **13**: 497–500.
[41] GREGG DE, GREEN HD (1940) Registration and interpretation of normal phasic inflow into a left coronary artery by an improved differential manometric method. *Am. J. Physiol.* **130**: 114–125.
[42] HANLEY FL, GRATTAN MT, STEVENS MB, HOFFMAN JIE (1986) Role of adenosine in coronary autoregulation. *Am. J. Physiol.* **250** (*Heart Circ. Physiol.* **19**): H558–H566.
[43] HEINEMAN FW, GRAYSON J (1985) Transmural distribution of intramyocardial pressure measured by micropipette technique. *Am. J. Physiol.* **249** (*Heart Circ. Physiol.* **18**): H1216–H1223.
[44] HESLINGA G, STASSEN HG, SPAAN JAE (1991) Evalutation of the control function of interstitial osmolarity in coronary autoregulation. *J. Med. Biol. Eng. Comp.* In press.
[45] HIRAMATSU O, WADA Y, YAMAMOTO T, YANAKA M, KIMURA A, OGASAWARA Y, TSUJIOKA K, KAJIYA F (1989) Similar phasic characteristics of artery inflow into and vein outflow from myocardium between left and right ventricles. *Circulation* **80** *Suppl.* IV: II-549.
[46] HOFFMAN JIE, SPAAN JAE (1990) Pressure-flow relations in the coronary circulation. *Physiol. Rev.* **70**: 331–390.
[47] HOFFMAN JIE, BAER RW, HANLEY FL, MESSINA LM, GRATTAN MT (1985) Regulation of transmural myocardial blood flow. *J. Biomech. Eng.* **107**: 2–9.
[48] HOLTZ J, FÖRSTERMANN U, POHL U, GIESLER M, BASSENGE E (1984) Flow-dependent, endothelium-mediated dilation of epicardial coronary arteries in conscious dogs: effect of cyclo-oxygenase inhibition. *J. Cardiovasc. Pharmacol.* **6**: 1161–1169.
[49] IGNARRO LJ, BUGA GM, WOOD KS, BYRNS RE, AND CHAUDHURI G. (1989) Endothelium-derived relaxing factor produced and released from artery and vein is nitric oxide. *Circ. Res.* **65**: 1–21.
[50] KAJIYA F, TSUJIOKA K, OGASAWARA Y, HIRAMATSU O, WADA Y, GOTO M, YANAKA M (1989) Analysis of the characteristics of the flow velocity waveforms in the left atrial small arteries and veins in the dog. *Circ. Res.* **65**: 1172–1181.
[51] KAJIYA F, KLASSEN GA, SPAAN JAE, HOFFMAN JIE (1990) *Coronary circulation. Basic mechanism and clinical relevance.* Springer-Verlag, Tokyo.
[52] KATZ SA, FEIGL EO (1988) Systole has little effect on diastolic coronary

blood flow. *Circ. Res.* **62**: 443–451.
[53] KING RB, BASSINGTHWAIGHTE JB (1989) Temporal fluctuations in regional myocardial flow. *Pflügers Arch.* **413**: 336–342.
[54] KLOCKE FJ, MATES RE, CANTY JM JR, ELLIS AK (1985) Response to the article by Spaan on 'Coronary diastolic pressure-flow relation and zero flow pressure explained on the basis of intramyocardial compliance.' (*Circ. Res.* (1985) **56**: 293–309) *Circ. Res.* **56**: 791–792.
[55] KLOCKE FJ, MATES RE, CANTY JM JR, ELLIS AK (1985) Coronary pressure-flow relationships. Controversial issues and probable implications. *Circ. Res.* **56**: 310–323.
[56] KRAMS R, SIPKEMA P, ZEGERS J, WESTERHOF N (1989) Contractility is the main determinant of coronary systolic flow impediment. *Am. J. Physiol.* **257** (*Heart Circ. Physiol.* **26**): H1936–H1944.
[57] KRAMS R, SIPKEMA P, WESTERHOF N (1989) Varying elastance concept may explain coronary systolic flow impediment. *Am. J. Physiol.* **257** (*Heart Circ. Physiol.* **26**): H1471–H1479.
[58] KRAMS R (1988) *The effect of cardiac contraction on coronary flow. Introduction to a new concept.* PhD Thesis. Free University of Amsterdam, The Netherlands.
[59] KROLL K, FEIGL EO (1985) Adenosine is unimportant in controlling coronary blood flow in unstressed dog hearts. *Am. J. Physiol.* **249** (*Heart Circ. Physiol.* **18**): H1176–H1187.
[60] KUO L, DAVIS MJ, CHILIAN WM (1988) Myogenic activity in isolated subepicardial and subendocardial coronary arterioles. *Am. J. Physiol.* **255** (*Heart Circ. Physiol.* **24**): H1558–H1562.
[61] LIE M, SEJERSTED OM, KIIL F (1970) Local regulation of vascular cross section during changes in femoral arterial blood flow in dogs. *Circ. Res.* **27**: 727–737.
[62] LOWENSOHN HS, KHOURI EM, GREGG DE, PYLE RL, PATTERSON RE (1976) Phasic right coronary artery flow in conscious dogs with normal and elevated right ventricular pressures. *Circ. Res.* **39**: 760–766.
[63] MARCUS ML (1983) *The coronary circulation in health and disease.* McGraw-Hill, New York.
[64] MARCUS ML, KERBER RE, ERHARDT JC, FALSETTI HL, DAVIS DM, ABBOUD FM (1977) Spatial and temporal heterogeneity of left ventricular perfusion in awake dogs. *Am. Heart J.* **94**: 748–754.
[65] MARZILLI M, GOLDSTEIN S, SABBAH HN, LEE T, STEIN PD (1979) Modulating effect of regional myocardial performance on local myocardial perfusion in the dog. *Circ. Res.* **45**: 634–640.
[66] MEER JJ VD, RENEMAN RS (1973) The relation of intramyocardial pressure (IMP) to coronary blood flow (CBF). 7th Eur. Conf. Microcirculation, Aberdeen (1972), Part I Bibl. Basel, Karger. *Anat.* **11**: 151–157.

[67] MOHRMAN DE, FEIGL EO (1978) Competition between sympathetic vasoconstriction and metabolic vasodilation in the canine coronary circulation. *Circ. Res.* **42**: 79–86.
[68] OLSSON RA, BUGNI WJ (1986) The coronary circulation. In: *The Heart and Cardiovascular System: Scientific Foundations.* Eds. FOZZARD HE, HABER E, JENNINGS RB, KATZ AM, MORGAN HE. Raven Press, New York: 987–1037.
[69] PORTER WT (1898) The influence of the heart beat on the flow of blood through the walls of the heart. *Am. J. Physiol.* **1**: 145–163.
[70] RENEMAN RS Personal communication.
[71] VONRESTORFF W, HOLTZ J, BASSENGE E (1977) Exercise induced augmentation of myocardial oxygen extraction in spite of normal coronary dilator capacity in dogs. *Pflügers Arch.* **372**: 181–185.
[72] ROULEAU J, BOERBOOM LE, SURJADHANA A, HOFFMAN JIE (1979) The role of autoregulation and tissue diastolic pressures in the transmural distribution of left ventricular blood flow in anesthetized dogs. *Circ. Res.* **45**: 804–815.
[73] RUITER JH, SPAAN JAE, LAIRD JD (1977) Transient oxygen uptake during myocardial reactive hyperemia in the dog. *Am. J. Physiol.* **232** (*Heart Circ. Physiol.* **1**): H437–H440.
[74] SABISTON DC JR, GREGG DE (1957) Effect of cardiac contraction on coronary blood flow. *Circulation* **15**: 14–20.
[75] SCARAMUCCI J (1695) De motu cordis, theorema sextum. In: *Theoremata familiaria de physico-medicis lucubrationibus Iucta leges mecanicas.*: 70–81.
[76] SESTIER FJ, MILDENBERGER RR, KLASSEN GA (1978) Role of autoregulation in spatial and temporal perfusion heterogeneity of canine myocardium. *Am. J. Physiol.* **235** (*Heart Circ. Physiol.* **4**): H64–H71.
[77] SPAAN JAE (1985) Coronary diastolic pressure-flow relation and zero flow pressure explained on the basis of intramyocardial compliance. *Circ. Res.* **56**: 293–309.
[78] SPAAN JAE (1985) Response to the article by Klocke *et al.* on 'Coronary pressure-flow relationships: controversial issues and probable implications' (*Circ. Res.* (1985) **56**: 310–323) *Circ. Res.* **56**: 789–791.
[79] SPAAN JAE, BREULS NPW, LAIRD JD (1981) Forward coronary flow normally seen in systole is the result of both forward and concealed back flow. *Basic Res. Cardiol.* **76**: 582–586.
[80] SPAAN JAE, BRUSCHKE AVG, GITTENBERGER-DE GROOT AC (1987) *Coronary circulation, from basic mechanisms to clinical implications.* Martinus Nijhoff, Dordrecht, The Netherlands.
[81] SPAAN JAE, BRUINSMA P, LAIRD JD (1983) Coronary flow mechanics of the hypertrophied heart. In: *Cardiac left ventricular hypertrophy.* Eds. TERKEURS HEJD, SCHIPPERHEIJN JJ. Martinus Nijhoff, Dordrecht, The

Netherlands: 171–191.
[82] SPAAN JAE, VERGROESEN I, DANKELMAN J, STASSEN H (1987) Local control of coronary flow. In: *Coronary circulation, from basic mechanisms to clinical implications*. Eds. SPAAN JAE, BRUSCHKE AVG, GITTENBERGER-DEGROOT AC. Martinus Nijhoff, Dordrecht, The Netherlands: 45–58.
[83] SPAAN JAE, BREULS NPW, LAIRD JD (1981) Diastolic-systolic coronary flow differences are caused by intramyocardial pump action in the anesthetized dog. *Circ. Res.* **49**: 584–593.
[84] STEENBERGEN C, DELEEUW G, BARLOW C, CHANCE B, WILLIAMSON JR (1977) Heterogeneity of the hypoxic state in perfused rat heart. *Circ. Res.* **41**: 606–615.
[85] VANBAVEL E (1989) *Metabolic and myogenic control of blood flow studied on isolated small arteries*. PhD Thesis. University of Amsterdam, The Netherlands.
[86] VANWINKLE DM, SWAFFORD AN, DOWNEY JM (1990) The subendocardial extravascular resistance in dog hearts is independent of ventricular lumenal pressure. *FASEB J.* **4**: A946.
[87] VERGROESEN I, NOBLE MIM, WIERINGA PA, SPAAN JAE (1987) Quantification of O_2 consumption and arterial pressure as independent determinants of coronary flow. *Am. J. Physiol.* **252** (*Heart Circ. Physiol.* **21**): H545–H553.
[88] VERGROESEN, I (1987) *Local regulation of coronary flow*. PhD Thesis. University of Amsterdam, The Netherlands.
[89] WESTERHOF N (1990) Physiological hypotheses-Intramyocardial pressure. A new concept, suggestions for measurement. *Basic Res. Cardiol.* **85**: 105–119.
[90] WIGGERS CJ (1954) The interplay of coronary vascular resistance and myocardial compression in regulating coronary flow. *Circ. Res.* **2**: 271–279.
[91] WÜSTEN B, BUSS DD, DEIST H, SCHAPER W (1977) Dilatory capacity of the coronary circulation and its correlation to the arterial vasculature in the canine left ventricle. *Basic Res. Cardiol.* **72**: 636–650.
[92] YANAGISAWA M, KURIHARA H, KIMURA S, TOMOBE Y, KOBAYASHI M, MITSUI Y, YAZAKI Y, GOTO K, MASAKI T (1988) A novel potent vasoconstrictor peptide produced by vascular endothelial cells. *Nature* **332**: 411–415.
[93] YIPINTSOI T, DOBBS WA JR, SCANLON PD, KNOPP TJ, BASSINGTHWAIGHTE JB (1973) Regional distribution of diffusible tracers and carbonized microspheres in the left ventricle of isolated dog hearts. *Circ. Res.* **33**: 573–587.

Chapter 2

Structure and function of the coronary arterial tree

THE PURPOSE OF THE CORONARY ARTERIAL TREE, a branching network of vessels, is to distribute blood over the capillary bed and to regulate coronary flow. Regulation is exercised by the smooth muscle cells in the vessel walls, especially of the smaller arteries and arterioles. These smooth muscle cells are under the control of tissue metabolism and are able to adapt perfusion to local needs independently of the structure of the arterial tree. However, the architecture of the arterial tree determines the potential for the distribution of blood flow, which then is modulated by control. The magnitude by which vessels of certain diameter may contribute to the control of flow depends on their contribution to overall resistance. This can be inferred from the pressure distribution over the coronary arterial tree. If the drop of pressure over vessels with a certain diameter is negligible, their potential to alter flow significantly will also be very slight. Theoretically, the resistance of a vessel can readily be estimated from its length and diameter, applying Poiseuille's law and neglecting entrance effects and peculiarities of rheology. However, the vessel's contribution to the overall resistance and its potential to alter flow distribution depends strongly on the structure of the network and the position of the vessel in it. A good test of whether the relation between structure and function of the arterial tree is understood follows from the comparison between the experimentally determined pressure distribution and its prediction on the basis of the structure of the arterial tree.

For understanding coronary flow mechanics the amount of volume in the coronary arterial tree and its distribution is of importance. Both volume and resistance are determined by geometrical factors and hence bear relation to each other. As with pressure, volume distribution can be predicted from the structure of the tree. Such a prediction should match the measurements reported.

Because of the rather straightforward dependence of volume and resistance on geometrical vessel properties, the task of predicting their distribution over the tree should not be too difficult. However, the arterial tree contains many segments and their positions in the tree do not follow a regular deterministic ordering. In a heart weighing 100 g, arterial diameter can taper from several mm to 7 μm over as many as 10 bifurcations. Moreover, very small vessels branch off from very large ones, adding a complication to the ordering scheme. Since it is impossible to achieve an exact reconstruction of the complete coronary tree, understanding volume and pressure distributions may be attempted from such morphometrically, obtained stochastic relations as variation of vessel diameter, vessel segment length as a function of diameter, and diameter ratios at branch nodes. Obviously, the distribution of flow should be predicted as well. At this moment, there is no model that describes all three distributions satisfactorily.

This chapter provides a stochastic description of the anatomy of the coronary arterial tree and will emphasize the strengths and shortcomings of a dichotomous symmetric branching network which often is implicitly used to describe the distribution function of the coronary arterial tree.

2.1 Basic anatomy

The arterial tree consists of large arteries, small arteries and arterioles. Arterioles are the very small arteries with one to three layers of smooth muscle cells in the wall and diameters which tend to be smaller than 100 μm [9]. The distinction between large and small arteries is arbitrary and in this book all arteries with diameters larger than 400 μm are referred to as large arteries and those with diameters smaller than 400 μm are considered small arteries.

All arteries, large and small, take part in the distribution function. However, the control function is restricted to the arteries smaller than about 400 μm. Those vessels are referred to as control vessels. Hence, not only arterioles but also the other small arteries belong to the category of control vessels.

There is a large variability in the anatomy of the coronary system. However, this may be simplified in the following terms. Two major coronary arteries originate from the aortic valve region. Each of the three leaflets of the aortic valve is attached to the lower rim of a semispherical structure called the sinus of Valsalva. A major coronary artery springs from the top of two of these sinuses, to become the right and the left coronary arteries respectively. The latter is also referred to as the left main stem. Usually the right ventricular wall is mainly perfused by the right coronary artery and the left coronary artery primarily perfuses the left ventricular wall and septum. However, in humans and pigs an important part of the left ventricular wall may be perfused from the right coronary artery as well, a condition which is referred to as right dominant [20].

2.2 Basic anatomy

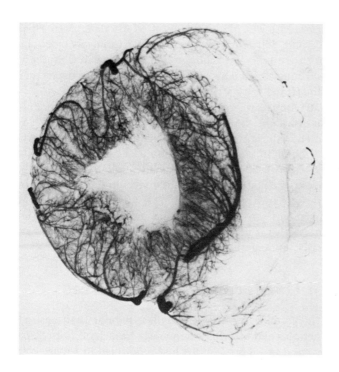

Figure 2.1: Angiogram of a slice of dog myocardium with the arterial tree filled with barium-gelatine mixture showing transmural arteries and their branching into arterioles. Small arterial volume is higher at the subendocardium than in the subepicardium [42]. (This photograph was kindly provided by Dr. W. Chilian, Dept. of Physiology, A & M University, Texas.)

The coronary arteries branch into large arteries coursing over the surface of the heart. The two main branches of the left main stem are: the left anterior descending artery (LAD) and the left circumflex artery (LCX). The LAD runs in the interventricular groove. The LCX runs in the atrio-ventricular groove. Septal arteries penetrate straight into the septum between left and right ventricles and are, apart from the very beginning, completely surrounded by tissue, unlike the epicardial arteries. As is shown in Figure 2.1, transmural arteries branch from the epicardial arteries into the myocardial wall. From the transmural arteries, small arteries and arterioles branch off to perfuse the capillary bed.

The branching of the coronary arterial system can be compared to the branching of a tree. This implies that each branch or segment thereof can only be reached from the stem by a single pathway. This is not entirely true, because collaterals and anastomoses occur at almost all levels of vessel diameter.

2.2 Collaterals

Collaterals are vessels connecting arterial branches from different parent branches in one region of the heart to the other. Their function is to bypass obstructions in arterial branches and to perfuse tissue that otherwise would be ischemic, or in other words, would receive too low a blood supply. Collaterals are a normal occurrence in many species and will start to function if arterial obstructions become significant. A quantitative analysis of collateral flow is given in Chapter 5. The reader interested in their function and growth is referred to other books and literature, e.g., the richly illustrated work written by Schaper [31].

Schaper [31] (pages 4–10) states, referring to Schoenmackers [32] and Fulton [18], that in humans and pigs the majority of the arterial collaterals are located subendocardially and endomurally. However, in the normal canine heart, most of the collaterals are found in the subepicardium. These latter vessels generally have diameters of between 20 and 80 μm. When collateral growth is stimulated by ischemia, epicardial collaterals with a diameter similar to the more distal large epicardial arteries are seen.

When coronary flow mechanics are studied and the imbalance between the perfusion pressures of main arteries is not excessive, the effect of collaterals can be ignored. This will generally be done in this book.

2.3 Structure of the coronary arterial tree

The branching pattern of the coronary arterial tree is less regular than desired for model purposes. Small arteries and arterioles frequently branch off from large parent vessels. This is illustrated in Figure 2.2 [37] and quantified in Figure 2.4. To continue the tree analogy, this pattern is very like the twigs and shoots which sprout from the larger branches and provide a denser foliage.

Recently, some work on the quantification of the arterial structure was done in our laboratory. Measurements were done on casts obtained with Batson's #17 corrosion compound. Pig and goat hearts were first perfused according to Langendorff using a Tyrode solution containing adenosine. Then perfusion was switched to a solution containing 2.0% glutaraldehyde to fix the vascular bed. The vascular tree was filled with a cast compound having a viscosity of 260 cP at 4 °C for approximately 45 minutes. Filling pressure was maintained at 50 mm Hg. These conditions prevented the capillaries from filling with cast material. After hardening, the tissue was dissolved by a strong base. Branches were broken from the structure for analysis. The length and diameter of unbranched segments were measured under the microscope. These segments are defined by a proximal and distal sidebranch, regardless of the side branch diameter.

The branching was found to be dichotomous in 99% of the bifurcations. Only in about 1% of the arteries did a proximal branch split into three or more side

2.3 Structure of the coronary arterial tree

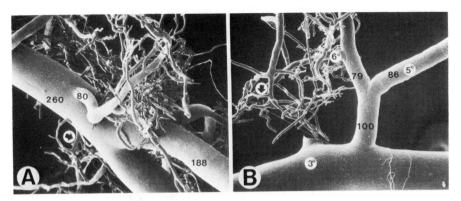

Figure 2.2: Branching of very small arteries from larger coronary branches. Pictures were taken from coronary casts of rabbit left ventricle. In A, arterial and arteriolar diameters are given. Terminal arterioles are indicated by arrows. In B, the order of branches is given with LAD = 1. The vessels were obtained from the epicardial half of the myocardium. On purpose, just enough casting material was injected to show the branches from the arterial main branch. (From Tomanek [37] by his permission and that of Martinus Nijhoff.)

branches at the same location. These branch points were not included in the analysis.

2.3.1 Ratios between diameters of mother and daughter branches

The symmetry of branching, S, in our measurements was defined as

$$S = \frac{d_s/d_l - d_{\min}/d_l}{1 - d_{\min}/d_l} \qquad [2.1]$$

where:

d_s is the diameter of the smaller daughter branch,
d_l is the diameter of the larger daughter branch,
$d_{\min}$ = 9 μm is the minimum diameter measured in the cast.

The factor $d_{\min}$ was introduced to compensate for the increase in symmetry with decreasing diameter that would otherwise have been found because of the lower limit of measured diameters.

The symmetry as a function of the diameter of the mother vessels is depicted in Figure 2.3. A value of 1 for the symmetry factor reflects perfect symmetry

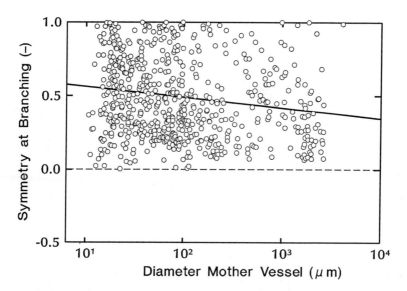

Figure 2.3: Symmetry of branching of the coronary arterial tree in the pig. Symmetry is defined according to Equation [2.1]. Perfect symmetry is reflected by the value 1. A symmetry value of zero corresponds to the diameter of the smaller branch equal to $d_{\min}$. Note that the branching pattern is not symmetrical. Symmetry increases slightly with decreasing diameters. The heavy line illustrates the curve of best fit. (Data from VanBavel [38].)

while zero occurs when the diameter of the smaller daughter vessel equals $d_{\min}$. Sometimes negative values may occur due to the fact that some vessels have a diameter of less than $d_{\min}$. The results of symmetry quantify the observations discussed with Figure 2.2, i.e., that small arterioles may branch from larger vessels.

A different picture of the branching characteristic of the coronary arterial tree is obtained when the diameters of the larger and smaller side branches are separately plotted versus the diameter of the mother branch. This is done in Figure 2.4. The diameter of the larger daughter branch correlates nicely with the diameter of the mother branch, d_m. As reference, the identity line is given as well as the line corresponding to the ratio of 50% in diameter reduction. The variation in the ratio between smaller diameter and mother diameter is much larger but decreases as the mother diameter decreases. This is to be expected because of the lower limit of diameters occurring in the data set. Note that the variation in the ratio of d_s/d_m is about a factor of 10 in vessel diameters above 100 μm.

2.3 Structure of the coronary arterial tree

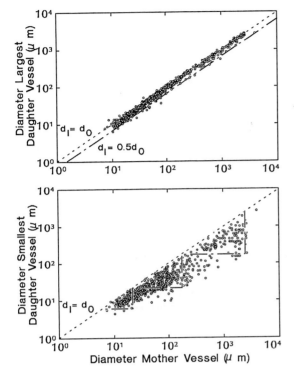

Figure 2.4: Diameters of the daughter branches at bifurcations as a function of the diameter of the mother branch. Top panel: Larger daughter diameter. Bottom panel: Smaller daughter diameter. The dotted lines are lines of identity. The dash-dotted line in the top panel reflects a diameter reduction of 50%. The staircase line in the bottom panel illustrates that a main artery of 3 mm may bifurcate to a diameter of 7 μm in 3 steps. (Data from VanBavel [38].)

The number of branching nodes between the main coronary artery and the arteriolar level can be inferred. From the bottom panel of Figure 2.4., starting at a vessel with a large diameter, the daughter with the smallest possible diameter is selected. A daughter vessel may, in turn, spring from this, which vessel can have the smallest diameter given by this plot. By repeating this procedure it is possible to arrive at a diameter of 7 μm in only 3 steps. If, on the other hand, it is assumed that at each branching node, the daughter branch will have approximately the average of the smaller daughter diameter, the level of smallest arterioles is reached in about 8 steps. When taking the larger possible value of the smaller diameter at each selected node, quite a number of nodes can come in between the origin of the arterial tree and the smallest nodes.

2.3.2 Growth of arterial cross-sectional area

A different way of characterizing the branching structure is the growth, G, of cross-sectional area at each bifurcation. The growth function is defined as

$$G = \left[\frac{d_s}{d_m}\right]^2 + \left[\frac{d_l}{d_m}\right]^2 \qquad [2.2]$$

These results are depicted in Figure 2.5. It can be noted that the cross-sectional area decreases at a significant number of bifurcations. On the average, the cross-sectional area is increasing, more at smaller diameters than at higher diameters. Although the growth in cross-sectional area is small per bifurcation, the growth between the coronary entrance arteries and the capillary bed can still be considerable, since growth occurs repeatedly at consecutive vascular nodes. This total growth can only be estimated if information on the number of nodes in the coronary bed is available.

In physiology, Murray's law [27] predicts that the sum of the cubes of radii of the daughter vessels should be equal to the cube of the radius of the mother vessel. As is clear from Figure 2.5 and Equation [2.2] a square law holds for vessels of about 1 mm in diameter, $G = 1$, in stead of the cube law. For the vessels around 50 μm growth is stronger and the exponent describing the relation between the radii of mother and daughter vessels for symmetrically branching nodes is about 2.55, still lower than the cubic law predicts.

2.3.3 Length distribution in the arterial tree

Data on vessel length distribution in the coronary bed are hard to find in the literature. The length distribution for different organs has been discussed by McDonald [25]. Some work on the heart has been reported by Suwa [34, 35] and Zamir [43]. In our cast, the lengths of the segments, determined by two branching points, were determined [43]. The relation between segment length and segment diameter is depicted in Figure 2.6. Note the wide variation in segment length. Segments with a given diameter vary in length over two orders of magnitude.

The definition of segment length is clear but one may wonder whether this is an optimal definition. When a vessel of 400 μm gives rise to a side branch of 10 μm, flow in the parent vessel will be less disturbed than when a vessel with a diameter of 300 μm branches off. In the former example one may consider the large vessel to continue at the node while in the latter example one should consider the vessel to end at that node. Hence, in functional terms it makes sense to define vessel length in a different way. Quite arbitrarily, we defined a functional length by ignoring a side branch for vessel length estimation when the ratio between the two distal segments at the bifurcation exceeded 2. This did not change the correlations very much. Segment length at a diameter of 400 μm increased, on the average, by about 50%.

2.3 Structure of the coronary arterial tree

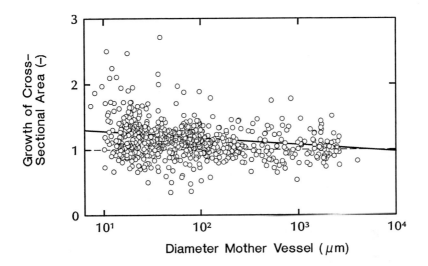

Figure 2.5: *Relative growth of arterial cross-sectional area at branch points as function of diameter of the mother branches. For a value 1 (dashed line) the cross-sectional area will remain constant. For values higher than one, the total cross-sectional area increases at each branch point. (Data from VanBavel [38].)*

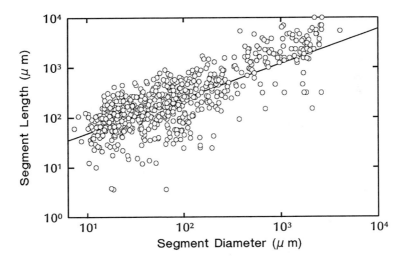

Figure 2.6: *Relation between segment length and diameter measured in a cast of the coronary arterial tree. Also shown is the regression line of segmental length as a function of segmental diameter. (Data from VanBavel [38].)*

2.3.4 Arterial density applying symmetrical branching networks

The data from our casts clearly demonstrate that the coronary arterial tree is not a symmetrical branching tree. However, a practical alternative different from such a network is not readily at hand. Moreover, most of us have a symmetric branching tree model in mind when thinking about the distribution of resistance over the coronary arterial bed. Therefore, this section will interpret some anatomical data by applying a symmetrical branching model.

Arts *et al.* [1, 2] made casts from the large coronary arterial branches and removed all arteries smaller than 400 µm. Then they counted the number of branches with diameters of approximately 400 µm which were situated distal to a branch with larger diameter. The larger the diameter of the reference branch, the more vessels with diameters of 400 µm belonged to the perfusion area of this branch. This resulted in a relation between segment diameter and number of segments of 400 µm diameter as depicted in Figure 2.7. Their results can be rewritten to yield a relation between diameter and the number of 400 µm diameter segments

$$N(d) = \left[\frac{d_0}{d}\right]^s \qquad [2.3]$$

where:

    d is diameter of an artery,
    $N(d)$ is number of arterial segments with diameter d,
    d_0 is diameter of the most proximal arterial segment,
    s is parameter estimated from the results.

The value of s for the arterial tree of the dog was found to equal 2.55. For a heart of about 100 g, d_0 was 3.5 mm. In this way the data of Arts can be transformed into a plot showing the relation between diameter and the number of vessels per unit weight. This is depicted in Figure 2.8.

For a symmetrical and dichotomous branching tree it can be shown that a similar exponential relation between N and d exists (see Equation [2.4] and [2.5] below). From this it can be concluded that the ratio between mother and daughter vessels should be $2^{1/s}$. This ratio follows directly from Equation [2.3] for the first bifurcation of the vessel with $d = d_0$. In that case $N(d) = 2$. Hence, the experimental relation of Figure 2.7 is consistent with a tree in which vessels branch symmetrically in two distal vessels with the ratio of 1.31 between proximal and distal diameters.

An estimate of the density of smaller arteries in the rat heart was obtained by Wieringa *et al.* [41]. Experiments were done in a Langendorff perfused potassium arrested rat heart. Coronary smooth muscle tone was removed by adenosine. The

2.3 Structure of the coronary arterial tree

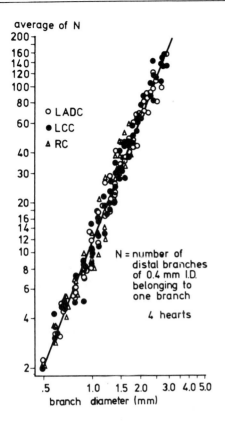

Figure 2.7: Branching pattern of the large coronary arteries after removal of vessels smaller than 400 μm diameter. The number of vessels of 400 μm diameter, N, fed by an artery of a certain diameter were counted. The number of 400 μm diameter vessels are plotted on the vertical axis and the corresponding artery diameter on the horizontal axis. Note that N here is defined differently from the way this is used in the text. (From Arts et al. [2] by permission of the author and the American Physiological Society.)

coronary flow reduced gradually after switching to a perfusion solution containing a small concentration of pollen to obstruct arterioles. The fraction of obstructed arterioles was calculated from the reduction in flow. The amount of injected pollen was known and hence an estimate could be made of the number of arteries of a certain diameter. The pollen had diameters of 15 μm, 25 μm and 50 μm. Equation [2.3] was fitted to these data and a value of $s = 2.35$ was obtained, close to the value found by Arts [2] for the larger arteries. If this is interpreted in the same way as the data of Arts et al. [2] we might conclude that these data on arteriolar density are compatible with a symmetrical dichotomous tree model for the small arteries with a ratio between proximal and distal diameters of 1.34.

The data relating to number and diameter of vessel segments are compiled in Figure 2.8. The data of Arts et al. [2], expressed as number of vessels per 100 g tissue, are indicated by the bottom heavy line over the measurement range and is extrapolated by a dash-dotted line to smaller diameters. The upper dash-dotted line is the extrapolation from Wieringa's data to larger diameters using the exponents in Equation [2.3] found by Arts et al. [2].

The density of arterioles in the dog heart can also be inferred from the amount

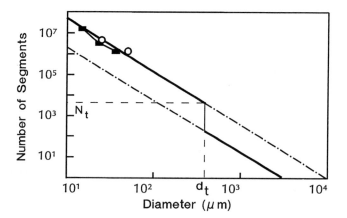

Figure 2.8: Number of vessels per 100 g as function of diameter. Data on small arteries (■) are from Wieringa et al. [41]. Heavy line for $d > d_t$ reflects the data on large arteries from Arts et al. [2] as shown in Figure 2.7. The dash-dotted lines are extrapolations. Open circles (○) are arteriolar densities calculated from necrotic areas after microsphere embolization of arterioles [15]. d_t is the diameter at which a breakpoint is assumed between the region where the large artery correlation ends and small artery correlation commences. N_t is the number of small arteries with diameter d_t. N_t and d_t are used in the branching model explained in Subsection 2.6.1.

of tissue made necrotic by obstruction of single arterioles by 50 μm beads. These experiments were done by Eng et al. [15]. The dimensions of these necrotic areas were approximately 700 μm × 325 μm × 325 μm = 0.074 mm³. Assuming a specific mass of 1 g · ml^{-1} for heart tissue, a total of 13×10^5 arterioles per 100 g is arrived at. In a similar way, one can calculate the density of 25 μm arterioles, resulting in a value of 43×10^5 per 100 g. These numbers agree reasonably with the data on arteriolar density in the rat provided by Wieringa et al. [41].

Figure 2.8 shows that with extrapolation of the experimental relation of the large arteries to the very small arteries, the number of small arteries would be underestimated more than tenfold. On the other hand, extrapolation of the data on small arteries would result in an overestimate of the diameter of the artery feeding a piece of heart tissue of 100 g. This discrepancy can easily be explained. Arts removed all small arteries from the large arteries analyzed, which obviously results in an underestimate of the number of small arteries from their correlation, especially after extrapolation outside the range of measurements. Moreover, the arterial trees analyzed by Arts et al. [2] were mainly epicardial structures combined with the larger transmural arteries. However, the inner half of the heart tissue is mainly supplied by arteries smaller than 400 μm as Figure 2.1 shows. Larger arteries are absent in the subendocardium, whereas the volume of small arteries at this location is larger than at the subepicardium [42].

That analysis of the data by means of a symmetrical network is an oversimplification is clear from the data on symmetry provided in Figure 2.3. The error made by interpreting microsphere data as obtained by Wieringa et al. [41] applying models with symmetry was assessed by Pelosi et al. [29] and can easily be about factor of two.

2.4 Data on filling volume of the coronary arterial tree

To determine the volume of the larger arteries in the dog, Douglas and Greenfield [14] blocked the perfusion area of the left main stem with 200 μm diameter beads and subsequently injected it with silicone. A correlation between arterial volume and total heart weight was found: 1.25 ml per 100 g tissue. In dog hearts weighing 123 g Arts [1] found 1.12 ml of volume for the left anterior descending and circumflex arteries together, including vessels with diameters down to 400 μm. If, as an estimate, these arteries perfuse 60% of the heart weight, the volume for arteries down to 400 μm is 1.5 ml per 100 g tissue. The volume of small intramural arteries was estimated by Wüsten et al. [42] as 3.6 ml per 100 g tissue. It was explicitly stated in their study that the larger epicardial and intramural arteries were excluded from the analysis. Wüsten et al. [42] also reported a larger small artery volume at the subendocardium than at the subepicardium.

2.5 Pressure distribution in the coronary arterial tree

Measurements show that pressure drops gradually from larger to smaller arterioles in the coronary arterial tree. Pressure distributions in the left coronary arterial tree have been reported on by Tillmanns [36] for the rat and by Chilian [12] for the cat. Nellis [28] reported on the pressure distribution in the right coronary arterial tree of the rabbit. Pressure distribution in arterial trees of other organs can be found in the literature [13, 26, 33, 44].

Measurements of the pressure distribution and also alteration by control actions or by pharmacological interventions in the beating left ventricle are extremely difficult and require special techniques. However, these measurements are very important for a proper understanding of the determinants of coronary flow.

Some data on pressure distribution in the left coronary arterial tree were kindly provided by Chilian and are reproduced in Figure 2.9. The left panel depicts the measured pressure distribution in control conditions with vasomotor

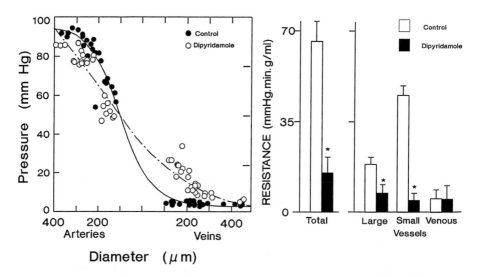

Figure 2.9: *Pressure and resistance distribution in the cat epicardial vasculature as established by Chilian. Left panel: Distribution of pressure with local control intact (●) and after vasodilation with dipyridamole (○). Right panel: The distribution of resistance and the effect of dipyridamole on it. The resistance was calculated for three compartments, which are defined in the text. (Redrawn from Chilian et al. [11].)*

tone intact and after the administration of dipyridamole. Dipyridamole is a vasodilator and believed to function by releasing endogenous adenosine [8]. In control conditions, flow amounted to 1.8 ml · min^{-1} · g^{-1}; following the infusion with dipyridamole, a fourfold increase in flow was observed. The mean pressure in the different vessels is provided as a function of diameter. Aortic pressure was maintained at constant levels during experimentation and was independent of the intervention. The results on pressure distribution and changes invoked by dipyridamole infusion can best be interpreted in conjunction with the changes in calculated resistance of the different levels of vessels. For these resistance calculations, the data were grouped in ranges of diameters. Each group formed a compartment. The arterial compartment contained the arteries with diameters above 170 μm, and the venous compartment, the venules and veins with diameters larger than 150 μm. The small vessel compartment contained arteries smaller than 170 μm and the capillaries and venules smaller than 150 μm. The average pressure drop over these ranges was then divided by coronary flow as measured by microspheres to estimate resistance. It should be noted that this calculation of resistance assumes symmetry of the arterial tree. The calculated resistance distribution is provided in the right panel of Figure 2.9.

Most of the resistance during autoregulation is within the microvessels although a significant resistance, about 25% of the total, is within arteries with diameters larger than 170 μm. Dipyridamole induced tremendous changes. The contribution of the small vessels to total resistance decreased to the level of the resistance of the venous system. The resistance of the upstream arterial tree was reduced by more than a factor of two. Hence, a contribution to local control of the coronary resistance by these vessels is potentially present. The resistance distribution in the dilated state is fairly even over the compartments. Clearly, the most important site of action is within the arterioles with diameters of less than 170 μm.

The site of resistance control is a point of general physiological discussion. From experimentation on other vascular beds, the idea has been established that the site of flow control is in the smallest arterioles or even in precapillary sphincters. As Chilian's results show, this statement is probably too general. It might be true at a very low metabolic state of the perfused tissue, where the flow per gram of tissue is low and the arterioles are close to being maximally constricted. However, measurement on other microvascular beds reveal gradual pressure drops as well [13, 26, 33].

The data presented in Figure 2.9 leaves a wide possible range for the average capillary pressure. In the vasodilated heart and at an aortic pressure of 100 mm Hg, this pressure must be between 30 and 45 mm Hg, being the highest measured venular and lowest measured arteriolar pressure respectively. With autoregulation this range is much wider: between 7 and 50 mm Hg. Data on pressure in smaller arterioles and veins are required to narrow this range. Knowledge of capillary pressure is required to make inferences on the water balance in the myocardium (e.g., Chapter 10).

2.6 Symmetrical, dichotomous branching network model

In this section, the volume and pressure distribution in a symmetrical and dichotomous branching network will be analyzed. One may wonder why such an attempt is undertaken when the experimental data on the structure of the arterial bed seem to lack any systematic ordering which would justify such an assumption. The reasons are pragmatic ones. The assumption of symmetry makes it possible to describe pressure distribution over the tree by a simple chain of resistances, each resistance having the equivalent magnitude of the vessels of certain order in parallel. A nonsymmetrical model would require a much more detailed analysis of how the vessels are interrelated. The second reason is that in many studies, implicitly or explicitly, this symmetry is assumed in interpreting data and consequently, it is worth quantifying the consequences of this assumption.

2.6.1 Definition of model structure

The quantitative basis for the model is provided by the Figures 2.6 and 2.8 defining the relations between diameter and length of vessel segments and number and diameter of vessel segments. Figure 2.8 illustrates that the relations between number and diameter of the arterioles and larger coronary arteries are not simply each other's extrapolation. This was explained by the observations that the larger segments, disregarding the branches of 400 μm and smaller, do follow a certain system, but that small arteries may be connected at arbitrary places to the large arteries. Therefore, in the model, the distinction between the large branching structure and small branching structure is emphasized. Tissue units are defined, each being fed by a small artery with diameter d_t. There are N_t of these tissue units and N_t is determined by the number–diameter relation for the arterioles as indicated in Figure 2.8. The vessels with diameter d_t are connected randomly to vessels from the large branching structure. Hence, within the regular branching pattern, a breakpoint is assumed at arteries with diameter d_t. It is further assumed that both the large arteries and arteries with a diameter smaller than d_t branch dichotomously according to the respective relationships depicted in Figure 2.8, implying that the ratio between diameters of mother and daughter vessel segment is constant and equal to 1.31.

For the calculation of volume distribution (and later pressure distribution) an ordering system for the vessel segments in the larger and small artery branching structure will now be defined. The ordering for the large branching structure starts with one vessel having order 0 and diameter d_0. This vessel branches into two segments of order 1 with diameter d_1. These segments branch further and so on. Hence, in general, a vessel of order i has a diameter d_i. The number of vessels with order i is obviously:

$$N_i = 2^i \qquad [2.4]$$

The diameter of the vessel segments with order i follows from the number–diameter relation for the large branch structure:

$$d_i = d_0 N_i^{-1/s} \qquad [2.5]$$

The branching of the larger vessel structure stops on reaching a diameter where further branching would result in a diameter equal to or smaller than d_t. The order at which this happens is I. The order $I+1$ reflects the first arteries with diameter smaller than d_t. The number of vessels of this order are:

$$N_{I+1} = \left[\frac{d_t}{d_{0,t}}\right]^{-s} \qquad [2.6]$$

where $d_{0,t}$ is the intercept with the diameter axis of the diameter-number relationship for the smaller arteries in Figure 2.8.

2.6 Symmetrical, dichotomous branching network model

The arteries with diameter d_t branch further dichotomously with the same ratio between mother and daughter segments as in the large branching structure. Hence:

$$\text{for } i > I, \quad N_i = N_{I+1} 2^{(i-I)} \qquad [2.7]$$

and

$$d_i = d_{0,t} N_i^{-1/s} \qquad [2.8]$$

Obviously, branching has to end somewhere. It was assumed that no arterioles with diameters smaller than 7 μm occur.

2.6.2 Prediction of volume

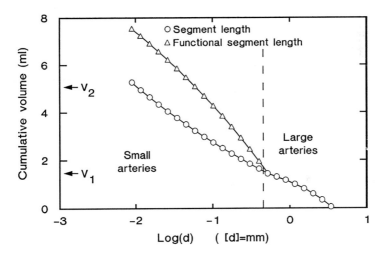

Figure 2.10: *Cumulative volume as function of vessel diameter for the large and small artery structure. V_1 (= 1.5 ml) and $V_2 - V_1$ (= 3.6 ml) are the experimental volumes determined for the large and small artery structure respectively. The effect of definition of segment length on small artery volume is shown as well. The functional segment lengths are longer since they may consist out of segments in series. For the large arteries only functional segment lengths were used and V_1 was used as boundary condition.*

Having defined the number of segments with known length and diameters of a certain order, the total vascular volume of segments of this order can be easily calculated, assuming a cylindrical shape of the segments. Figure 2.10 depicts the calculated volume as a function of diameter for the large and small artery structures. The cumulative volume as function of diameter d_i is the total volume of the part of the bed containing all segments from zero order to the order i. The prediction for the large artery structure only yields new information with respect to the distribution of volume over the vessels of different diameter. Since total volume of the arterial tree was provided by Arts et al. [2] but not the length–diameter relationship, an estimate for the length distribution was made by an exponential function using the tree volume as boundary condition. For the small artery structure, the volume distribution and cumulative volume are dependent on the length–diameter relation used. If the distribution of unbranched segments was used, the cumulative volume will have been accurately predicted; however, this will have been overestimated if functional segment length was used (Figure 2.10). The difference in predicted values will be discussed in more detail after the presentation of predicted pressure distributions.

2.6.3 Prediction of pressure

The application of the two-stage model complicates the prediction of pressure distribution in the small arteries. A significant pressure drop in the larger coronary arteries would make the inlet pressure for the different tissue units dependent on the diameter of the segment of the large artery structure to which it is connected. This would cause the symmetry of the small artery structure to be lost. In order to preserve symmetry, it will be assumed that the inlet pressure of the small artery structure equals the aortic pressure. Hence, the pressure drop in the large artery structure is ignored when it comes to predicting pressure distribution in the small artery structure.

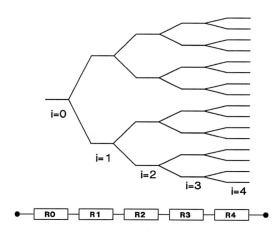

Figure 2.11: Schematic of branching tree model (top) and equivalent schematic (bottom) for calculation of the pressures at the branching points (see Appendix A).

Ignoring the pressure drop in the large artery system accentuates the distribution function of the larger coronary arteries and emphasizes the role of the small artery system in controlling perfusion of the myocardium. In addition to

2.6 Symmetrical, dichotomous branching network model

an even distribution of inlet pressure of tissue unit supply arteries (diameter = d_t), the outflow pressures of the smallest arterioles are also assumed to be equal.

The above assumptions make the pressure distribution symmetrical, which means that all segments of the same order have equal inlet and outlet pressures. This enables pressure distribution to be calculated by means of the schematic illustration in Figure 2.11. The large artery structure and small artery structure can each be represented by a series of resistors. Each resistor represents a vessel order and its value equals the parallel equivalent of the resistances of that order (the correctness of this statement will be proven in Appendix A). Hence,

$$R_i = \frac{1}{N_i} R_{si} \qquad [2.9]$$

where:

R_{si} is resistance of one segment of the order i,
N_i is the number of segments of order i.

According to Poiseuille's law, the resistance of each segment can be written as

$$R_{si} = \frac{128 \mu_i L_i}{\pi d_i^4} \qquad [2.10]$$

where:

L_i is the length of a segment i,
d_i is the diameter of a segment i,
μ_i is viscosity of blood in segment i.

Because of the Fåhraeus-Lindquist effect [8] the viscosity will depend on vessel diameter and on the average shear rate in the vessels. This latter effect will be neglected but the implications of the first will be considered.

The pressure distribution in the branching tree model can be evaluated in several ways by using the equivalent circuit of Figure 2.11. The relative pressure distribution follows directly from the distribution of resistances without further definition of flow or outflow pressure. Note that the relative distribution is insensitive to errors in, e.g., N_t the number of tissue units. Absolute pressures at the different nodes can be calculated after definition of flow through the tree and this forms a test of the choice of absolute numbers. Relative pressure distribution has been calculated for the small arterial structure only, absolute pressure distribution for both the small and large artery structure. For the estimation of absolute pressure drop in the small arterial structure, the pressure drop over the larger arteries is ignored.

The relative pressure distribution was calculated for two different length distributions and two viscosity properties for each distribution. The first length distribution is the unbranched segment length as a function of diameter. For the

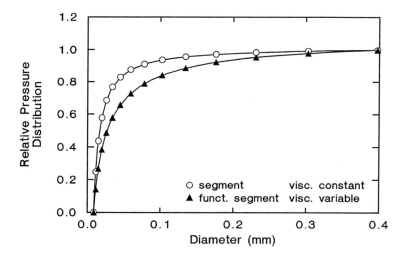

Figure 2.12: *Relative distribution of pressure over the branching points in the small artery tree model as function of proximal diameter for two extreme conditions. The open circles are the results when applying the segment length definition (short segments) and constant viscosity. Closed triangles are the results when the functional segment length-diameter relation is used and the Fåhraeus-Lindquist effect is taken into account. Note that for both the pressure drop is predicted to be within vessels having much smaller diameter than can concluded from data of Chilian et al. [11] (Figure 2.9).*

second length distribution the functional segment length was used as a function of diameter. For the first viscosity property it was assumed that viscosity was constant and equal to the high shear rate wide tube diameter viscosity, which is in the order of 4 mPa s (4 cP). For the second viscosity property, the pressure distribution was corrected for the diameter dependency of viscosity, the so-called Fåhraeus-Lindquist effect [10]. The two extremes for the relationships found are depicted in Figure 2.12.

The branching tree model predicts that the steepest pressure gradient will be found in the smaller arteries and that the major pressure drop will occur in the range between 50 and 10 μm. This prediction is in contrast to the experimental data presented in Figure 2.9. If the diameter dependency of viscosity is taken into account the drop of relative pressure shifts to larger vessels since the resistance in the smaller arterioles is diminished. However, the discrepancy with the experimental data is not materially reduced.

Up to now, the branching tree model was only evaluated for the pressure distribution. However, since all the resistances in Figure 2.11 are defined, absolute pressure at the nodes can be calculated if the total flow through the tree is

2.6 Symmetrical, dichotomous branching network model

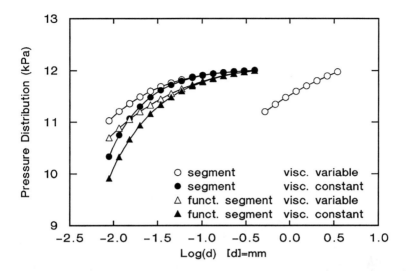

Figure 2.13: Distribution of pressure over the branching nodes in the large and small artery tree model. Pressure decreases progressively with smaller diameters. The pressure drop is smaller if the Fåhraeus-Lindquist effect is taken into account (open symbols). Pressure drop over small arterial structure is too small compared to experimental data.

defined. This number is clearly directly related to the amount of tissue that the branching tree is supposed to feed. Flow in the subepicardium of the cat hearts in which Chilian measured the pressure distribution was 10.7 ml $\cdot$ s^{-1} $\cdot$ [100 g]$^{-1}$. The quantitative pressure distribution predicted for the large and small vessel structures is depicted in Figure 2.13. The predicted pressure difference for the large coronary arteries is in the order of 10 mm Hg, which is small but significant and agrees with some experimental findings [16]. Such a pressure would imply that input pressure may not be equal for all small arterial subunits, but this is neglected in the present analysis.

The cumulative pressure drop over the small artery tree structure is low compared to the estimated total pressure drop from large coronary artery to the small arterioles. This holds especially true when blood rheology has been taken into account. As illustrated, this discrepancy is quite sensitive for the assumed length distribution for the small artery tree model.

The predicted pressure drop can be increased if the same branching structure is assumed but with longer vessels than measured. However, increased length of vessels also increases their volume. Hence, the measure to be taken to improve the prediction of pressure reduction increases the disparity between experimental and predicted data for vascular volume. The two constraints provided by experiments, cumulative pressure drop over the arterial tree and the total filling volume, are therefore incompatible with a symmetrical branching tree model applying realistic stochastic relations between variation of vessel diameter, vessel segment length as a function of diameter, and diameter ratios at branch nodes.

2.7 Nonsymmetrical dichotomous branching network analysis

2.7.1 Strahler ordering

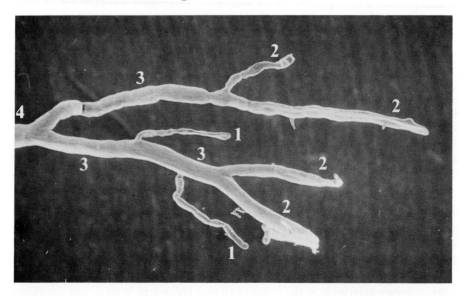

Figure 2.14: EM photograph of a cast of a small branching structure of the coronary arterial tree showing the smallest arterioles filled with casting material. The ordering indicated is according to the method of Strahler. A vascular part has been chosen illustrating the jumps in segment order number.

Strahler ordering was developed in the field of earth sciences for classifying river structures, but has also been applied to classify the ordering in arterial trees. In the Strahler system of classification, the branching pattern is described starting at the terminal segments in the tree. These segments are assigned the order one: the order of any nonterminal segment is taken equal to the highest of the orders of its branches, if these latter orders are unequal. If the branches have equal order, then the order of the proximal segment is one higher than that of both its branches. Successive segments of equal order together form vessels, with length equal to the sum of the segmental lengths, the diameter equal to the mean

2.7 Nonsymmetrical dichotomous branching network analysis

diameter of the segments. The more the order of the vessels increases, the further upstream these vessels occur. However, a situation may arise in which a vessel of, say, order j is connected to a parent vessel which was already assigned order $j + 2$ because of earlier confluencing of vessels with order $j + 1$; thus there will be a jump in vessel order of 2. The Strahler ordering is illustrated by an E.M. photograph of the smallest arteries in our cast in Figure 2.14. A vascular part was chosen in which the order jumps from 1 to 3 to illustrate the above.

Strahler ordering is virtually impossible to apply to casts of the coronary arterial tree. It requires the vascular tree to be observed from the smallest arterioles up to the large arteries. However, measurements of physical dimensions on the smallest vessels require breaking of the cast, which then prevents an easy localization of the smaller vessels with respect to the larger ones. In order to evaluate the potential of the Strahler ordering to the coronary arterial tree we generated a stochastic network based on the measurements reported on in Figures 2.3–2.6 [38, 39]. The tree generation started with a vessel segment with a diameter of 400 μm. Its length was decided on by chance according to the measured distribution (Figure 2.6). The segment was then branched into daughter segments, again according to chance, but in agreement with the measured branching distribution. This process was then repeated for each of the generated side branches, resulting in four segments, and so on. No further branching was carried out on segments with diameters less than 13.5 μm. In this way, a theoretical network was generated which had the same statistical behavior with respect to distribution of segment length and diameter as the cast on which the measurements were made. The Strahler analysis could be performed in this theoretical network as all segments were defined. Quite arbitrarily, end-segments with a diameter of less than 11.5 μm were assigned order 1 and larger than 11.5 μm order 2. The results of 30 simulations were averaged and are documented in Table 2.1.

The statistical models have an average of about 10 Strahler orders.

The geometry of the arterial tree is quantified by the bifurcation ratio RB (also referred to as Horton's bifurcation ratio), the diameter ratio RD and the length ratio RL. These ratios are defined as

$$\left. \begin{array}{rcl} RB(j) & = & N(j) \; / \; N(j+1) \\ RD(j) & = & d(j+1) \; / \; d(j) \\ RL(j) & = & l(j+1) \; / \; l(j) \end{array} \right\} \quad [2.11]$$

where j refers to the order number, $N(j)$ to the number, $d(j)$ to the diameter and $l(j)$ the length of the vessels with order j.

As the results in Table 2.1 illustrate, the Strahler ordering shows a rather striking similarity at different orders, except at order 1. This, however, is most probably due to the artificial definition of the first two orders in the model. On the average each vessel of a certain order gives rise to approximately 3 to 4 vessels of a lower order. The average diameter ratio between vessels of succeeding orders is 1.5. Only the length ratio reduces progressively with decreasing vessel order.

Table 2.1: *Strahler ordering in a stochastic tree model of the coronary arterial tree. The model generation started at a segment diameter of 400 μm and was repeated 30 times. The Strahler ordering started at terminal model segments, where segments with a diameter smaller than 11.5 μm were assigned order 1. Diameter and length refer to complete vessels, rather than individual segments. Errors are SD. RB = bifurcation ratio, RD = diameter ratio and RL = length ratio.*

Order	N	Diameter [μm]	Length [μm]	RB	RD	RL
1	329590	10.3 ± 0.7	67.2 ± 46.1	1.100	1.305	1.842
2	299700	13.5 ± 1.3	123.7 ± 100.9	3.357	1.435	2.088
3	89284	19.3 ± 2.7	258.0 ± 219.7	3.435	1.488	1.838
4	25996	28.8 ± 4.8	474.0 ± 416.2	3.453	1.506	1.721
5	7529	43.4 ± 8.0	816.3 ± 709.5	3.457	1.511	1.600
6	2178	65.4 ± 12.9	1306.7 ± 1146.7	3.372	1.534	1.435
7	646	100.3 ± 21.3	1873.8 ± 1690.6	3.365	1.582	1.357
8	192	158.6 ± 33.7	2542.1 ± 2226.6	3.254	1.550	1.495
9	59	245.9 ± 54.6	3800.8 ± 3238.4	3.278	1.499	1.215
10	18	368.9 ± 38.4	4617.3 ± 4536.2	—	—	—

Obviously, when the network is generated in this way, the volume and pressure distribution can be predicted since the whole network is defined. The models, indeed, resulted in a more even pressure distribution; however, the total pressure drop predicted by the network was also too small. We will not further elaborate on these issues.

Strahler ordering based models have been applied by Popel [30] and Fronek and Zweifach [17] to the arteriolar beds of mesentery and tenuissimus muscle. Their analysis, however, included only a limited number of orders of branching.

2.7.2 Fractal models

Fractal analysis has been brought to the field of coronary circulation by Bassingthwaighte [3, 4, 5, 7, 6]. Led on by his interest in describing the heterogeneity of flow distribution over the myocardium, he injected radioactive microspheres to measure regional flows. The heart was cut into little pieces and its radioactivity measured. He discovered that the standard deviation of the regional flow measurement was related to the number of pieces into which the myocardium was divided in a way that could not be explained by a pure statistical error. When plotting the coefficient of variation[1], being the standard deviation divided by the

---
[1]Often the term dispersion is applied instead of coefficient of variation. However, dispersion has a different definition in statistics [22].

2.7 Nonsymmetrical dichotomous branching network analysis

mean, as a function of the number of pieces in a logarithmic plot; the curve thus obtained could be described by a fractal equation and hence connections with other fractal systems are being sought.

A structure can be called fractal if it consists of fragments of varying size and orientation but similar shape (self-similarity). Different physiological structures have been described by a fractal systematic, such as the airways of the lung. A nice popular description of the application of fractal analysis to physiological structures and functions has been given by Goldberger et al. [19].

The term 'fractal' is related to fraction and its introduction can be understood from the following. If a geometrical figure, say square, is scaled, its perimeter will be proportional to the length of a leg to the power one and its area to the length of a leg to the power two. In both cases the exponent is a whole number. In case of fractals, the quantity to be scaled is not related to the reference measure to the power of a whole number but to the power of a fraction. A different example is the the measurement of the length of the coast line of England from a map with a yardstick by repeatingly moving the yardstick by one length. The smaller the length of the yardstick, the larger the length of the measured coastline becomes since more irregularities are taken into account. The relation between 'coast line length' expressed by the number of repeated measurements and the length of the yardstick should have an exponent one if the coastline consisted out of straight lines each having a length equal to a whole number of the yardstick length. However, the exponent differs from unity and is a fraction. The value of this exponent contains information on the stochastic nature of the coastline.

The idea of fractional exponents in the scaling of structures goes back to Hausdorff [21] in 1919. However, the name fractal is more recent and its application became rather popular by the computer generation of geometrical figures using fractal equations [24].

From our results on the structure on the coronary arterial tree, both in the raw data as well as from the Strahler analysis, we may conclude that this structure also fulfills the condition of self-similarity. Both mean and variation around the mean of the growth and symmetry functions point in that direction. The bifurcation ratio and diameter ratio are quite independent of the level in the ordered tree used as observation point for the more distal vascular bed. It is not clear yet whether such an observation is just a peculiarity or may really contribute to a better understanding of the functioning or genesis of the coronary arterial tree. It should be noted in this respect that also Fibonacci series have been popular as a mathematical description biological structures[2].

A fractal model for the prediction of heterogeneous distribution of myocardial perfusion has been developed by VanBeek et al. [40]. This concerns a dichotomous bifurcating model. At each node the flow is divided into two different fractions,

---

[2]The discussions with my colleague prof. Jan Strackee on the topic of physiological scaling rules were very helpful in understanding its history and mathematical framework.

in which aspect it differs from the symmetrical dichotomous branching model discussed above. It appeared that the fractal behavior of flow distribution as measured by Bassingthwaighte *et al.* [4] could be described adequately. Only a slight asymmetry (5%) of flow deviation at branch points was needed to explain the coefficient of variation in microsphere flow measurement. Obviously, the dispersion in the model at the end-vessel level was raised due to the multiple branch points in succession. The model of VanBeek *et al.* [40] provides insight into the propagation of asymmetry at different branch points. However, it does not relate the flow distribution to the anatomical structure of the vascular bed. In fact, it did not define an anatomical structure at all and hence does not predict a pressure and volume distribution over the coronary arterial tree.

2.8 Discussion on structure and function of the arterial tree

This chapter could not provide a satisfactory quantitative relation between structure and function of the coronary arterial tree. There is little doubt that when a detailed description of a vascular branching tree is provided, the distribution of volume over the branch segments and the distribution of pressure over the branching nodes will be able to be calculated. Such a description should be as detailed as a road map. However, such an analysis has little practical value. One would like to have a simple model relating volume and/or pressure to, for example, vessel diameter. Obviously, it should be possible to derive an empirical model, based on a series of resistances each of which describes the pressure drop over vessels of a certain diameter. By measuring pressure as a function of vessel diameter, values of these resistances can be calculated. However, the relation between the resistances in such an empirical model and the physical resistance of vessels with a certain diameter remains obscure.

The symmetrical dichotomous model analysis above did predict that the major pressure drop occurs over vessels with a diameter of less than 50 μm. This has been assumed for a long time. However, recent experimental results do not support this prediction. The discrepancy between the model predictions and experimental outcome is striking. Hence, the major conclusion to be drawn from the exercise above is that the asymmetry in the coronary arterial tree may not be ignored.

Fractal models aimed at the description of pressure and volume distribution have not yet been developed. Such a model requires the description in fractal mathematics of the anatomical structure of the coronary arterial tree.

The conceptual problem one generally faces is the assumption of the arterial tree being a structure which is generated starting from the main branch and bifurcating along certain rules [23]. This probably is so for the larger arterial structure but need not to be so for the small arteries. The ultimate structure of the vascular bed is probably the result of a rather stochastic growth of vessels depending on local oxygen needs. Hence, the arterial bed is the consequence of tissue growth and not the result of an independently expanding arterial tree. Indeed, the comparison to the river structure is appropriate. Surface bound water is generated within a large area and the distribution of this generating process is independent of the river structure. The river structure is the consequence of the confluencing small branches. Obviously, the conceptual difference between the arterial bed and a river structure is that in the former the direction of flow is toward the smaller vessels, while in the latter water flows in the direction of larger segments. The consequence of this line of reasoning is that models based on the concept of a branching tree are bound to fail and that, indeed, one should think along the lines of confluencing arterial segments. The ordering found in the coronary arterial tree as, for instance, can be described by the Strahler ordering is then the result of the process as a whole rather than a rule which was followed when the tree was actually bifurcating.

An extra complication in describing the coronary arterial tree is the difference between subendocardium and subepicardium. The transmural arteries probably branch differently from the arteries parallel to the heart's surface. Hence, a systematic neglect of the distribution of vascular function over the myocardial wall is a gross oversimplification.

2.9 Summary

The primary channels for blood supply to the myocardium are formed by a system of branching arteries running over the heart surface. From these epicardial arteries, transmural arteries branch off and penetrate the myocardial wall. There is regularity in the branching pattern of the arterial tree if only diameters above 400 μm are considered. A similar regularity for the small arteries might be inferred from measurements on density of arterioles of different diameter. However, the analysis of the structure of the arterial tree with diameters ranging in between 400 and 10 μm from casts reveal that a consistent branching system is not present. The continuation of the branching pattern from larger to the very small arteries is not consistent. Very thin arteries may branch from very thick ones.

For model purposes, the arterial tree can be considered as two independent branching systems: one large and one small. The former is considered to have a distribution function only, the latter as the structure for pressure reduction and resistance control. At present, no model can adequately describe the gradual pressure reduction over arteries with diameters of less than 400 μm. A dichotomous model fails to obey absolutely the two boundary conditions with respect to pressure drop and cumulative volume.

The model predicts the pressure distribution experimentally found better when the Fåhraeus-Lindquist effect for blood viscosity is included and a length distribution neglecting the branching of very small arteries from large ones is applied. Additional anatomical data are required for constructing more realistic models based on structure of the arterial tree. An important factor complicating the interpretation of and balance between experimental results is the pressure dependency of the diameters of microvessels.

A mathematical reconstruction of the coronary tree from the data on length distribution and distribution of diameter ratios at branch points allowed the application of Strahler ordering. The ratio between number of vessels of successive orders was about 3.4. Average ratio between diameters of successive orders was 1.55

References

[1] ARTS MGJ[3] (1978) *A mathematical model of the dynamics of the left ventricle and the coronary circulation.* PhD Thesis. University of Limburg, Maastricht, The Netherlands.

[2] ARTS T, KRUGER RTI, VANGERVEN W, LAMBREGTS JAC, RENEMAN RS (1979) Propagation velocity and reflection of pressure waves in the canine coronary artery. *Am. J. Physiol.* **237** (*Heart Circ. Physiol.* **6**): H469–H474.

[3] BASSINGTHWAIGHTE JB (1988) Physiological heterogeneity: fractals link determinism and randomness in structure and function. *New Physiol. Sci.* **3**: 5–10.

[4] BASSINGTHWAIGHTE JB, KING RB, ROGER, SA (1989) Fractal nature of regional myocardial blood flow heterogeneity. *Circ. Res.* **65**: 578–590.

[5] BASSINGTHWAIGHTE JB, VANBEEK JHGM (1988) Lightning and the heart: fractal behavior in cardiac function. *Proc. IEEE* **76**: 693–699.

[6] BASSINGTHWAIGHTE JB, MALONE MA, MOFFETT TC, KING RB, LITTLE SE, LINK JM, KROHN KA (1987) Validity of microsphere depositions for regional myocardial flows. *Am. J. Physiol.* **253** (*Heart Circ. Physiol.* **22**): H184–H193.

[7] BASSINGTHWAIGHTE JB, MALONE MA, MOFFETT TC, KING RB, CHAN IS, LINK JM, KROHN KA (1990) Molecular and particulate depositions for regional myocardial flows in sheep. *Circ. Res.* **66**: 1328–1344.

[8] BECKER BF, BARDENHEUER H, OVEEHAGE DE REYES I, GERLACH E (1985) Effects of theophylline on dipyridamole-induced coronary venous adenosine release and coronary dilation. In: *Adenosine: Receptors and modulation of cell function.* Eds. STEVANOVICH V, RUDOLPHI K, SCHUBERT K. IRL Oxford: 441–449.

---

[3] Arts MGJ is the same person as Arts T [2].

[9] BROWN RE (1965) The pattern of the microcirculatory bed in the ventricular myocardium of domestic mammals. *Am. J. Anat.* **116**: 335–374.
[10] CHIEN G, DORMANDY J, ERNST E, MATRAI A (1987) *Clinical hemorheology.* Martinus Nijhoff, Dordrecht, The Netherlands.
[11] CHILIAN WM, LAYNE SM, KLAUSNER EC, EASTHAM CL, MARCUS ML (1989) Redistribution of coronary microvascular resistance produced by dipyridamole. *Am. J. Physiol.* **256** (*Heart Circ. Physiol.* **25**): H383–H390.
[12] CHILIAN WM, EASTHAM CL, MARCUS ML (1986) Microvascular distribution of coronary vascular resistance in beating left ventricle. *Am. J. Physiol.* **251** (*Heart Circ. Physiol.* **20**): H779–H788.
[13] DAVIS MJ, FERRER PN, GORE RW (1986) Vascular anatomy and hydrostatic pressure profile in the hamster cheek pouch. *Am. J. Physiol.* **250** (*Heart Circ. Physiol.* **19**): H291–H303.
[14] DOUGLAS JE, GREENFIELD JC JR (1970) Epicardial coronary artery compliance in the dog. *Circ. Res.* **27**: 921–929.
[15] ENG C, CHO S, FACTOR SM, SONNENBLICK EM, KIRK ES (1984) Myocardial micronecrosis produced by microsphere embolization. Role of α-adrenergic tonic influence on the coronary microcirculation. *Circ. Res.* **54**: 74–82.
[16] FAM WM, MCGREGOR M (1969) Pressure-flow relationships in the coronary circulation. *Circ. Res.* **25**: 293–301.
[17] FRONEK K, ZWEIFACH BW (1975) Microvascular pressure distribution in skeletal muscle and the effect of vasodilation. *Am. J. Physiol.* **228**: 791–796.
[18] FULTON WFM (1965) *The coronary arteries.* CHARLES C. THOMAS, Springfield III.
[19] GOLDBERGER AL, RIGNEY DR, WEST BJ (1990) Chaos and fractals in Human Physiology. *Scientific Am.* **262**(2): 34–41.
[20] GREGG DE, FISHER LC (1963) Blood supply to the heart. *Handbook of Physiology. Circulation.* **2**. Sect. **2**. Am. Physiol. Soc., Washington D.C.
[21] HAUSDORFF F (1919) Dimension und aüszeres Mass. *Math. Analen* **79**: 157–197.
[22] KENDALL MG, STUART A (1958) *The advanced theory of statistics.* vol. 1 Distribution Theory. Charles Griffin & Company Limited, London.
[23] LABARBERA M (1990) Principles of design of fluid transport systems in zoology. *Science* **249**: 992–1000.
[24] MANDELBROT B (1977) *Fractals: From chance, and dimensions.* Freeman, San Francisco.
[25] MCDONALD N (1983) *Trees and networks in biological models.* JOHN WILEY & SONS, New York.
[26] MEININGER GA, FEHR KL, YATES MB (1987) Anatomic and hemodynamic characteristics of the blood vessels feeding the cremaster skeletal muscle in the rat. *Microvasc. Res.* **33**: 81–97.

[27] MURRAY CD (1926) The physiological principle of minimum work. I. The vascular system and the cost of blood volume. *Proc. Nat. Acad. Sci.* **12**: 207–214.
[28] NELLIS SH, LIEDTKE AJ, WHITESELL L (1981) Small coronary vessel pressure and diameter in an intact beating rabbit heart using fixed-position and free-motion techniques. *Circ. Res.* **49**: 342–353.
[29] PELOSI G, SAVIOZZI G, TRIVELLA MG, L'ABBATE A (1987) Small artery occlusion: A theoretical approach to the definition of coronary architecture and resistance by a branching tree model. *Microvasc. Res.* **34**: 318–355.
[30] POPEL AS (1980) A model of the pressure and flow distribution in branching networks. *Trans. ASME. J. Appl. Mechan.* **102**: 247–253.
[31] SCHAPER W (1971) The collateral circulation of the heart: *volume* I, *Clinical Studies.* Ed. BLACK DAK North Holland Co., Amsterdam, London.
[32] SCHOENMACKERS J (1958) *Zur Anatomie und Pathologie der Coronargefasse.* Bad Oeynhausener Gespräche **II**: 133.
[33] SHAPIRO HM, STROMBERG DD, LEE DR, WIEDERHELM CA (1971) Dynamic pressures in the pial arterial microcirculation. *Am. J. Physiol.* **221**: 279–283.
[34] SUWA N, NIWA T, FUKASAWA H, SASAKI Y (1963) Estimation of intravascular blood pressure gradient by mathematical analysis of arterial casts. *Tohoku J. Exp. Med.* **79**: 168–198.
[35] SUWA N, TAKAHASHI T (1971) *Morphological and Morphometrical Analysis of Circulation in Hypertension and Ischemic Kidney.* Eds. URBAN & SCHWARZENBERG. Heidelberg, FRG.
[36] TILLMANNS H, STEINHAUSEN M, LEINBERGER H, THEDERAN H, KÜBLER W (1981) Pressure measurements in the terminal vascular bed of the epimyocardium of rats and cats. *Circ. Res.* **49**: 1202–1211.
[37] TOMANEK RJ (1987) Microanatomy of the coronary circulation. In: *Coronary circulation, from basic mechanisms to clinical implications.* Eds. SPAAN JAE, BRUSCHKE AVG, GITTENBERGER-DEGROOT AC. Martinus Nijhoff, Dordrecht, The Netherlands.
[38] VANBAVEL E (1989) *Metabolic and myogenic control of blood flow studied on isolated small arteries.* PhD Thesis. University of Amsterdam, The Netherlands.
[39] VANBAVEL E, SPAAN JAE (1990) Branching characteristics of the coronary circulation. *FASEB J.* **4**(4): A850.
[40] VANBEEK JHGM, ROGER SA, BASSINGTHWAIGHTE JB (1989) Regional myocardial flow heterogeneity explained with fractal networks. *Am. J. Physiol.* **257** (*Heart Circ. Physiol.* **26**): H1670–H1680.
[41] WIERINGA PA, STASSEN HG, LAIRD JD, SPAAN JAE (1988) Quantification of arteriolar density and embolization in rat myocardium. *Am. J. Physiol.* **254** (*Heart Circ. Physiol.* **23**): H636–H650.

[42] WÜSTEN B, BUSS DD, DEIST H, SCHAPER W (1977) Dilatory capacity of the coronary circulation and its correlation to the arterial vasculature in the canine left ventricle. *Basic Res. Cardiol.* **72**: 636–650.

[43] ZAMIR M, CHEE H (1987) Segment analysis of human coronary arteries. *Blood vessels* **24**: 76–84.

[44] ZWEIFACH BW, LIPOWSKY HH (1977) Quantitative studies of microcirculatory structure and function III. Microvascular hemodynamics of cat mesentery and rabbit omentum. *Circ. Res.* **41**: 380–390.

Chapter 3

Structure and perfusion of the capillary bed

3.1 Structure of capillary bed

THE CAPILLARY BED is not simply the continuation of the arterial tree. It does not have a branching structure; however, it forms an interconnected network of vessels of more or less equal diameters [28]. A good impression of the capillary network in the dog's heart is supplied by Figures 3.1 and 3.2. The picture of Figure 3.1 is from Bassingthwaighte *et al.* [2] and provides an overview over an area larger than 1 mm^2. Long, parallel capillaries (so-called main capillaries) are visible with a considerable number of interconnections, forming the capillary network. The myocytes are organized within the open spaces in this network. The main capillaries can run over several millimeters. Terminal arterioles are connected to the network. Because of this structure it is not a priori clear from which terminal arteriole the blood that runs through a specific capillary segment originates. The insert offers a closer look at how the small vessels spring from larger branches, an observation also emphasized in Figure 2.2.

A different picture, with basically the same information but over a smaller area, is given in Figure 3.2. This was made from the capillary bed of rat myocardium by Tomanek *et al.* [36] using Batson corrosion cast compound. Again, the structure of the capillary bed is that of long main capillaries with many interconnections. The arteriole at the bottom and venule at the top of the picture are connected to the capillary network at several locations. It is at this point useful to ask the reader for his impression of the main direction of net capillary flow in the network shown in Figure 3.2. Most students and colleagues answer that net flow would be in the length direction of the capillaries, hence parallel to the venule, and arteriole. However, since the net blood flow is from the arteriole to the venule it is more realistic to assume that the net flow direction is perpendicular to these vessels. The blood flow in the main capillaries may be in either direction and hence cancelled out when averaged flow in their direction is considered. Consequently, in this particular instance, the cross-capillary segments must be important to the transport of blood through the network.

The two photographs give the impression of a continuous capillary network. However, work from Okun et al. [26] shows that the capillary bed is not continuous at the boundary between the perfusion area of two larger coronary arteries. At these boundaries capillary endloops can be observed.

3.2 Capillary density and volume

Capillary density is usually defined as the number of capillaries found in a cross section of the tissue perpendicular to the direction of the main capillaries. Values for capillary density expressed in number per mm^2 vary widely. For rat hearts, the numbers 2100 and 2200 mm^{-2} were reported [4, 24]. The density reported for the human heart is considerably higher, namely 3343 mm^{-2} [29, 39]. This value is similar to those reported for the dog which vary between 3170 mm^{-2} [2] and 3600 mm^{-2} [14]. This latter source also reports a significantly lower capillary density for the subendocardium (3147 mm^{-2}) than for the subepicardium (3637 mm^{-2}) although this difference has not always been found in other studies. Obviously, the difference in number may be species dependent, but could also be due to differences in techniques used. For example the structure of the capillary bed makes it difficult to fill all the capillaries with a substance to enhance observability of the vessels. For the purpose of this book we will assume the value of 3200 mm^{-2}.

There are no reports on direct measurements of total capillary volume in the in vivo heart. In the post mortem heart, a capillary volume fraction of 27% [25] was reported which is larger than the total myocardial blood fraction measured by more direct means.

The total capillary cross-sectional area fraction in a plane perpendicular to the orientation of the main capillaries equals the product of capillary density and capillary cross-sectional area. The latter requires a measure of the capillary diameter. Published values vary between 4 and 9 μm [2, 5, 17, 26, 27, 33, 34, 36].

Since cross-sectional area is proportional to the square of the diameter, the range of about a factor 2 in diameter results in a range of factor 4 of the volume of the capillary bed, neglecting possible length changes. The large variations in capillary diameter must be due to techniques used. For example, the capillaries are distensible and the diameters to be measured pressure dependent. In further calculations we will assume a value of 5 μm if the capillary bed is perfused under control conditions. This value is in the range of the in vivo measurements.

3.2 Capillary density and volume

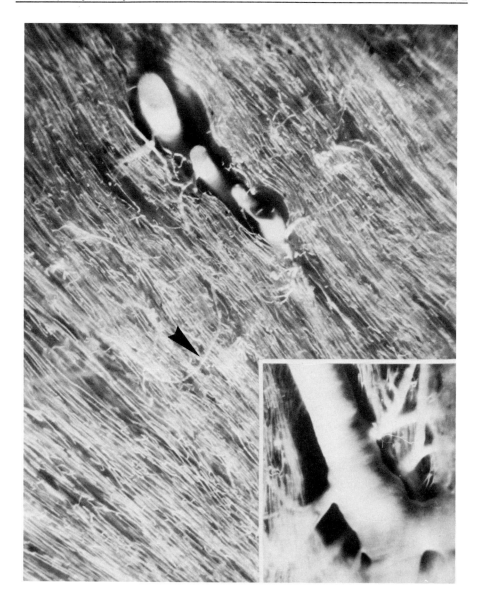

Figure 3.1: The capillary network of the dog's myocardium. The capillary bed was filled with silicone rubber. The tissue was made transparent by using methylsalicylate after dehydration with ethanol. The capillaries run continuously over many millimeters but are interconnected frequently. Unbranched segments are between 60 and 250 μm in length. Within the picture three larger vessels are shown. The middle one is an arteriole and the two outer ones are venules. Note the thin arteriole branching from the feeding arteriole (see arrow) and its connections to the capillary network. The insert (same scale) shows a 160 μm vein connected over a small distance with the parallel capillaries by small venules. (From Bassingthwaighte et al. [2], by permission of authors and Academic Press, Inc.)

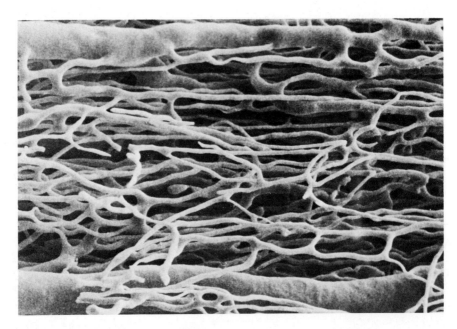

Figure 3.2: Corrosion cast of the capillary bed of the rat, at a higher magnification than in Figure 3.1. Also here the impression of parallel running capillaries with frequent interconnections is given. (From Tomanek et al. [36], by permission of the author and American Heart Association, Inc.)

The estimated volume fraction of the capillary bed is therefore about 0.063. Obviously, the volume fraction will be dependent on luminal pressure and outside compression.

3.3 Mechanical properties

Not much is known about the mechanical properties of myocardial capillaries. Hence, for the present, the best solution is to assume that they have mechanical properties similar to capillaries in other organs. It has been argued for a long time that capillaries can be described as rigid tubes [13]. This assumption was based on older measurements with a resolution which was probably too low. Smaje et al. [32] developed an elegant method to measure distensibility of single capillaries. The distensibility, D_S, of a vessel is defined by

3.3 Mechanical properties

$$D_s = \frac{1}{d}\frac{\mathrm{d}d}{\mathrm{d}P} \qquad [3.1]$$

and expresses the relative change of diameter, d, as a function of a change in pressure. The value found for capillary distensibility was 6×10^{-3} mm Hg^{-1} at an average capillary pressure of about 20 mm Hg. It should be realized that this distensibility is pressure dependent, as with all other blood vessels. For the small arteries this will be discussed in Chapter 8.

The capillaries are connected to myocytes by collagen struts [3]. Borg and Caulfield [3] concluded that these struts were less wavy if the heart was fixed in systole than when it was fixed in diastole. Therefore they suggested that the stress in these struts was higher in systole than in diastole and that this might reflect a mechanism to keep capillaries patent during systole. It is very hard to incorporate these effects in models of the coronary circulation, although attempts are being made.

The volume of the capillary bed will, of course, also be affected by compression due to contraction of the heart. Some reports on measurement of this effect can be found in literature. One should be very cautious with the interpretation of these data. Tillmanns et al. [34] reported that capillary diameter varied in his experiment from 5.3 μm in diastole to 4.1 μm in systole. These diameter differences imply a volume change of the capillary bed of 40%. This could even be an underestimate since the diameters were measured in the subepicardium where the compression effects on flow are surprisingly slight [18]. A cyclic volume variation of 40% of capillary volume is far above the value to be expected from the swing in coronary arterial and venous flow.

Recently, Levy et al. [22] measured capillary diameters in the subendocardium of hearts arrested with potassium or barium, hence in the relaxed and contracted state respectively. Mean subendocardial capillary diameter in the relaxed heart was 6.8 μm and in the contracted heart 5 μm. Their results are of importance since these show that capillary diameter depends on the contraction of myocytes. However, caution is required in extrapolating these data to the normal beating heart. First, the hearts were frozen, starting at the outside, thereby inhibiting suddenly flow into and out of the muscle via the transmural arteries and transmural veins, but allowing some time for redistribution of blood from vessel lumens with high pressure to those with low pressure. Hence, capillary blood may have been translocated to the venules. Second, a steady barium contracted heart might not be a good model for the systolic phase of a normally beating heart. The question is whether systole is normally too short to establish a steady state (Chapters 6 and 7). Hence, capillary volume squeezed during systole might be much smaller than the volume squeezed by a very long period of barium contraction.

3.4 Red cells in the capillary bed

3.4.1 Velocities

Observations on capillary blood velocities within the myocardium have been reported by several groups [1, 33, 34, 43]. Most of these studies must be considered preliminary, in the sense that the number of observations are small (about 10–20) and the locations of these measured capillaries within the capillary bed are not well documented. The range of velocities reported is between 900 and 4000 μm $\cdot$ s^{-1}. These velocities were measured in autoregulating vascular beds and hence typical perfusion rates averaged over the whole myocardium were probably about 1 ml $\cdot$ min^{-1} $\cdot$ g^{-1}. Tillmanns et al. [35] reported variation of epicardial capillary red cell velocities through the cardiac cycle. However, the variation measured by Ashikawa et al. [1] is much less. Phasic red cell velocity of the capillaries is compared with those in small arterioles and venules in Figure 3.3.

The data provided by Ashikawa et al. [1] illustrate velocity signals quite different from the phasic flow pattern in the large coronary artery as demonstrated in Figure 1.1. Flow becomes retrograde in all three vessel types at the occurrence of the QRS-complex. Apart from this stagnation of flow, capillary red cell velocity is relatively steady. However, the difference between velocities in the capillaries and the arterioles and venules is much smaller than one would expect on either the basis of the difference in diameters of these vessels or the number of these vessels. This must be due to the structure of the whole vascular tree and the capillary bed in particular. The reported capillary red cell velocities for the myocardium are high compared to velocities reported for striated muscle [37], especially when the fact that the myocardial data were obtained during autoregulation is taken into account. Damon and Duling [6] reported data for the hamster tibialis anterior muscles. Mean capillary red cell velocity was 145 μm $\cdot$ s^{-1} at rest and 675 μm $\cdot$ s^{-1} when the muscle was stimulated at a frequency of 4 Hz, with a standard deviation equal to half of the mean at both frequencies. This is about twice as high as compared to the standard deviation reported by Tillmanns et al. [34, 35] for heart muscle.

3.4.2 Red cell distribution at bifurcations

At the level of the microcirculation, blood can no longer be treated as a homogenous fluid. At branching points, the plasma flow and red cell flow are not necessarily distributed proportionally. Krogh [21] described the disparity between red cell and plasma distribution, which is particularly apparent when a small vessel branches from a larger one at a right angle. Mostly plasma flows into this side branch since it drains almost exclusively from the plasma boundary layer in the larger vessel. Such a plasma boundary layer is the result of plasma skimming, as was noted by Krogh in 1921 [20], and is due to the tendency of

3.4 Red cells in the capillary bed

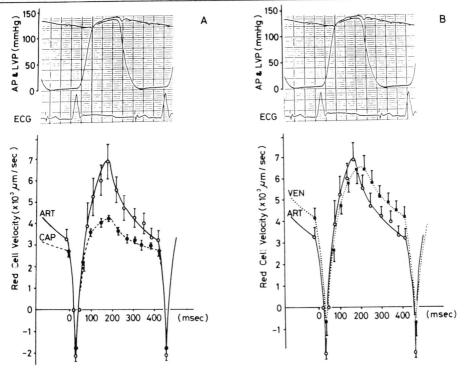

Figure 3.3: Results on red cell velocity in arterioles (diameter 12.8 ± 4.1 μm, mean ± SD), capillaries and venules (diameter 16.5 ± 6.5 μm, mean ± SD) in the subepicardium of the dog. Measurements were done with a fluorescence microscope with floating objective. (From Ashikawa et al. [1], by permission of the author and American Heart Association, Inc.)

red cells to move to the center of a vessel. Within the capillary bed, red cells seem to show a stochastic behavior in choosing direction at bifurcations. When flow is distributed evenly at a symmetrical branch point it is almost impossible to predict how the red cells will distribute themselves. However, the in vitro observations on the distribution of red cells and plasma can be described reasonably well by mathematical models [12, 23]. Yen and Fung [44] observed that if the difference in branch flows was great enough, all cells entered the branch with the greatest amount of flow. In vivo measurements on muscle tissues reveal that red cell velocities and hematocrits vary among the branches of a capillary network [31].

3.4.3 Hematocrit

One of the biggest anomalies in microvascular physiology involves the capillary hematocrits [7]. The anomaly becomes immediately evident in Figure 3.4 [9]. The illustrated capillary network shows a realistic preparation such as hamster cheek pouch and cremaster muscle. The network is supplied by an arteriole connected to an arterial system which is filled with blood with an hematocrit of 50% and is drained by a venule into a larger vein having the same hematocrit. With vasoconstriction of arterioles, the capillary bed seems almost empty (low hematocrit) while the picture obtained at vasodilation shows a degree of occupied space which is compatible with the systemic hematocrit. The difference in observation reflected by the left and right panels are not surprising if red cells can go through parallel channels. However, such parallel vessels must have high hematocrits which were never found. Despite the difference in hematocrit, blood withdrawn from the collecting venule showed the same hematocrits for both the vasoconstricted and vasodilated states.

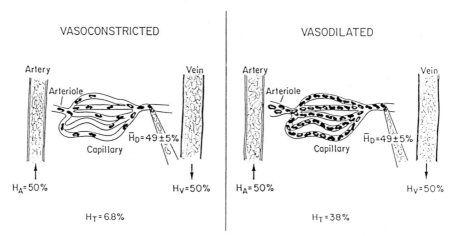

Figure 3.4: Capillary hematocrit as in the hamster cremaster muscle in vasoconstricted (left) and vasodilated state (right) of the feeding arterioles. Since a low capillary hematocrit can also be explained by a filtering effect at the inlet of the microvessels the venule, draining a well-defined part of the capillary network observed, was cannulated. Hematocrit in the collecting venule was independent of the state of vasodilation. (From Duling and Desjardins [9], by permission of authors and American Physiological Society.)

In itself, the tube hematocrit needs not to be the same as the discharge hematocrit. The tube hematocrit is defined as the volume fraction of the capillaries occupied by the red cells. The discharge hematocrit is the volume fraction of the blood flowing out of the tube and collected in a container. Fåhraeus [11] previously noted the difference between tube hematocrit and discharge hematocrit and related this to the higher red cell velocity compared to plasma velocity. The effect of lower hematocrit in microvessels is referred to as 'Fåhraeus effect'[1]. It has been calculated however that the Fåhraeus effect cannot explain the observed low tube hematocrits illustrated in the left panel of Figure 3.4.

One would expect the conditions controlling the tube hematocrit of the capillaries to be closer to the vasodilated state indicated in Figure 3.4 for the heart, because the working myocardium has a relatively high basal perfusion. This may indeed be concluded from a study of Vetterlein [38]. In slices of rat heart made in the length direction of the main capillaries, the fraction of capillary length free of red cells was measured. The mean of this fraction was roughly between 44% in the subepicardium and 54% in the subendocardium. The subepicardial-subendocardial difference, however, was only statistically significant if the animals had been subjected to respiratory arrest. There was no significant effect of hypoxia or asphyxia on this distribution. Moreover, there was no significant difference between capillaries having a high flow versus low flow. The difference between high and low flow was determined by the distribution of RB200-globulin within one second of injection. The study of Vetterlein et al. [38] shows a more or less normal distribution of red cell free length fraction ranging between zero and one. A fraction of zero corresponds to a tube hematocrit of zero. A fraction of one does not correspond to a tube hematocrit of 1 since red blood cells, even if they touch, do not fill the capillary space completely.

3.5 Model of parallel and homogeneous perfused capillary bed

If the capillary bed consisted of parallel capillaries of equal length which were perfused homogeneously in direction (cocurrent only) and magnitude, a simple model would relate capillary flow to whole organ flow. As, in our system, estimates of capillary velocity are available but capillary length is hard to define from the network, this length can be estimated from such a model on the basis of capillary blood velocities and whole organ flow.

The model for homogeneous perfusion is illustrated in Figure 3.5. Consider a piece of tissue with a length L and cross-sectional area A. The flow per unit mass equals Q_m while the length L would equal the capillary length. The connections to the arterial and venous systems are at opposite ends of the tissue piece as illustrated in Figure 3.5. The number of capillaries N_c in the cross section can be calculated from cross-sectional area and capillary density, C_D:

---

[1] For a review of the Fåhraeus effect the reader is referred to a recent tribute to Fåhraeus by Goldsmith et al. [16].

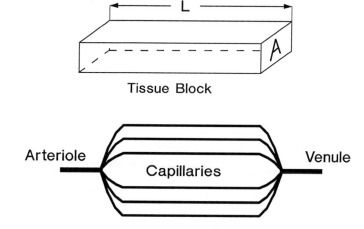

Figure 3.5: Model of homogeneous distribution of flow in a parallel capillary network without interconnections. A = the cross-sectional area of the tissue element. L = length of the capillary segments. It is assumed that blood flow is distributed evenly over the capillaries. See the text for the theoretical relations between overall blood flow and red cell velocities in this model.

$$N_c = C_D A \qquad [3.2]$$

If q_c is the flow per capillary, then the relation between the flow through the piece of tissue, $Q_m \times A \times L$, and capillary flow assuming a specific mass of $1 \text{ g} \cdot \text{ml}^{-1}$, is simply:

$$q_c = \frac{Q_m A L}{N_c} = \frac{Q_m L}{C_D} \qquad [3.3]$$

Hence, in this simple model, capillary flow and flow per unit mass are proportionally related, the proportionality being the ratio between capillary length and capillary density.

In general it is not capillary flow that is measured, but red cell velocity. Assuming that red cell velocity, v_c, equals average capillary blood velocity, one arrives at the following equation:

$$v_c = \frac{4q_c}{\pi d_c^2} = \frac{4Q_m}{\pi d_c^2} \frac{L}{C_D} \qquad [3.4]$$

From the continuous nature of the coronary capillary bed it is impossible to estimate a value of L. However, a functional value of L can be derived from Equation [3.4] and the values for the different parameters discussed above. For $C_D = 3200 \text{ mm}^{-2}$, $d_c = 5 \times 10^{-3}$ mm, $Q_m = 1 \text{ ml} \cdot \text{min}^{-1} \cdot \text{g}^{-1}$ and v_c in the range of 1 to 4 mm · s^{-1}, a range is arrived at for L between 3.8 and 15.1 mm. These values are large compared to reported capillary lengths for other vascular beds: 0.262 mm ± 0.166 (SD) for hamster cremaster muscle [19] and about half that for striated muscle [10].

Because of the interconnectedness of the capillary vascular bed depicted by Figures 3.1 and 3.2, it is impossible to define an anatomical capillary length for the coronary microcirculation. The length of the path to be travelled by the red cells from arteriole to venule was estimated to be about 1.5 mm for regions at the junction of two cognate beds supplied by the left anterior descending artery and circumflex artery respectively [2]. This is also much shorter than calculated by the simple model of Figure 3.5. A similar model analysis has been made by Duling et al. [8] for capillary beds of cremaster (hamster), gracilis (dog) and tenuissimus (cat, rabbit). In that study capillary blood velocities were calculated from bulk flow. Predicted capillary velocities were about 4.4 times lower than measured ones. This is in accordance with our conclusion on capillary length for the coronary microcirculation. Duling et al. [8] analyzed several possible explanations for the discrepancy and showed that the assumption of a stabilized plasma boundary layer at the capillary wall of 1 μm would explain the discrepancy. There is at present not much evidence for such a thick, unmovable layer in the capillaries.

The conclusion is unavoidable that the model for homogeneous perfusion of the capillary bed is too simple to relate capillary flow to total organ flow. Apart from rheological properties, the analysis of myocardial capillary flow should account for the interconnectedness of the capillary bed and thereby include the function of capillary anastomoses.

3.6 A model for the heterogeneous perfusion of the capillary bed

A mathematical three-dimensional model of the capillary perfusion, taking into account the interconnectedness of the capillary bed, has been made by Wieringa et al. [41] and its structure is illustrated by Figure 3.6. The model consisted of 11 by 11 capillaries hexagonally stacked. Interconnections between the main capillaries were simulated in equidistant planes perpendicular to the main capillary direction. The distance between these planes represents a length of about 30 μm. The location of the cross capillaries was such that the distribution of unbranched capillary segments was close to that measured by Bassingthwaighte et al. [2]. Three arterioles and five venules were connected at arbitrary nodes in the network. The arterioles were considered as flow sources. The venules were considered to have zero pressure. The capillary segments had a resistance proportional to their length. By applying the network theory developed for electronic

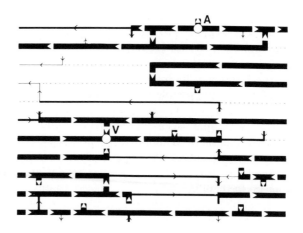

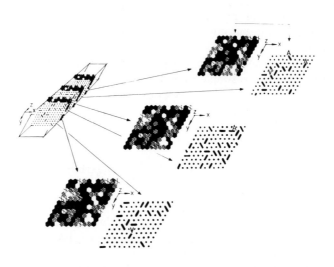

Figure 3.6: Length section and cross section of a three-dimensional model of the capillary network according to Wieringa et al. [41]. There are 11 × 11 main capillaries. Each main capillary consists of segments of constant length connected to each other at nodes. At some nodes the main capillaries are interconnected. Top: In lengthwise direction, the direction of the predicted flow is indicated by the arrows. The thickness of the lines indicates the level of capillary flow. Cross segments only partly shown, are connected to main capillaries in adjacent planes. Bottom: Cross section through the model. The cross sections at the node planes show the interconnections. The grey level in the cross sections through the middle of the segments indicate the flow levels in the capillary segments. (From Wieringa et al. [41] , by permission of Marcel Dekker, Inc..)

3.6 A model for the heterogeneous perfusion of the capillary bed

circuits the flow distribution in such a network can be calculated.

The model network dimensions were restricted by the power of the computer to solve the matrix equations. This restriction is rather rigorous; Figure 3.1 shows that the capillary network can comprise quite a large area. Without extra measures, the model does not allow flow over the boundary planes, whereas this will occur with a piece of tissue of the same size. To compensate for this shortcoming, the main capillaries at the opposite boundary side planes of the network were mathematically treated as if they were neighbors. Moreover, heads and tails of capillaries were mathematically treated as if they were connected. In this way, it is theoretically possible, although highly unlikely, that flow can circulate through the network in length direction five times without passing the same main capillary. Example simulation results are illustrated in Figure 3.6.

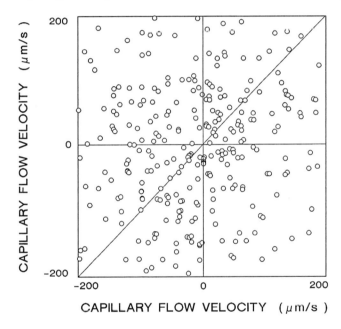

Figure 3.7: *The relation between flows in adjacent segments of main capillaries within a heterogeneous model. Note the absence of any significant correlation. (Redrawn from Wieringa [40].)*

The predicted capillary flow distribution is heterogeneous and very capricious. Capillaries with high flow rates are adjacent to capillaries with low flow rates. Functional capillary endloops are predicted, as well as co- and counterflow capillaries. The low flow in some of the model capillaries is due to a condition that is also created in a Wheatstone bridge. The current in the side branches of the Wheatstone bridge can be high but the voltage difference over the galvanometer can be zero. True mean capillary flow in the model is about zero because the flow magnitudes in all directions cancel out.

The heterogeneity of capillary flow in the model is also illustrated in Figure 3.7, where the relation between flows in adjacent capillary segments is plotted. As is obvious from this figure, there is no correlation. The characteristics of such a model for predicting oxygen transfer to tissue are analyzed in Chapter 11.

3.7 Capillary recruitment in the heart

One has to distinguish between anatomical recruitment and functional recruitment. Anatomical recruitment is the growth of the capillary bed to compensate for a continuous shortage of blood supply to a certain region. For the dog heart, it has been shown that in the first weeks after birth, the capillary bed grows with the number of myocytes. If at a later age the myocytes grow due to hypertrophy, the number of capillaries of the heart remain the same, capillary density is reduced and intercapillary distance increases [15, 25]. However, long term bradycardial pacing [42] may induce an increase of capillary density.

Functional recruitment is defined from the observation that not all capillaries are perfused continuously. The number of capillaries perfused may increase when needed or capillaries may alternately be perfused or show stagnation of blood. Rheological factors may play a role in this dynamic process. Functional recruitment, defined as the changing number of capillaries with red cell flow, has been observed in resting muscle and organs like the mesentery. However, in a carefully designed experiment Damon and Duling [6] observed the maximal variation of capillaries perfused at the surface of hamster tibialis anterior muscles to be between 71 and 99%. Mean red cell velocities varied in the same experiment between 89 and 675 μm $\cdot$ s^{-1}, hence over a much wider range.

Martini and Honig [24] measured intercapillary distance in the subepicardium of the isolated rat heart using a fluorescence technique and concluded that intercapillary distance decreased with ischemia, and hence that capillary density increased. These authors related these changes to capillary recruitment; however, other mechanisms may also account for their results. Their numbers are statistical and may have been affected by altered patterns of red cell perfusion of the capillary bed. Decrease in capillary distance could not be induced by hypoxia during vital microscopic studies [33]. Recently Vetterlein and colleagues [38] pointed out that hypoxia elongates fibers which increases both capillary and fiber density and hence decreases intercapillary distance.

It is believed by some authors that functional recruitment is part of the regulatory mechanism for organ blood supply. This assumption is in agreement with the results from experiments on tracer response curves of diffusible and nondiffusible tracers injected in the coronary arterial blood. From these measurements, it was concluded that the product of permeability and surface area of the capillary bed increased with coronary flow. The increase of product of permeability and surface area, the PS product, was explained as an increase of surface area and hence by the increase of the number of perfused capillaries [30]. The recruitment found, based on these experiments, is much higher than observed by Martini and Honig [24] and observed in striated muscle. It should be noted that the estimate of PS product is strongly based on a model of the microcirculation in which parallel perfused capillaries were assumed. As discussed above, this model is a considerable oversimplification of the structure and perfusion of the myocardial capillary bed. A more realistic model of coronary capillary perfusion could possibly provide an alternative explanation for the tracer response curves.

Capillary recruitment is often related to the presence and action of precapillary sphincters. The presence of precapillary sphincters in the heart is still a matter of debate and may vary with species. The action of precapillary sphincters would result in a compensation of spatial heterogeneity by temporal heterogeneity. It is, however, questionable whether such an extrapolation from observations on resting muscle to the highly metabolic active myocardium is justified. Oxygen extraction by the heart is high and substantial changes in oxygen consumption must be met by changes in flow. In resting muscle, oxygen extraction is low and changes in oxygen consumption can be accommodated by changing extraction. This difference in oxygen extraction may point to a difference in control mechanism. It may be concluded that the applicability of the concept of capillary recruitment to control of flow through the heart has yet to be proven.

3.8 Summary

The capillary bed of the myocardium is a continuous network of main capillaries running parallel to the myocardial fibers and continuous for over a few millimeters. These main capillaries are interconnected by capillary interconnections. The average unbranched capillary segment is about 100 μm long. Capillary density in a cross section perpendicular to the fiber orientation is about 3200 mm^{-2}. Capillary diameter is approximately 5 μm but may be affected by transmural pressure or other factors related to cardiac contraction. A model of parallel capillaries, homogeneously perfused, results in either an underestimate of capillary blood velocity or overestimate of capillary length. A model taking into account the capillary topology predicts heterogeneous capillary perfusion and may be more realistic. Capillary recruitment is a concept of which the use in coronary physiology is as yet still unclear.

References

[1] ASHIKAWA K, KANATSUKA H, SUZUKI T, TAKISHIMA T (1986) Phasic blood flow velocity pattern in epimyocardial microvessels in the beating canine left ventricle. *Circ. Res.* **59**: 704–711.

[2] BASSINGTHWAIGHTE JB, YIPINTSOI T, HARVEY RB (1974) Microvasculature of the dog left ventricular myocardium. *Microvasc. Res.* **7**: 229–249.

[3] BORG TK, CAULFIELD JB (1981) The collagen matrix of the heart. *Fed. Proc.* **40**: 2037–2041.

[4] BUSS DD, WÜSTEN B, SCHAPER W (1978) Effects of coronary stenoses and ventricular loading conditions on coronary flow. *Basic Res. Card.* **73**: 571–583.

[5] CONLEY KE, KAYAR SR, RÖSLER K, HOPPELER H, WEIBEL ER, TAYLOR CR (1987) Adaptive variation in the mammalian respiratory system in relation to energy demand. IV. Capillaries and their relation to oxidative capacity. *Resp. Physiol.* **69**: 47–64.

[6] DAMON DH, DULING BR (1985) Evidence that capillary perfusion heterogeneity is not controlled in striated muscle. *Am. J. Physiol.* **249** *(Heart Circ. Physiol.* **18**): H386–H392.

[7] DESJARDINS C, DULING BR (1987) Microvessel hematocrit: measurement and implications for capillary oxygen transport. *Am. J. Physiol.* **252** *((Heart Circ. Physiol.* **21**): H494–H503.

[8] DULING BR, SARELIUS IH, JACKSON WF (1982) A comparison of microvascular estimates of capillary blood flow with direct measurements of total striated muscle flow. *Int. J. Microcirc. Clin. Exp.* **1**: 409–424.

[9] DULING BR, DESJARDINS C (1987) Capillary hematocrit-what does it mean. *NIPS* **2**: 66–69.

[10] ERIKSSON E, MYRHAGE R (1972) Microvascular dimensions and blood flow in skeletal muscle. *Acta Physiol. Scand.* **86**: 211–222.

[11] FÅHRAEUS R (1929) The suspension stability of the blood. *Physiol. Rev.* **9**: 241–274.

[12] FENTON BM, CARR RT, COKELET GR (1985) Nonuniform red cell distribution in 20 to 100 µm bifurcations. *Microvasc. Res.* **29**: 103–126.

[13] FUNG YC, ZWEIFACH BW, INTAGLIETTA M (1966) Elastic environment of the capillary bed. *Circ. Res.* **19**: 441–461.

[14] GERDES AM, KASTEN FH (1980) Morphometric study of endomyocardium and epimyocardium of the left ventricle in adult dogs. *Am. J. Anat.* **159**: 389–394.

[15] GERDES AM, CALLAS G, KASTEN FH (1979) Differences in regional capillary distribution and myocyte sizes in normal and hypertrophic rat hearts. *Am. J. Anat.* **156**: 523–532.

[16] GOLDSMITH HL, COKELET GR, GAEHTGENS P (1989) Robin Fåhraeus: Evolution of his concepts in cardiovascular physiology. *Am. J. Physiol.* **257**

(*Heart Circ. Physiol.* **26**): H1005–H1015.
[17] HENQUELL L, ODOROFF CL, HONIG CR (1978) Coronary intercapillary distance during growth: relation to PtO$_2$ and aerobic capacity. *Am. J. Physiol.* **231**: 1852–1859.
[18] HOFFMAN JIE, SPAAN JAE (1990) Pressure-flow relations in the coronary circulation. *Physiol. Rev.* **70**: 331–390.
[19] KLITZMAN B, JOHNSON PC (1982) Capillary network geometry and red cell distribution in hamster cremaster muscle. *Am. J. Physiol.* **242** (*Heart Circ. Physiol.* **11**): H211–H219.
[20] KROGH A (1921) Studies on the physiology of capillaries. II. The reactions to local stimuli of the blood vessels in the skin and web of the frog. *J. Physiol. Lond.* **55**: 412–422.
[21] KROGH A (1930) *The anatomy and physiology of capillaries.* Yale University Press, New Haven. Mrs. Hepsa Ely Silliman Memorial Lectures.
[22] LEVY BI, SAMUEL JL, TEDGUI A, KOTELIANSKI V, MAROTTE F, POITEVIN P, CHADWICK RS (1988) Intramyocardial blood volume measurement in the left ventricle of rat arrested hearts. In: *Cardiovascular dynamics and models.* Eds. BRUN P, CHADWICK RS, LEVY BI, INSERM, Paris: 65–76.
[23] LEW HS, FUNG YC (1969) On the low-reynolds-number entry flow into a circular cylindrical tube. *J. Biomech.* **2**: 105–119.
[24] MARTINI J, HONIG CR (1969) Direct measurement of intercapillary distance in beating rat heart in situ under various conditions of O$_2$ supply. *Microvasc. Res.* **1**: 244–256.
[25] O'KEEFE DD, HOFFMAN JIE, CHEITLIN R, O'NEILL MJ, ALLARD JR, SHAPKIN E (1978) Coronary blood flow in experimental canine left ventricular hypertrophy. *Circ. Res.* **43**: 43–51.
[26] OKUN EM, FACTOR SM, KIRK ES (1979) End-capillary loops in the heart: an explanation for discrete myocardial infarctions without border zones. *Science* **206**: 565–567.
[27] POTTER RF, GROOM AC (1983) Capillary diameter and geometry in cardiac and skeletal muscle studied by means of corrosion casts. *Microvasc. Res.* **25**: 68–84.
[28] RAKUSAN K (1971) Quantitative morphology of capillaries of the heart. Number of capillaries in animal and human hearts under normal and pathological conditions. *Methods Achiev. Exp. Pathol.* **5**: 272–286.
[29] ROBERTS JT, WEARN JT (1941) Quantitative changes in the capillary-muscle relationship in human hearts during normal growth and hypertrophy. *Am. Heart J.* **21**: 617–633.
[30] ROSE CP, GORESKY CA, BELANGER P, CHEN MJ (1980) Effect of vasodilation and flow rate on capillary permeability surface product and interstitial space size in the coronary circulation. *Circ. Res.* **47**: 312–328.

[31] SARELIUS IH, DAMAN DN, DULING BR (1981) Microvascular adaptations during maturation of striated muscle. *Am. J. Physiol.* **241** (*Heart Circ. Physiol.* **10**): H317–H324.
[32] SMAJE LH, FRASER PA, CLOUGH G (1980) The distensibility of single capillaries and venules in the cat mesentery. *Microvasc. Res.* **20**: 358–370.
[33] STEINHAUSEN M, TILLMANNS H, THEDERAN H (1978) Microcirculation of the epimyocardial layer of the heart. I. A method for in vivo observation of the microcirculation of superficial ventricular myocardium of the heart and capillary flow pattern under normal and hypoxic conditions. *Pflügers Arch.* **378**: 9–14.
[34] TILLMANNS H, IKEDA S, HANSEN H, SARMA JSM, FAUVEL JM, BING RJ (1974) Microcirculation in the ventricle of the dog and turtle. *Circ. Res.* **34**: 561–569.
[35] TILLMANNS H, STEINHAUSEN M, LEINBERGER H, THEDERAN H, KÜBLER W (1981) Coronary microcirculation hemodynamics during myocardial ischemia. *European Heart J.* **2** (abstract 303) *Suppl. A*: 159.
[36] TOMANEK RJ, SEARLS JC, LACHENBRUCH PA (1982) Quantitative changes in the capillary bed during developing peak and stabilized cardiac hypertrophy in the spontaneously hypertensive rat. *Circ. Res.* **51**: 295–304.
[37] TYML K, ELLIS CG, SAFRANYOS RG, FRASER S, GROOM AC (1981) Temporal and spatial distribution of red cell velocity in capillaries of resting skeletal muscle, including estimates of red cell transit times. *Microvasc. Res.* **22**: 14–31.
[38] VETTERLEIN F, HEMELING H, SAMMLER J, PETTIO A, SCHMIDT G (1989) Hypoxia-induced acute changes in capillary and fiber density and capillary red cell distribution in the rat heart. *Circ. Res.* **64**: 742–752.
[39] WEARN JT (1928) The extent of the capillary bed in the heart. *J. Exp. Med.* **47**: 273–292.
[40] WIERINGA PA (1985) *The influence of the distribution and control of local blood.* PhD Thesis. Technical University of Delft, The Netherlands.
[41] WIERINGA PA, SPAAN JAE, STASSEN HG, LAIRD JD (1980) Heterogeneous flow distribution in a three dimensional network simulation of the myocardial microcirculation; a hypothesis. *Microcirc.* **2**: 195–216.
[42] WRIGHT AJA, HUDLICKA O (1981) Capillary growth and changes in heart performance induced by chronic bradycardial pacing in the rabbit. *Circ. Res.* **49**: 469–478.
[43] YAMAKAWA T, NIIMI H (1984) Behavior of blood cells flowing through capillaries of atrial heart muscle in acute ischemia-intravital microscopic study. *Int. J. Microcirc. Clin. Exp.* **3**: A332–437
[44] YEN RT, FUNG YC (1978) Effect of velocity distribution on red cell distribution in capillary blood vessels. *Am. J. Physiol.* **235** (*Heart Circ. Physiol.* **4**): H251–H257.

Chapter 4

Structure and function of coronary venous system

THE CORONARY VENOUS SYSTEM is like a three-dimensional river bed draining the blood from the myocardial capillary system and channeling it to the right heart. This system forms almost a mirror image of the coronary arterial tree.

From a mechanistic view the role of the venous bed may be very subtle and has received much less attention than the function of the coronary arterial tree. However, studies have been performed on the beneficial effects of coronary sinus occlusion and coronary venous retroperfusion on ischemic parts of the myocardium [8, 12, 13]. In the larger epicardial veins a Starling resistor mechanism is active, which uncouples venous pressure from right atrial pressure under certain circumstances. The intramural veins and venules are under the influence of tissue pressure and may act as regulators of the hydrostatic pressure difference over the capillary wall, which is important for keeping these vessels patent and maintaining transcapillary water transport (see Chapter 10). This chapter forms a general introduction to the structure and function of the coronary venous system in so far as this relates to the theme of this book.[1]

4.1 Basic anatomy

Blood from the capillary bed is drained into venules, confluencing into larger veins. Some authors report that, especially at the level of small veins and venules, two venous vessels accompany small arteries and arterioles [3]. There may be a

---
[1]Those interested in a more detailed look at the coronary venous circulation are recommended to read 'The Coronary Sinus' [10].

difference between species since this is also the case with epicardial veins. Epicardial arteries are often accompanied by two veins in the dog but only by one in the human. Transmural veins conduct the blood to the epicardial venous structure. A large number of these epicardial veins drain into the coronary sinus that empties into the right atrium. Epicardial veins of the free wall of the right ventricle drain directly into the right atrium. Characteristic of the epicardial venous system are the numerous anastomoses that can readily be seen at the surface of the heart as illustrated by Figure 4.1 (left panel) [11]. Small venous anastomoses with diameters in the order of 100 μm can also be found intramurally. The posterior and anterior veins are connected by anastomoses around the apex of the heart. When the great cardiac vein is perfused retrogradely with barium-gelatin mixture, the large anastomoses around the apex become visible as illustrated in Figure 4.1 (right panel). Venous anastomoses might be important because with the low pressure in the epicardial veins, flow in them is easily obstructed. The anastomoses offer alternate venous pathways if such an obstruction occurs.

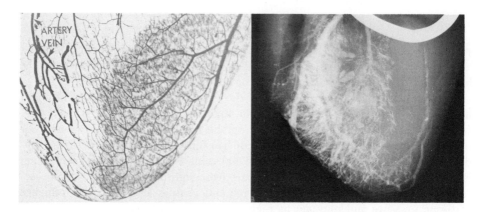

Figure 4.1: *Structure of epicardial venous system with anastomoses. Left: Photograph of a cast of the dog's epicardium eliciting the small diameter anastomoses. (From Grayson et al. [11], by permission of the author and Academic Press, Inc.) Right: X-ray photograph eliciting the large apical anastomoses between anterior and posterior veins. The great cardiac vein was injected retrogradely with barium-gelatine mixture. The posterior vein was clearly filled via the apical anastomoses. The smaller interconnections are not visible. Curved structure in top is a cannula.*

Not all the coronary venous blood drains via the coronary sinus. Some blood drains directly into the atria or ventricles; these flow channels are called Thebesian veins. Some studies report arterial-venous anastomoses [17]; however, these cannot be numerous or functional or must be otherwise of very small diameter. Radioactive microspheres 15 μm in diameter are almost all captured in the myocardial microcirculation and can barely be detected in coronary venous blood [14].

4.2 Distribution of coronary venous flow

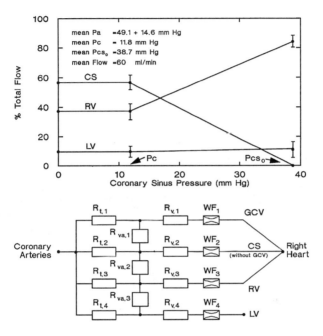

Figure 4.2: *Partition of coronary venous outflow as a function of coronary sinus pressure. Top: Results obtained in a Langendorff preparation. (Redrawn from Scharf et al. [18].) The vertical axis represent the percentage of total flow via the coronary sinus, CS, the right ventricle, RV and left ventricle, LV respectively. RV flow is right Thebesian flow plus flow from anterior veins draining directly into the right atrium. LV flow is presumably Thebesian flow only. Bottom: Model of the coronary venous outflow. The sum of arterial and capillary resistances of tissue units are represented by $R_{t,i}$ and the resistances of the venous outflow channels by $R_{v,i}$. The critical pressures are thought to be caused by Starling resistances, WF_i. Resistances of the anastomoses between venous channels are indicated by $R_{va,i}$.*

Because of the venous anastomoses, the distribution of flow over the outflow channels may change when the venous outflow pressure is altered. This issue has been studied by Scharf *et al.* [18]. In an isolated heart preparation the coronary system was perfused according to Langendorff. The coronary sinus was cannulated and the right and left ventricles drained. The relative distribution of flow over these outflow channels was as a function of the coronary sinus pressure which was manipulated in the experiment. Elevation of coronary sinus pressure did not affect this outflow distribution as long as this remained under 10 mm Hg. Above this threshold, coronary sinus flow decreased but flow in the alternative pathways increased. Their results are summarized in Figure 4.2 (top panel).

A model suitable for interpreting the results of Scharf et al. [18] is provided in Figure 4.2 (bottom panel). The myocardial wall is subdivided in units represented by a resistance $R_{t,i}$. In the experiment of Scharf et al. [18], i varies between 1 and 3. The tissue units are drained by venous channels with a resistance $R_{v,i}$ and a Starling resistance. The Starling resistance elements (WF_i) are responsible for the critical pressure below which alterations to venous outflow pressure have no effect on flow. The model differs from that of Scharf et al. [18] by the subdivision of resistances proximal to the venous channels and the resistance of the anastomoses. Scharf et al. [18] suggested the presence of a Starling resistor behavior within the coronary venous system because of the plateau phase in the flow–venous pressure curves.

Some years ago, I tried to identify the magnitude of the resistances of the venous anastomoses by altering the pressure in the great cardiac vein. The great cardiac vein of six anesthetized open chest dogs was cannulated and the blood from it was drained into a container in which the pressure could be controlled. The left main coronary artery was also cannulated and artificially perfused by a perfusion system. The coronary bed was fully dilated by the infusion of adenosine. Coronary arterial pressure and great cardiac venous pressure after clamping the venous drainage line were measured as function of coronary arterial flow. As is shown in Figure 4.3, the relation between mean perfusion pressure and mean occluded venous pressure on the one hand, and flow on the other hand is nonlinear. According to the model in the bottom panel of Figure 4.2, the pressure in the great cardiac vein during venous occlusion must equal the proximal pressure of the outflow resistance of the tissue normally drained by the great cardiac vein. With constant resistances the pressure proximal of the patent part of the venous system should be equal to the pressure in the occluded vein and proportional to flow. Since this is clearly not so, either the resistances of the venous circulation are pressure dependent or the distribution of venous flow is also altered by a redistribution of critical pressures. Either way, the nonlinearity of these curves hampers the quantification of resistance distribution in the schematic of Figure 4.2.

Regardless of the problems related to the nonlinearity of the flow–pressure relations in applying linear analysis, such analysis still may be helpful in interpreting data as demonstrated by Cohen et al. [9]. The relation between great cardiac venous flow and left anterior descending flow was studied by a model as given in the bottom of Figure 4.2. The interaction of only two tissue units was considered, fed by the left circumflex artery, LCX, and left anterior descend-

4.2 Distribution of coronary venous flow

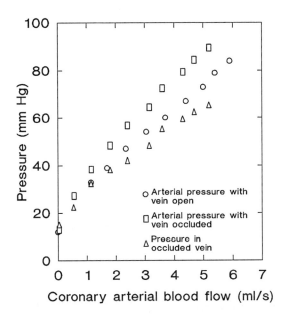

Figure 4.3: *Coronary arterial pressure and great cardiac venous pressure during obstruction of outflow as function of coronary arterial flow in the anesthetized open chest dog. The left main coronary artery was cannulated and perfused artificially. Note the nonlinear relation between obstructed venous pressure and coronary arterial flow indicating a nonlinear behavior of resistances in the unobstructed coronary veins and venous anastomoses.*

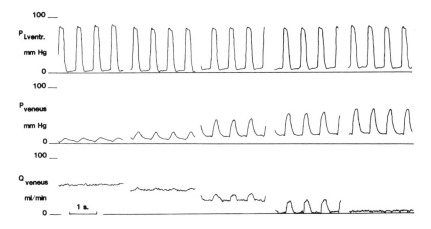

Figure 4.4: *Effect of mean epicardial venous pressure on phasic nature of this pressure and the flow through a cannula in the great cardiac vein of the dog. The outer right panels were obtained by occluding the cannula. Note that pulsatility of flow and pressure is increasing with the time average of epicardial venous pressure.*

ing artery, LAD, respectively. Important additional information was obtained by these authors by measuring regional flows. The disparity of flow changes measured in great cardiac vein and left anterior descending artery could well be described assuming a venous collateral resistance of only 10% of the LAD tissue resistance. Schematics like the one in Figure 4.2 are also being applied in studies of the effect of coronary sinus occlusion on coronary flow redistribution during ischemia [4].

4.3 Flow and pressure waves in the epicardial veins

In anesthetized open chest animals the coronary venous flow signal is about 180^0 out of phase with the coronary arterial flow signal, as venous flow is high in systole and low in diastole. The increased systolic venous flow is caused by the squeezing effect of heart contraction on intramyocardial blood volume. In the early days the increased systolic venous flow was observed from spurts of blood from incisions in the epicardial veins as reported by Porter [16]. Phasic venous flow signals are reported by among others Wiggers [24], Chilian and Marcus [7] and Tomonaga *et al.* [21]. Recently coronary venous phasic flow in the great cardiac vein and coronary sinus of the conscious dog were reported by Canty and Brooks [5]. Important differences between the two sites of measurements were reported when autoregulation was intact. The wave form in the great cardiac vein was similar to these found in the acute experiments. However, the flow wave in the coronary sinus was much more flat, with a peak reduction in flow coinciding with atrial contraction. The difference between great cardiac venous and coronary sinus flow waves was attributed to the large epicardial venous compliance. However, if vasomotor tone was abolished, Canty and Brooks found also a predominant systolic coronary sinus flow, probably because of reduced compliance at higher flows inducing an increase in coronary venous pressure.

The interpretation of coronary venous flow signals must be done with care. Because of the relatively low pressures in the venous system, the diameters of the veins are much more variable than those of the coronary arteries. Geometrical changes of epicardial veins may be considerable. In a quietly beating heart held within a cradle in the open chest of an anesthetized dog, the epicardial veins can be seen to flatten during diastole and to fill during systole. Because the veins operate under conditions in which the geometry changes from round to flat and vice versa, the compliance of these vessels under normal conditions is large. The pressure and flow waves in the coronary veins are therefore less well defined than in the coronary artery and depend strongly on the pressure level in the veins. In a series of studies Klassen *et al.*analyzed the effects of different interventions on pressure measured in the larger epicardial veins [1, 2, 15, 25]. Since in some

4.3 Flow and pressure waves in the epicardial veins

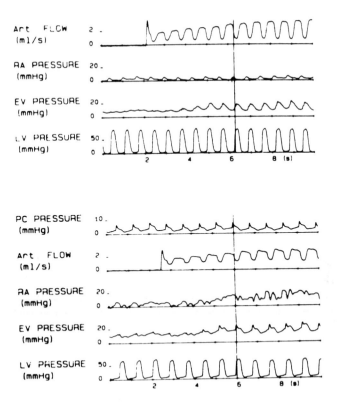

Figure 4.5: The effect of pericardium and flow on the phasic pressure signal in the epicardial vein alongside the LAD. Measurement was done in an anesthetized goat with open chest. The left main coronary artery was cannulated and perfused artificially. The top half of the figure was obtained with open pericardium, the bottom half with pericardium closed. Note the effect of flow on pressure. With pericardium and flow present the venous pressure wave is different from when the pericardium is absent. RA = right atrium, EV = epicardial venous, LV = left ventricular, PC = Pericardial. Note that without pericardium, the pulse in EV pressure increases with the level of pressure. The EV pressure is affected by the radial stress of the pericardium.

of these studies the pressure was measured with a catheter inserted upstream the absolute pressure levels measured might have been overestimated because of flow obstruction. However, from these studies it may be concluded that the venous pressure wave forms are under direct influence of the strength of cardiac contraction.

The effect of coronary venous pressure on flow and pressure wave forms in the great cardiac vein is illustrated in Figure 4.4. These results were obtained in an open chest anesthetized dog with cannulated great cardiac vein. Blood was drained into a reservoir with constant pressure. Epicardial venous pressure was measured with a thin catheter and increased by increasing reservoir pressure. As is clear from Figure 4.4 the pulsatility of venous cannula flow and epicardial venous pressure increased with the mean epicardial venous pressure. These increases are consistent with decreasing epicardial venous compliance caused by increasing pressure and the assumption of a constant blood pressure pulse generated by tissue compression. However, the results are also consistent with the time varying elastance concept [23] discussed in Chapters 1, 6 and 7. This concept predicts larger pulse pressure generation inside intramural blood vessels when the volume of these vessels is increased. Such a volume increase is to be expected with a higher epicardial venous pressure. Hence, the increase in pulsations of epicardial venous pressure and flow may also reflect these increased intramyocardial pressure pulsations. This explanation is also consistent with the observed increase of epicardial venous pressure pulsations induced by positive inotropic stimuli [1].

The effect of the pericardium and flow on the pressure in the vein along the LAD is illustrated in Figure 4.5. The experiment was done in the anesthetized open chest goat with cannulated left main stem. However, the coronary veins were not cannulated. A catheter was introduced in the vein along the LAD. This catheter has an outside diameter of 1 mm within a vessel of about 3 mm. More importantly, the open end of the catheter pointed in the outflow direction and hence the pressure pulsations could not be the result of obstruction of coronary venous flow. The panels in the top half of the figure were obtained with the pericardium open and in the bottom half with the pericardium closed. The radial stress exerted by the pericardium was qualitatively measured by the insertion of a fluid filled bag between epicardium and pericardium [19]. The bag was at a different position than the epicardial vein in which pressure was measured.

Without the pericardium, an epicardial venous pressure signal is flat during cessation of flow but pulsatile with flow. Systolic pressure is higher because blood is squeezed into the epicardial veins from the intramyocardial vessels. The pericardial pressure is pulsatile as well. This pressure increases during diastole due to filling of the left ventricle, and the epicardium is pushed against the pericardium. Pericardial pressure decrease starts at the peak of left ventricular pressure and hence can be explained by reducing left ventricular volume.

Note that pericardial pressure is not affected by coronary arterial flow and is hardly transmitted to epicardial venous pressure during arterial occlusion. Lack of transmission of the pericardial pressure pulse to epicardial venous pressure in the absence of flow is probably due to the fact that the epicardial veins in the goat are partly submerged into the heart muscle, providing protection against pericardial stress.

With flow, the pulsatility in the epicardial venous pressure is altered compared to when the pericardium is absent. In theory it is possible that the effects of the squeezing of blood from the intramyocardial blood space are cancelled out by the compressive force from the pericardium which is almost 180^0 out of phase with the blood flow coming from the transmural veins. This interaction between epicardial venous pressure and pericardial stress has not yet been studied extensively.

Note also in Figure 4.5 that epicardial venous pressure is dependent on coronary flow but that this effect is small. This makes it unlikely that the epicardial venous pressure as such plays an important role in determining the magnitude of myocardial perfusion. However, the collapse behavior of these vessels may be an important determinant in maintaining patency of intramyocardial blood vessels.

4.4 Waterfall behavior of coronary epicardial veins

A discussion of epicardial venous pressure is incomplete without discussing the waterfall behavior of the coronary veins. The waterfall model as such will be discussed in Chapter 6. For the time being, it is sufficient to know that when a vessel collapses, the proximal pressure and distal pressure are no longer coupled by a simple resistance. The flow through such a vessel will depend on the one hand on the outside pressure and vessel wall stresses combining to cause the collapse, and on the other hand on proximal pressure. The distal luminal pressure has no effect on flow. This waterfall behavior is clear from Figure 4.3. At a certain low level of outflow cannula pressure, this pressure can be further decreased without increasing venous outflow.

Uhlig et al. [22] showed that waterfall behavior could be demonstrated in the coronary sinus, also without cannulation of this vessel. These authors also showed that the waterfall pressure, the pressure below which the venous pressure and right atrial pressure are uncoupled, increases with increasing end-diastolic left ventricular pressure. In a series of experiments on goats, we measured the epicardial venous pressure as a function of left ventricular diastolic pressure with and without the pericardium. In both situations, the two pressures were well correlated.

The coronary venous system does not act entirely as a waterfall or Starling resistor since epicardial venous pressure is slightly flow dependent as was discussed above.

4.5 Coronary venous compliance

Not much is known about the compliance of the coronary venous vessels. In other organs, distensibility of venules is similar to those of capillaries and about

0.005 ml · mm Hg^{-1} at a pressure of around 20 mm Hg. Pressure diameter relations of veins with a diameter of the order of that of the larger coronary veins have been reported [6]. Based on a transmural pressure–distensibility relationship, estimated coronary venous volume and pressure distribution, a compliance of 0.04 ml · mm Hg^{-1} · [100 g]$^{-1}$ has been estimated [20].

4.6 Summary

The coronary venous system is a mirror image of the coronary arterial system, albeit with some differences. In the dog, small arteries are often accompanied by two small veins. There are numerous intramyocardial and epicardial anastomoses. The coronary venous system lacks a unique outflow track. The coronary sinus drains about 55% of coronary arterial flow and 35% is drained directly into the right heart. About 10% drains into the left ventricular cavity via Thebesian channels. Because of venous anastomoses, the distribution of flow over these venous channels depends on the pressures in these channels. Quantitative analysis of the venous circuit is hampered by nonlinear behavior of the vessel resistances involved. Epicardial veins do exhibit a waterfall behavior but epicardial venous pressure is slightly affected by flow. Pressure and flow waves in the epicardial veins are easily affected by the level of epicardial venous pressure because these vessels operate at low transmural pressures. The pericardium does affect the venous flow and pressure waves, especially at low heart frequencies.

References

[1] ARMOUR JA, KLASSEN GA (1984) Pressure and flow in epicardial coronary veins of the dog heart: response to positive inotropism. *Can. J. Physiol. Pharmacol.* **62**: 38–48.

[2] ARMOUR JA, KLASSEN GA (1981) Epicardial coronary venous pressure. *Can. J. Physiol. Pharmacol.* **59**: 1250–1259.

[3] BASSINGTHWAIGHTE JB, YIPINTSOI T, HARVEY RB (1974) Microvasculature of the dog left ventricular myocardium. *Microvasc. Res.* **7**: 229–249.

[4] BEYAR R, GUERCI AD, HALPERIN HR, TSITLIK JE, WEISFELDT ML (1989) Intermittent coronary sinus occlusion after coronary arterial ligation results in venous retroperfusion. *Circ. Res.* **65**: 695–707.

[5] CANTY JM JR, BROOKS A (1990) Phasic volumetric coronary outflow patterns in conscious dogs. *Am. J. Physiol.* **258** (*Heart Circ. Physiol.* **27**): H1457–H1463.

[6] CARO CG, PEDLEY TJ, SCHROTER RC, SEED WA (1978) *The mechanics of the circulation.* Chapter 14, The systemic veins. Oxford, UK, Oxford University Press: 434–475.

[7] CHILIAN WM, MARCUS ML (1984) Coronary venous outflow persists after cessation of coronary arterial inflow. *Am. J. Physiol.* **247** (*Heart Circ. Physiol.* **16**): H984–H990.
[8] CIUFFO AA, GUERCI AD, BUKLEY G, CASALE A, WEISFELDT ML (1984) Intermittent obstruction of the coronary sinus following coronary ligation in dogs reduces ischemic necrosis and increases myocardial perfusion. In: *The Coronary Sinus.* Eds. MOHL W, WOLNER E, GLOGAR D. Steinkopff Verlag Darmstadt, Springer-Verlag New York: 454–464.
[9] COHEN MV, MATSUKI T, DOWNEY JM (1988) Pressure-flow charateristics and nutritional capacity of coronary veins in dogs. *Am. J. Physiol.* **255** (*Heart Circ. Physiol.* **24**): H834-H846.
[10] *The Coronary Sinus.* (1984) Proceedings of the 1st International Symposium on Myocardial Protection via the Coronary Sinus. Eds. MOHL W, WOLNER E, GLOGAR D. Steinkopff Verlag Darmstadt, Springer-Verlag New York.
[11] GRAYSON J, DAVIDSON JW, FITZGERALD-FINCH A, SCOTT C (1974) The functional morphology of the coronary microcirculation in the dog. *Microvasc. Res.* **8**: 20–43.
[12] GROSS L, BLUM L, SILVERMAN G (1935) Experimental attempts to increase the blood supply to the dog's heart by means of coronary sinus occlusion. *J. Exp. Med.* **65**: 91–106.
[13] GUNDRY SR (1982) Modification of myocardial ischemia in normal and hypertrophied hearts utilizing diastolic retroperfusion of the coronary veins. *J. Thor. Cardiovasc. Surg.* **83**: 659–669.
[14] HOF RP, SALZMANN R, WYLER F (1981) Trapping and intramyocardial distribution of microspheres with different diameters in cat and rabbit hearts in vitro. *Basic Res. Cardiol.* **76**: 630–638.
[15] KLASSEN GA, ARMOUR JA (1983) Canine coronary venous pressures: responses to positive inotropism and vasodilation. *Can. J. Physiol. Pharmacol.* **61**: 213–221.
[16] PORTER WT (1898) The influence of the heart beat on the flow of blood through the walls of the heart. *Am. J. Physiol.* **1**: 145–163.
[17] RATAJCZYK-PAKALSKA E, KOLFF WJ (1984) Anatomical basis for the coronary venous outflow. In: *The Coronary Sinus.* Proceedings of the 1st International Symposium on Myocardial Protection via the Coronary Sinus. Eds. MOHL W, WOLNER E, GLOGAR D. Steinkopff Verlag Darmstadt, Springer-Verlag New York: 40–46.
[18] SCHARF SM, BROMBERGER-BARNEA B, PERMUTT S (1971) Distribution of coronary venous flow. *J. Appl. Physiol.* **30**: 657–662.
[19] SMISETH OA, FRAIS MA, KINGMA I, SMITH ER, TYBERG JV (1985) Assessment of pericardial constraint in dogs. *Circulation* **71**: 158–164.
[20] SPAAN JAE (1985) Coronary diastolic pressure-flow relation and zero flow pressure explained on the basis of intramyocardial compliance. *Circ. Res.*

56: 293–309.

[21] TOMONAGA G, TSUJIOKA K, OGASAWARA Y, NAKAI M, MITO K, HIRAMATSU O, KAJIYA F (1984) Dynamic characteristics of diastolic pressure-flow relation in the canine coronary artery. In: *The Coronary Sinus*. Eds. MOHL W, WOLNER E, GLOGAR D. Steinkopff Verlag Darmstadt, Springer-Verlag New York: 79–85.

[22] UHLIG PN, BAER RW, VLAHAKES GJ, HANLEY FL, MESSINA LM, HOFFMAN JIE (1984) Arterial and venous coronary pressure-flow relations in anesthetized dogs. *Circ. Res.* **55**: 238–248.

[23] WESTERHOF N (1990) Physiological hypotheses-Intramyocardial pressure. A new concept, suggestions for measurement. *Basic Res. Cardiol.* **85**: 105–119.

[24] WIGGERS CJ (1954) The interplay of coronary vascular resistance and myocardial compression in regulating coronary flow. *Circ. Res.* **2**: 271–279.

[25] WONG AYK, ARMOUR JA, KLASSEN GA, LEE B (1984) The dynamics of the coronary venous system in the dog. *J. Biomech.* **17**: 173–183.

Chapter 5

Linear system analysis applied to the coronary circulation

THE CORONARY CIRCULATION IS A COMPLEX SYSTEM of vascular channels through which flow is determined by driving pressure, adjustable hydraulic resistances, and mechanical factors such as compression and geometrical variations. Gaining understanding the way this functions is hampered by the limited possibilities of observing the details of this complex system. It is obvious that help is sought from the theories and techniques which have been developed to design and describe man-made complex systems to analyze biological systems.

A conglomerate of entities that function in relation to each other can be defined as a system. In a linear system, each cause and effect relation is linear. By ensuring that linear subsystems are used in the design of a system, the final complex system can be described by a linear set of equations. The field of linear system analysis has evolved up to a high level of sophistication and, therefore, very useful since many techniques for manipulating and analyzing data have been developed.

In general, biological systems deserve the qualification complex and are often nonlinear. Moreover, they are not designed by a human engineer and hence the structure and function of subsystems are badly defined. As a result of these properties, linear system analysis cannot be applied to them without using the utmost care. Behavior of nonlinear systems can be studied by linearizing their relations around what is called a reference or working point. Hence, for small variations around this working point, the linear analysis techniques may again be applied. The value of linear system analysis to the understanding of biological systems is significant in that it provides a framework for interpretation of relationships and acts as a structural aid in developing experiments (e.g., [12]).

As regards the general theory of system analysis, this chapter only provides a simple introduction, meant to familiarize those without an engineering background with some elementary definitions. Furthermore, the strengths, dangers and shortcomings of linear system analysis as applied in some experimental studies on coronary arterial pressure–flow relations will be illustrated. In accordance with the philosophy of this book, only the material necessary to the understanding of the mechanisms under study is discussed. The reader is encouraged to read a more detailed work on signal and system analysis (e.g., [9]).

5.1 Definitions

5.1.1 System

A general definition of a system is 'a process that can be considered isolated from its surroundings, possessing a certain degree of ordering, and is related to its surroundings. The relationship with the environment that can be described by input, output and disturbance signals whereby these signals have a functional relationship'. The notion signal is quite abstract and the adjectives input and output do not necessarily relate to physical concreteness. For example, when relating coronary arterial flow to coronary arterial pressure and the latter is the independent variable, the coronary circulation can be considered as a system whereby coronary arterial pressure is the input signal and coronary flow is the output signal. Hence, although coronary arterial flow enters the coronary vascular bed and physically flows into the coronary vascular tree, it may be the output signal in terms of signal analysis. The coronary flow signal depends not only on arterial pressure but also on venous pressure and heart rate. These same factors also affect the coronary outflow. Hence, the coronary circulation may be considered as a system with many input and output signals.

It is customary to represent input, output and noise signals relevant to a certain problem as in Figure 5.1. Note that there is relatively free choice of input and output signals, although there are restrictions. For example, since arterial flow and pressure are related by the input impedance of the arterial system, only one can be chosen as input signal. The other then automatically becomes the output signal. Normally, the number of input and output signals will be restricted depending on the question under study. For example, if one is interested only in the input impedance, the coronary circulation as physical reality can be considered as a single input, single output system. Note that all the other signals involved are treated as noise signals and should be kept as constant as possible. A nice demonstration of the application of these principles to the coronary circulation has been presented by Saint-Felix and Demoment [13].

5.1 Definitions

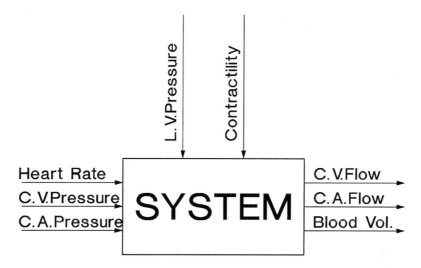

Figure 5.1: *Schematic representation of the coronary circulation as a system with multiple inputs (left hand arrows) and outputs (right hand arrows). The number of input and output signals to be taken into account depends on the scientific question that is posed. The arrows pointing downward are uncontrollable signals, referred to as noise signals.*

5.1.2 Linearity

The relation between an independent and dependent variable is linear if the following criterion is fulfilled. Denote the independent and dependent variables with x and $y(x)$, respectively. The relation is linear if the following property holds:

$$y(x_1 + x_2) = y(x_1) + y(x_2) \qquad [5.1]$$

In short, the relation is only linear if there is a proportionality between the dependent and independent variable. In the graphical representation this is a straight line passing through the origin. Hence, x and y are not linearly related in the following equation:

$$y(x) = ax + b \qquad [5.2]$$

Still, this equation is known as a linear equation. Hence the definition of linearity for a system and for mathematical expressions exhibits a discrepancy.

The nonlinearity described by Equation [5.2] is a special example. By introducing a simple substitution, e.g., $y(x) = y'(x) - b$ the relation between $y'(x)$ and x has become linear. A relevant example for coronary studies is the diastolic pressure–flow relation (e.g., Chapters 6 and 7). This relation may be straight but because there is an intercept on the pressure axis, the relation between coronary flow and coronary pressure is not linear.

Signal analysis deals mainly with time varying input and output signals. The input signal can then be split into a time dependent and time independent part. It is very practical to define the time independent part as the time average of the signals and the time dependent part as the difference between the original signal and the time averaged signal. Very often the time average parts of the signals are not linearly related but the time varying parts are.

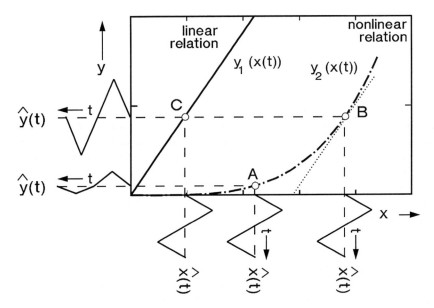

Figure 5.2: Illustration of input (x) - output (y) relations for a linear and nonlinear system. Note that around the working point B for the nonlinear system, $y = y_2(x)$, the curve is quite straight and the time varying output signal, $\hat{y}(t)$, is almost linearly related to the input signal, $\hat{x}(t)$. The transfer is the same as by the linear system $y = y_1(x)$ since the slopes at B and C of the respective curves are the same. Note the distortion of the transfer of the input signal at working point A because of the high curvature of $y = y_2(x)$ in working point A. See text for further explanation.

The transfers of an input signal by a linear and nonlinear system are illustrated in Figure 5.2. The input signal, $\hat{x}(t)$, is a function of time with average value zero and varies around a reference value. The output signal is $\hat{y}(t)$ and varies around its reference value. The reference values for x and y together define the working point of the system. In Figure 5.2 these different working points are indicated. A and B are working points on the nonlinear relation and C on the linear relation. For the linear system the ratio between $y(t)/x(t)$ is constant and independent of the position on the working point. For the nonlinear system the transfer of the input signal is dependent on the working point. The amplitude of the output signal at working point A is much smaller than at working point B because the slope of the relation y versus x is much smaller at A than at B. Note also that the output signal at A is distorted with respect to the shape of its input signal. This is because the input signal has a large amplitude compared to the range around the working point over which the curve can be linearized. The curvature of $y(x)$ is larger at A than at B. Note that because of the nonlinear transfer at A, the time average of the output signal $\hat{y}(t)$ has become different from zero.

5.1.3 Time and frequency domains

The important consequence of linearity is the applicability of the superposition principle. An output signal can be described as a linear combination of functions which are related to a linear combination of functions forming the input signal. Since it is possible to describe arbitrary functions, e.g., step functions, delta functions or exponentials, by the superposition of elementary time dependent functions, the output signal of a system can be reconstructed from the input signal if the way in which the elementary functions are transferred by the system is known. Such an analysis describes the transfer of signals in the time domain.

Physiological signals often are periodic and analysis in the frequency domain is very useful. This analysis is based on Fourier analysis. An arbitrary signal can be represented by a series of sine waves. If the transfer of each sine wave is defined, by calculating the amplitude and the phase spectra of the inflow signal, the outflow signal can be reconstructed from the amplitude and phase spectra after application of the transformation rules to the inlet spectra. Hence, the characteristics of a system can be described by a transfer function in the frequency domain. The transfer function $H(\omega)$ is in the frequency domain and defines how harmonic output and input functions are related by amplitude and phase. These notions will be clarified in more detail when discussing input impedance of the coronary system[1].

5.1.4 Models

A model is an analog of a reality. In a physical model, reality is mimicked by a material system. For example, it is possible to study the fluid dynamic behavior of elastic blood vessels in tissue by studying the dynamics of flow through elastic tubes surrounded by air or by some other fluid. The similarities in fluid dynamic

---

[1] A book that may be helpful to the reader without engineering background is from Rubin [11].

behavior between the model and the real system depend on how well the vessel wall mechanics and suspension in tissue are mimicked by the model system. In a mathematical model one attempts to describe the properties of variables using quantitative relationships, i.e., mathematical equations.

One may distinguish between two different mathematical models: descriptive and predictive. In a descriptive model the primary aim is not to understand the underlying physical principles, but to provide a mathematical set of equations describing the behavior and relations between variables. A special class of descriptive models is those used in linear system analysis. Such models consist of elements that fit into a generalized approach. For example, one may estimate a transfer function for the input impedance of the coronary circulation and describe this with one or more first order elements. The advantage of this type of analysis is that complicated systems can be analyzed using formalisms developed for totally different physical systems. Predictive models are based on some physical principles applicable to the real system and the consequence of these principles for behavior of variables can be studied. Take, for example, the relation between flow through and pressure drop over a tube. A descriptive model consists simply of a resistance. The predictive model would be based on length and diameter of the tube and the rheology of the fluid flowing through the tube. This model would then predict the relation between flow and pressure drop, which prediction can then be tested by measurements. In addition to physical models and mathematical models, there are also the relational models. These models are limited to indicating qualitative relations between several processes. For example, one may state that there is a relation between adenosine production and coronary resistance. Such a statement can be indicated as a relational model, which becomes a mathematical model when this relation is quantified.

Amongst physiologists there is some dislike of models and use of the word is avoided. Often the notion index is used instead which, however, is mostly interpreted to mean a model which is not explicitly defined. A classic example is the end-diastolic resistance index which is mostly defined as the ratio between coronary arterial pressure and flow at the end of diastole. A change of the index induced by an intervention is subsequently explained as a change in vasomotor tone, which in turn is intuitively interpreted as a change in resistance.

Almost always, the biological system is too complex to be fitted into a predictive model predicting the relation between all variables involved. Hence the way to work is to develop models emphasizing the processes under study and therefore to restrict the number of variables and parameters involved (e.g., [1, 6]).

5.1.5 Load line analysis

The theorem of Thevenin in electrical engineering is a valuable one worth knowing [14]. This theorem states that the input-output relation of a complex circuit with impedances and other 'active elements' can be described by an equivalent

5.1 Definitions

circuit consisting of a power source with internal resistance. Active elements are elements that can generate energy. In hydrodynamic terms: for a complex system of vessels, in some of which pressure is generated, the input-output relation can be described by a pump consisting of an ideal pressure source with an impedance in series. This is illustrated in the left panel of Figure 5.3. The flow delivered by the system as well as the output pressure depend on the external load of the pump. By changing the load the relation between output pressure and flow of the pump can be varied and plotted in a diagram. The relation between these two quantities is linear and is called a 'load line'. The load obtained from the left panel in Figure 5.3 is shown in the right panel.

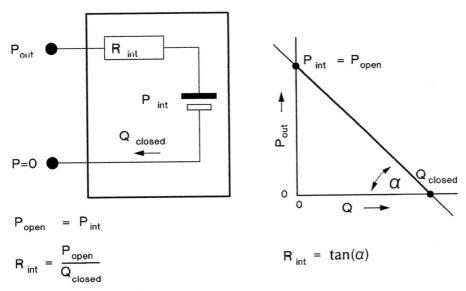

Figure 5.3: *Illustration of Thevenin's theorem and the load line analysis. Left: A 'black box' showing the pressure source having an internal impedance and the external load, P_{out}. Right: The load line that can be obtained by changing the external load. The heavy line is the trajectory that can be measured without the application of external pressure source.*

Where a physically complex system is to be described by a black box such as in Figure 5.3, one can, in theory, easily estimate the values to be attributed to the pressure source: internal pressure, P_{int}, and internal resistance, R_{int}. The simplest way to determine P_{int}, is to measure the so-called 'open clamp' pressure, P_{open}. This is the pressure at the outlet, or at the 'outs' of the black box, without external load. Since in this instance no flow passes through the resistance, there is no pressure loss across it and the open clamp pressure equals per definition the pressure of the equivalent source. The determination of internal resistance requires an additional measurement. A simple one is the 'closed circuit flow', Q_{closed}. It is not hard to see that the internal resistance of the black box can be calculated from the ratio between:

$$R_{int} = \frac{P_{open}}{Q_{closed}} \quad [5.3]$$

Note that R_{int} equals the inverse of the slope of the load line.

Because of the linearity of the load line, the equivalent pressure and internal resistance can be calculated by measuring two arbitrary points on the load line. However, a system should not a priori be assumed to be linear. The linearity of the system can be assessed by measuring the relation between outflow and outlet pressure over a wide range by either using an external pressure source or by varying the external load between zero and infinity. In the latter way the range indicated by the heavy line in Figure 5.3 (right panel) can be estimated. The load line can be constructed beyond this range by applying an external pressure source. This however implies the generation of either a negative value of pressure or negative value of flow.

5.2 Linear intramyocardial pump model

The intramyocardial pump model was designed on the assumption that systolic-diastolic flow variations in the coronary arteries were coupled to cyclic intramyocardial blood volume variations rather than to resistance variations or local vessel collapse. Obviously, volume variation of the coronary microcirculation might result in resistance variations as well. This will be discussed in Chapter 6.

The load line analysis was applied by Spaan et al. [15, 16] (Figure 5.4 and 5.5) to test whether the pulsations in coronary arterial flow and pressure could be ascribed to a pulsating pressure source with internal resistance. The experiments were performed in anesthetized open chest dogs with cannulated left main coronary artery. The flow pulsations can be attenuated by increasing the load for the pulsations by means of a out on the perfusion line. Of course, this resistance in the perfusion line would also affect the mean coronary arterial pressure. However, the pressure of the blood source proximal to the stenosis was increased to keep mean coronary arterial pressure constant and hence to compensate for the drop in mean pressure over the external load. Maintenance of mean coronary arterial pressure is important to minimize a response of the local coronary control mechanism. Local control is then assumed not to be activated by the pulse of either coronary arterial flow or pressure since these pulsations are influenced by the degree of stenosis.

Note that in the intramyocardial pump study the applicability of the superposition principle was assumed. The magnitudes of flow and pressure pulsations

5.2 Linear intramyocardial pump model

were considered separately from of the level of the mean values of pressure and flow.

The effect of the external stenosis on coronary arterial flow and pressure is shown in Figure 5.4. The increase of stenosis resistance reduces the pulsations in the flow signal and brings about the pulsations in coronary arterial pressure. It is practically impossible to eliminate all the flow pulses and maintain mean perfusion pressure at a fixed value. Because of the flat plateau in the autoregulation curve (see Figure 1.5) a deviation of 1% in flow results in a variation of 10 mm Hg in perfusion pressure. It is practically impossible to match the flow so exactly to the needs of the heart that a vasoconstrictive or vasodilatory response of the local coronary flow control mechanism is avoided [10].

Load lines can be defined to relate the pulsations in pressure and flow in the coronary artery (Figure 5.5), a finding which justifies the notion of an intramyocardial pump. Extrapolation of these load lines to the pressure axis results in an intercept that reflects the pressure pulsations at perfect constant flow and can be considered as the pressure source for pulsatile flow at constant pressure perfusion. The slope of the load lines represents the internal resistance of the intramyocardial pump. The question is what properties are reflected by the pressure source and internal resistance.

5.2.1 Interpretation of the coronary load lines

Regarding the interpretation of the coronary load lines, the obvious step is to look for a pressure source and resistance in the myocardial microcirculation. We will first consider the tissue pressure generated by ventricular contraction when this is taken as the pressure source. This is similar to what was assumed in the waterfall model. However, the concept of interaction with the microvessels is quite different. This is illustrated in Figure 5.6 for a vessel in a container where the outside pressure can vary. In the top panels, the condition in which both ends of the vessels are occluded is illustrated.

Because of the incompressibility of the fluid, the inside volume of the tube is constant whatever pressure is applied outside the vessel. Since the wall cannot deform, the stresses within the wall remain unchanged and hence transmural pressure, which is the difference between $P_{in} - P_{out}$, will remain constant regardless of the variations in P_{out}. The top panels illustrate that when P_{out} varies as a square wave, P_{in} will do so as well with the same amplitude.

The bottom panel of Figure 5.6 illustrates what will happen if fluid is able to leak out of the compartment. If a step change in outside pressure occurs, inside pressure will instantly follow the step by the same magnitude. However, the inside pressure will then decay because of fluid movement out of the compartment at a rate which depends on the inflow and outflow resistances of the vessel and vessel compliance. If resistances and compliance are constant, the decay is exponential with a time constant, T, equal to:

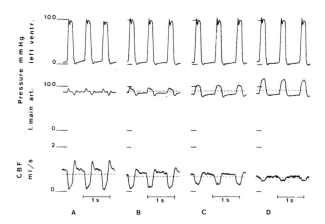

Figure 5.4: Effect of stenosis in the perfusion line on coronary arterial pressure and flow at constant mean coronary arterial pressure. Note that mean flow (dotted lines) is quite constant. The stenosis reduced the flow pulsations but increased the pressure pulsations. (Reproduced from Spaan et al. [15], by permission of the American Heart Association Inc.)

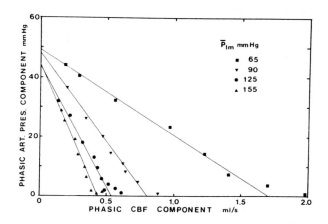

Figure 5.5: Load lines of the 'intramyocardial pump' at four different levels of mean arterial pressure in one dog. Because of the regulatory response of coronary smooth muscle tone it was impossible to measure the 'open clamp pressure' of the pump directly. Note, however, that the load lines intercept the pressure axis at similar values. As is indicated by the slopes of the load lines, the internal resistance of the pump depends on vasomotor tone as set by the mean coronary arterial pressure. (Reproduced from Spaan et al. [15], by permission of the American Heart Association Inc.)

5.2 Linear intramyocardial pump model

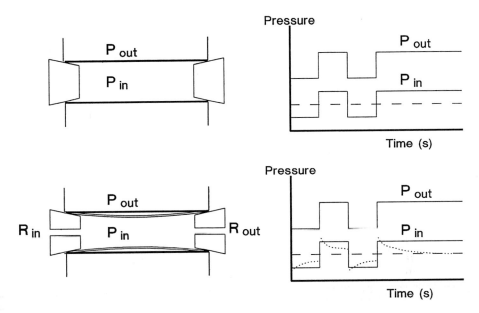

Figure 5.6: Relation between outside pressure, P_{out}, and inside pressure, P_{in}, of an elastic vessel in a container such that outside pressure can be varied. The top panels refer to the condition where no fluid can escape the vessel. The pulsations of pressure in the vessel are essentially equal to those outside the vessel. The bottom panels refer to the condition where vessel fluid volume may change because of variations in outside pressure; the rapid jumps in inside pressure equal those in outside pressure. However, P_{in} decays to the mean (- - -) because of fluid movement through R_{in} and R_{out}.

$$T = R_{eq}C = \frac{R_{in}R_{out}}{R_{in} + R_{out}}C \qquad [5.4]$$

where:

C is compliance,
R_{in} is inlet resistance,
R_{out} is outlet resistance,
R_{eq} is the equivalent resistance of R_{in} and R_{out} in parallel.

If P_{out} is a square wave, the wave form of P_{in} will resemble the one plotted at the bottom of Figure 5.6. The magnitude of the sudden jumps in pressure is equal to the amplitude of the square wave. In the periods when P_{out} is stable, P_{in} will drift exponentially to its mean value. However, if T is large enough compared to the periodic time of the square wave, it can never reach the mean because of the succeeding jump in outside pressure. The flow signals at the inlet and outlet of the vessel will mimic the shape of the inside pressure signal. Obviously, when volume is squeezed out of the tube, the tube radius will become smaller and the compliance value will change. We will consider this in the next chapter, but for now it is assumed that compliance remains constant.

When the tube is perfused at constant flow, the pressure variation inside the tube can be measured at the tube entrance since a loss of the pulsatile pressure component over R_{in} will occur. Hence, the pressure pulse is the equivalent driving pressure mentioned in Figure 5.3 and denoted there as P_{int}. If the tube is perfused with constant inlet pressure, the variation in pressure difference across R_{in} will cause the flow through R_{in} to be pulsatile. This situation equals the short circuit condition for pulsatile flow.

The 'tube in the box' model also shows that the outflow is pulsatile at all times. Inflow can even be retrograde if the superposition of the mean and the inside pressure becomes negative.

The interpretation of the physiological signals can now be made according to this tube in the box model. Tissue pressure is transmitted into the tube and the time constant for changing tube volume is much longer than the duration of systole and diastole. Indeed, the time for changing intramyocardial blood volume is in the order of 1.6 s. [19]. Hence, the volume variation during the heart cycle does not reach a steady state during systole or diastole. The driving pressure for the intramyocardial pump action equals the pressure pulse predicted by the extrapolation of the load line to zero flow pulse. This pressure pulse equals approximately half of the left ventricular systolic–diastolic pressure pulse. This is what one would expect if tissue pressure decreased linearly from ventricular pressure at the subendocardium to atmospheric at the subepicardium. If the load line were obtained from our tube in the box experiment, its slope would be equal to R_{int}. Hence, the slope of the coronary load lines reflect the inlet resistance of our model. This inlet resistance is dependent on the coronary arterial pressure because local coronary control dictates that arteriolar resistance is higher at higher coronary arterial pressure at constant oxygen consumption.

Obviously, the pressure of the intramyocardial pump might also be generated by the effect of fiber shortening on the vessels or elastance variations in the ventricular wall as suggested by Krams [7] and Westerhof [21]. The varying elastance as driving pressure of the intramyocardial pump will be discussed in Chapters 6 and 7.

From the intramyocardial pump experiments of Spaan *et al.* [15] it was concluded that the inlet resistance of the model was correlated to the total coronary resistance by the equation,

$$R_{in} = 0.63[R_{in} + R_{out}] - 12.9 \quad \text{mm Hg} \cdot \text{s} \cdot \text{ml}^{-1} \qquad [5.5]$$

This correlation illustrates that phasic flow variations are damped by only a part of the controllable resistance. In terms of the simple model of the bottom panel of Figure 5.6 this would imply that a significant part of the arterial tree, responsible for resistance control, has sufficient compliance to contribute to phasic flow by volume variations. However, it may be questioned whether the system of continuously decreasing diameters and increasing total cross-sectional area as a function of the level of branching can be approximated by a simple RCR-compartment.

5.2.2 Intramyocardial pump and the right coronary artery

The load line analysis has also been applied to the right coronary artery [5]. The pressure pulse was about half of the right ventricular pressure variations, which strongly supports the idea that the tissue pressures, responsible for the pulsations, are related to ventricular pressure. The pressure decay curve exhibited the same characteristic as in the left coronary artery and the compliance value deduced from it was also 0.75 ml · mm Hg^{-1} per 100 g tissue. The value of the ratio $R_{in}/[R_{in} + R_{out}]$ was 0.5, which is lower than in the left ventricle.

5.2.3 Shortcomings of the linear intramyocardial pump model

Low and even negative systolic flow values are well explained by intramyocardial pumping of blood. It all depends on the relative magnitudes of the mean flow and the flow pulse. However, the model can basically not explain the net reduction effect of cardiac contraction on time averaged coronary flow as seen in the pharmacologically dilated coronary bed, since in the model the mean signals are not affected by cyclic events. Such a reduction can be explained when the volume variations of the tube affect either one or both of the resistances (see Chapters 6 and 7).

The intramyocardial pump model has been tested by Spaan *et al.* [15] only in the autoregulatory range of the coronary bed with local control intact. Lee *et al.* [8] applied the load line analysis to the fully dilated bed and found that the pulsatile driving pressure was coronary arterial pressure dependent, contrary to the finding in the autoregulated bed. This will be discussed later as well.

5.3 Load line analysis of collateral flow

A nice illustration of linear analysis based on load lines has been presented by Wyatt *et al.* [22] for the analysis of the collateral system in the dog. In anesthetized dogs the left anterior descending artery, LAD, was cannulated and connected to an artificial perfusion system by which the LAD pressure could be manipulated. By lowering cannula pressure, retrograde flow can occur. This retrograde flow must be the result of collateral flow from the coronary arterial system, which continues to be directly fed by the aortic pressure, presumably from the circumflex coronary artery. The schematic suggested for the interpretation of retrograde flow and prediction of collateral flow is illustrated in Figure 5.7. The resistances of LAD and circumflex perfusion area are each represented by two resistances in series. The sum of these two resistances per area are presumably inversely proportional to the myocardial mass perfused by them. The two nodes are connected by a resistance, representing the collaterals between the two subsystems.

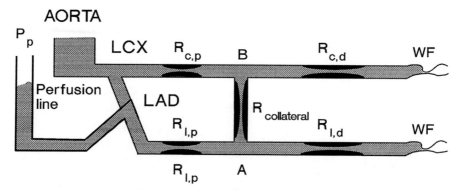

Figure 5.7: Schematic illustration of the model for the interpretation of collateral load lines and prediction of collateral flow. Normally both left anterior descending, LAD, and circumflex artery, LCX, are perfused at aortic pressure. $R_{\text{collateral}}$ is the resistance of the collaterals between LAD and LCX. A and B indicate the nodes of the collateral vessel with LAD and LCX respectively. $R_{c,p}$ and $R_{l,p}$ are the resistances of LCX and LAD respectively proximal to the nodes with the collaterals. $R_{c,d}$ and $R_{l,d}$ are the resistances distal of these nodes and are connected to waterfall elements. The collateral load lines were obtained by occluding all distal vessels of the LAD by microspheres and hence by making $R_{l,d}$ infinitely large. Hence, all flow through the collaterals is diverted into the proximal LAD which was cannulated and connected to a pressure source with pressure P_p. (Free according to Wyatt et al. [22].)

During occlusion of the LAD perfusion line a remaining pressure was measured which may be referred to as stop flow pressure, P_{zf}. If LAD pressure was reduced below stop flow pressure, flow became retrograde. By varying the LAD pressure between stop flow pressure and zero, a retrograde load line was obtained. The experiment was repeated after a period of anterograde perfusion of the LAD, during which microspheres about 25 μm diameter were lodged in the microcirculation perfused by the LAD until flow came to a complete stop. Then retrograde flow was measured again as a function of LAD cannula pressure, P_p. It appeared that the stop flow pressure was strongly increased while the maximal retrograde flow was unaltered. Results of these experiments on retrograde load line (open LAD microcirculation) and collateral load line (closed LAD microcirculation) are reproduced in figure 5.8.

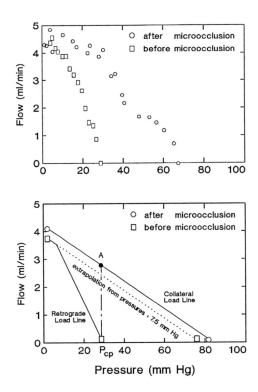

Figure 5.8: *Retrograde (□) and collateral (○) load lines from Wyatt et al. [22] obtained before and after LAD microvessel occlusion respectively. Flow is plotted versus cannula pressure. Top: Experimental curves. Bottom: Composite data of Wyatt et al. and their theoretical interpretation. P_{cP} equals the intercept of the retrograde collateral load line. Point A is determined by P_{cP} and is the pressure at node A from Figure 5.7 for both the conditions. Flow corresponding to this point will be the actual collateral flow without microvessel occlusion assuming $R_{l,p} = 0$. (Free according to Wyatt et al. [22].)*

Note that in absolute numbers the retrograde flow is quite small when compared to normal coronary flow values of 60 ml · min^{-1} measured in an LAD or circumflex of dogs in the weight range used by these authors.

The experimental results do fit the suggested model. The stop flow pressure, P_{zf}, represents the pressure at node A, since at the absence of flow there will be no pressure drop across the proximal LAD resistance. As is clear from the results, the collateral flow from the circumflex in these dogs was able to maintain a LAD perfusion pressure of an average 28 mm Hg. Most of the pressure drop from aortic to outflow pressure occurs in the proximal circumflex and collateral resistance in series. With total LAD microvascular occlusion the stop flow pressure increased to about 80 mm Hg on average. Since distal LAD flow and presumably also collateral flow were stopped because of proximal LAD occlusion, pressures at node A and B will be equal and hence the stop flow pressure will represent pressure at node B. In these circumstances, therefore, P_{cP} reflects the fraction of total circumflex resistance distal to where the collaterals tend to originate.

The retrograde load line exhibits a clear curvilinearity at low cannula pressure. This led the authors to distinguish two trajectories in these load lines, one below 10 mm Hg and one above this pressure. The slope of the part of the curve for pressure lower than 10 mm Hg had the same slope as the collateral load line. For the higher pressures the slopes were significantly different. One would have expected to find a straight curve departing from the flow intercept. The deviation from this behavior was explained by the existence of a waterfall in the distal part of the LAD bed. If cannula pressure is below the waterfall pressure, microvascular flow in the LAD region is stopped by the waterfall, which makes the retrograde load line coincide with the collateral load line; flow through the distal resistance was inhibited by microsphere occlusion. With a view to maintaining symmetry the waterfall element was also included in the LCX branch shown in Figure 5.7.

The stopped flow pressure without microvessel occlusion in combination with the collateral load line allows the prediction of true collateral flow without microvessel occlusion. This is illustrated in the bottom panel of Figure 5.8. To simplify matters it is assumed that the proximal LAD resistance can be neglected compared to the collateral resistance. Then the vertical line starting at $P = P_{cP}$ crosses the collateral load line at a point at which flow will be collateral flow without microvessel occlusion. This is the amount of flow that will be diverted through the LAD microcirculation when not this, but the proximal LAD is occluded. Assuming a waterfall pressure of 10 mm Hg the pressure drop over $R_{l,d}$ is on average 1/4 of the collateral perfusion pressure and hence collateral resistance must have been about 4 times the value of $R_{l,d}$. This rather simple analysis allowed the authors to predict collateral flow measured with microspheres with success.

In theory, the retrograde flow lines must contain more information on the distribution of resistances. However, because of the waterfall element which must be assumed, the absence of flow data other than the collateral flow data, and the uncertainty about the state of vasomotor control of the circumflex branch (one may assume that the LAD branch is vasodilated), further interpretation becomes overly speculative.

One has to realize that the type of analysis done above requires a linear behavior of the system. We will discuss the nonlinearities in the coronary circulation in more detail in the next two chapters. However, often a linear analysis may offer a framework for interpreting data. In fact, the analysis of Wyatt et al. for predicting collateral flow is quite independent of assumed linearity since it is based on the assumption that the collateral system will behave the same way as node A at the same pressure. However, it is worth reiterating that the experiment was designed on the base of linear system analysis.

5.4 Input impedance

Input impedance is a concept applied in electrical engineering and also in hydrodynamics. The concept is basically applicable to all linear systems. The basic assumption is that if coronary arterial pressure is perturbed harmonically coronary flow will respond in a harmonic way. The input impedance is then defined by two quantities: the modulus, being the magnitude of the pressure wave divided by the magnitude of the flow wave, and the phase lag between pressure and flow wave. Amplitude and phase will generally be frequency dependent. In terms of system analysis, the input impedance is the transfer function between pressure and flow. When a system is linear, the input impedance can be determined by applying any input function consisting of enough harmonic components. Fourier analysis is then applied to both input and output functions and the spectra are related to form the transfer function. The determination of a system's response to impulse and step functions can be done by well-established techniques. Below, we will report on the input impedance of the coronary circulation as determined through application of harmonic functions during a long diastole and an impulse function during normal diastoles and systoles.

In theory, when mechanical vessel properties and structure of the vascular bed are known, the input impedance can be predicted. The reverse may be true as well, as measurement of the input impedance does provide information on mechanics and structure of the vascular bed. The problems related to the interpretation of input impedance measurements in physical quantities are illustrated by analyzing the step response of a model of a nonlinear system.

5.4.1 Input impedance during long diastoles

Coronary input impedance applying harmonic pressure waves during long diastoles was estimated by Canty *et al.* [2, 3]. Hearts with a destroyed His bundle were paced and could be arrested by cessation of pacing. The circumflex artery was perfused artificially and pressure was varied sinusoidally with frequencies between 1 and 10 Hz. This frequency range was limited by practical considerations. A lower frequency was not possible since the method requires several periods of sinusoidal pressure within a single diastole. Moreover, in the autoregulated coronary bed, vasoconstriction may occur during a long diastole (e.g., Figure 7.9) and would alter the impedance of the vascular bed. Vasoconstriction restricted the lower boundary of frequency to 2 Hz at autoregulation. Frequencies higher than 10 Hz were not possible due to the construction of the spool valve.

The protocol was as follows. Mean circumflex pressure was set at the same mean value as aortic pressure when the heart was still beating. After the heart was arrested the pressure was changed to a new preset value. After 1 second and about 5 seconds, the response to a sinusoidal variation in perfusion pressure was measured.

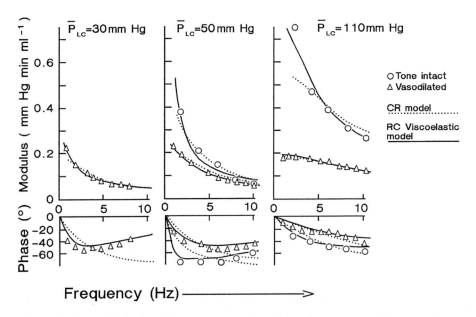

Figure 5.9: *Three panels showing modulus and phase of input compliance as a function of frequency from a representative experiment of Canty et al. [3]. Triangles represent data during vasodilation, circles during autoregulation. The average perfusion pressures, P_{Lc}, are the pressures at which impedance was measured. Before the induction of long diastoles prefusion pressures were equal to aortic pressure for all three panels. The solid curves represents the fits of a viscoelastic model and the dotted lines the fits from a CR model, (see Figure 5.11). With autoregulation, the data obtained after 1 second were used. (Redrawn from Canty et al. [3].)*

From the experimental results of Canty three panels were selected from a representative experiment to which the fit of the models was evaluated. These selected panels are reproduced in Figure 5.9. Coronary input impedance decreased with frequency at all mean test pressures and at vasodilation as well as at autoregulation. This frequency dependency of input impedance is common to all organs and reflects the compliance of the vessels. A typical example is the input impedance of the aorta where its low impedance to pulsatile flow, due to aortic compliance, minimizes the work of the heart. The modulus of the input impedance at autoregulation decreases with pressure. This cannot be attributed to the reduction of vasomotor tone induced by decreasing perfusion pressure. The authors report a reduction in mean flow between 1 and 5 seconds of cardiac arrest, which points in the direction of a vasoconstriction. Normally a reduction in perfusion pressure would induce vasodilation because of autoregulation. However, at cardiac arrest, vasomotor tone tends to increase because of the strong reduction in oxygen consumption (Chapter 9). Hence, the reduced input impedance at decreased pressure must be due to an increased compliance.

The strength of the approach of Canty et al., in which sinusoidal pressures were applied, is that linearity can be checked. The response of a nonlinear system to a perfect sine wave is the addition of higher harmonics to the response. Such an addition is absent when the system is linear. Canty et al. checked for linearity in this way. The coronary circulation appeared to be reasonably linear in the sense that the response of flow to a sine wave in pressure showed the addition of only 8% of a higher harmonics. Obviously this is not a check on linearity at frequency zero, because the lowest frequency studied was 1 Hz.

5.4.2 Coronary impulse response in diastole and systole

Van Huis et al. [18] measured the input impedance of the coronary arterial system by the impulse response technique. The coronary arterial system of the isolated cat heart was perfused according to Langendorff at constant flow. Suddenly, a flow pulse of short duration was applied and the response of pressure to that impulse was measured. The impulse response technique is powerful since in the Fourier spectrum of an ideal impulse, all frequencies are represented with the same amplitude. Hence, relating the spectrum of pressure to that of the flow provides the amplitude and phase spectra of the input impedance. The impulse response was measured during systole and diastole. By subtracting the pressure and flow wave of a preceding heart beat, the effect of the impulse could readily be analyzed. Results are shown in Figure 5.10.

In the frequency range up to 10 Hz the input impedance during diastole as measured by the impulse response showed the same behavior when this was measured using the sine wave technique. However, the responses started to oscillate at frequencies above 10 Hz, which the authors feel should be attributed to wave reflections in the coronary system. Theoretically, wave reflections in the coronary arterial tree are greatly reduced by the distributed and scattered nature of the termination of vessel segments [17]. Importance of reflections, however, were demonstrated by Van Huis et al. [18] by the effect of occlusion of a major branch on the input impedance.

It should be noted that the application of the impulse technique assumes a priori linearity of the system. An important advantage of the impulse technique, however, is that all frequencies are applied at once. Hence, only a short time is necessary to estimate the input impedance, although this applies solely to frequencies above $1/T$ where T equals the time that stationarity of the system can be assumed. Applying the impulse during systoles revealed that the input impedance measured during systole was precisely the same as when measured in diastole. This suggests that the physical parameters determining the input impedance are unaltered by cardiac contraction. One would expect intramy-

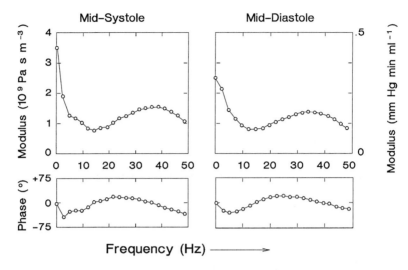

Figure 5.10: Input impedance derived from impulse responses in systole (left panel) and diastole (right panel). The systolic and diastolic responses are quite similar and resemble the diastolic amplitude and phase spectra of the responses depicted in Figure 5.9 for the frequency range of 2–10 Hz. The oscillations in the spectra at higher frequencies are due to wave reflection in the coronary circulation. (Redrawn from Van Huis et al. [18] .)

ocardial vascular compliance either to diminish because of increasing stiffness in surrounding muscle, or to increase as a result of the increased tissue pressure. Increased tissue pressure should reduce transmural pressure of the vessels which generally increases compliance as is illustrated in Figure 5.12. Hence, one may conclude that the impuls response does not provide information on a compliance of a significant part of the inramyocardial blood vessels. Since the diastolic input impedance derived from harmonic responses are similar to the impuls response results one may expect that a similar restriction holds for the data of Canty *et al.* [3].

5.4.3 Model interpretation of coronary input impedance

Interpretation of the data on input impedance in physical terms requires the definition of a model predicting the same relationships and allowing the estimation of parameters by curve fitting. Three models are of relevance. These three models are depicted in Figure 5.11. Two of these models, the CR model (left panel) and the viscoelastic model (middle panel), were evaluated by Canty *et al.* [3] and their predictions of modules and phase dependency on frequency are shown in

5.4 Input impedance

Figure 5.9. Both models fit the frequency dependency of the modules quite well. The phase is much better described by the viscoelastic model. The estimated mean values for compliance as a function of perfusion pressure resulting from these fits were provided by Canty et al. and are shown in Figure 5.12. From these values, the compliance values of the RCR model were derived by applying the equations provided by Westerhof and Krams [20]. Note that compliance is higher when estimated by the viscoelastic model. All models predict a decrease in compliance with increasing pressure, a property of all biological tissue. Tissue becomes stiffer when it is stretched.

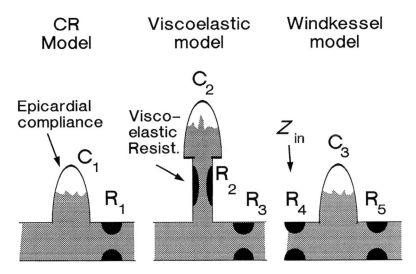

Figure 5.11: *Three lumped models by which input impedance data of Canty et al. [3] may be interpreted. The left hand panel is a simple CR model. The fit of this model to data is illustrated in Figure 5.9 by the dotted line. The middle panel is a viscoelastic compliance model. The viscoelasticity is accounted for by R_2 which, in combination with C_2, prevents vascular volume from increasing instantly when luminal pressure is increased. The fit of this model is illustrated by the heavy lines in Figure 5.9. The right panel illustrates the RCR model as suggested by Westerhof and Krams [20] and is in its behavior essentially equal to the middle panel. Hence, it fits as well as the viscoelastic model. The first resistance, R_4 (= Z_{in}, Equation [5.6]), accounts for inertance and compliance of the larger vessels.*

The fact that the CR model poorly predicts the phase frequency relation would in itself be a reason to reject the simple CR model. However, there are also physical grounds to doubt the correctness of the CR model. The fit of this model resulted in resistance values that increased with perfusion pressure, the opposite of what one would expect. Increasing perfusion pressure causes vessels to distend, thereby decreasing resistance. Hence, on the basis of physical factors, the viscoelastic model is the obvious choice, and indeed, the choice of the authors. However, as Westerhof and Krams [20] pointed out, the viscoelastic model is equivalent to the RCR model depicted in the right panel.

The similarity of the two models depicted in Figure 5.11, panels B and C, is well known in electrical engineering. Hence, the choice between the two models should not be made on the basis of input impedance measurements alone. Additional physical arguments must also be provided. Westerhof and Krams [20] expressed a preference for the RCR model, which also is referred to as the three-element windkessel model. This model has proven to be very valuable for the interpretation of the input impedance of the aorta. Its interpretation, however, needs some explanation since the first resistance does not represent a viscous resistance but describes effects related to wave transmission.

From wave analysis applied to elastic vessels of such a length that reflections may be ignored, the input impedance can be described by a real resistance independent of the length of the vessel. This follows from transmission line theory and is analogous with the coaxial antenna cable for television and FM-radio. There, too, the impedance of the cable is specified in units of a real resistance regardless of the length of the cable. This input impedance depends on the relative effects of capacitance and induction, both per unit length. For elastic vessels, the input impedance, Z_{in}, reflects the balance between vessel compliance and fluid inertance, both per unit length. For the elastic vessels, this yields

$$Z_{in} = \frac{1}{A}\sqrt{\frac{\rho}{D}} \qquad [5.6]$$

where:

ρ is mass density,
D is distensibility.

Since the presence of the first resistance in the three-element windkessel model, R_4, is assumed to account for the input impedance, it obscures the estimation of compliance of the vascular bed determined by dynamic methods described above. This may be assumed to lead to an underestimate since the large vessel compliance is partly accounted for by the first resistance. In Chapter 2, an estimate of large epicardial vessel compliance was given, calculated on the basis of distensibility of arterial walls. This was of the same order as the compliance estimated by the models.

As will be clear from the above, the interpretation of the coronary input impedance is not simple. The values for compliance are strongly dependent on the model chosen, with differences of about 50% between the two models, both of which fit the frequency dependency of impedance equally well. An extra complication is that input impedance may be totally independent of downstream

5.4 Input impedance 121

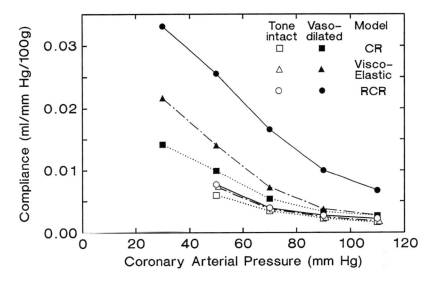

Figure 5.12: Input compliance of the coronary circulation as derived from the input impedance measurements of Canty et al. [3] . Open symbols are with tone, closed symbols without tone. The data with tone where obtained 1 s after the long diastole was induced. Moreover, perfusion pressure before decrease of pressure to the test pressure was the same for all 4 test pressures and hence tone was constant. The data obtained from the fit of the CR and viscoelastic models are from Canty et al. [3]. The values for the RCR model were derived from these data by applying the equations provided by Westerhof and Krams [20]. Note that with either model compliance decreases with perfusion pressure.

events. The most simple example is that of the elastic tubes without reflection. As was discussed, input impedance is essentially independent of the length of the tube. Total tube compliance, therefore, as estimated from static measurements of the ratio between change in volume and change in pressure, bears no relation to the input impedance.

Eng and Kirk [4] estimated a compliance of the arterial tree down to 25 μm to be about 0.016 ml · mm Hg^{-1} ·[100 g]$^{-1}$. This value is of the same order of magnitude of the input compliance at low perfusion pressure. Eng and Kirk combined their estimate by volume collection of retrograde arterial blood after obstruction of the microcirculation with 25 μm diameter microspheres. Hence, their compliance value should indeed hold at a low arterial pressure. From comparison of this number with input compliance, one may conclude that the input impedance measurement reflects the vascular space down to the small arterioles. The input compliance is however much smaller than the compliance of the myocardial capillary bed. It is hard to predict on theoretical grounds how total coronary compliance will relate to the input impedance.

Although the interpretation of the input impedance measurements in physical terms is not unique, its experimental quantification is not without value. It allows the quantitative interpretation of transients of the coronary arterial pressure and flow signals, but only in the frequency range where the impedance was measured. In the present example this applies only for frequencies above 1 Hz. However, transients in coronary arterial pressure after coronary occlusion as well as in venous outflow under other conditions exhibit time constants about 2 s. Hence, input impedance does not provide much insight into these events.

5.5 Nonlinear physical elements and linear system analysis

Because of the distensibility of vessels and, in turn, the pressure dependency of distensibility, the coronary system may be regarded as a highly nonlinear system. Although linearization may provide a reasonable outcome to some extent, it is not the answer to all the problems introduced by a nonlinear system. On the contrary, linear analysis may induce misleading conclusions when the interpretation is made on the basis of linear model components.

To illustrate the problem related to the application of linear analysis to a nonlinear system we will consider an RCR network as a model for a vascular bed. This model is depicted in Figure 5.13 (left panel) which is the electrical equivalent of the model of the right panel in Figure 5.11. This differs from the resistance–compliance models discussed above in assuming that the resistances are pressure dependent. This is not unrealistic because of the distensibility of the vascular bed. An increase in luminal pressure with respect to the surrounding pressure will increase vascular volume and decrease vascular resistance. The present model assumes that the two resistances have the same magnitude and that resistance is inversely related to the volume squared, which for a cylindrical vessel with Poiseuille flow would be

$$R(V) = R_0 + \frac{K}{V^2} \qquad [5.7]$$

where:

$R(V)$ is resistance as function of volume,
V is volume represented by the load on the capacitance,
K is constant determining the sensitivity of $R(V)$ on V.

A classical technique for system analysis is the step response. For linear systems, the step response provides essentially the same information as the harmonic and impulse responses discussed above. With the model, the response of

5.5 Nonlinear physical elements and linear system analysis

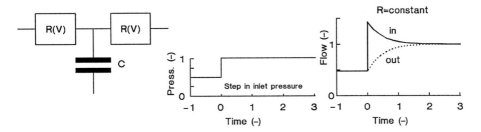

Figure 5.13: Left: RCR model for estimating the difference in response behavior of linear and nonlinear models depicts the model. The capacitance, (C), is kept constant. The resistances, R(V), are equal but depend on vascular volume which in the model is the load on C. Middle: The step response in pressure for which the model was tested. Right: The normal exponential response of inflow and outflow when the resistances are kept constant. Effect of changing resistance is illustrated in Figure 5.14.

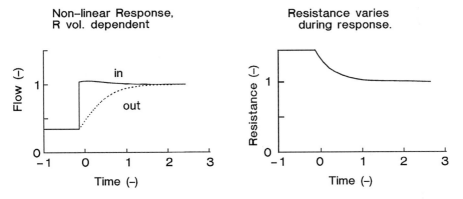

Figure 5.14: Predictions of the nonlinear model provided in Figure 5.13 and Equation [5.7]. Left: Simulated inflow and outflow response to a step change in inlet pressure. Inflow changes in an almost steplike manner while outflow changes more or less exponentially to a new steady state. Right: The change of resistance with time during the flow response.

flow was calculated as a function of a step change in inlet pressure, as shown in the middle panel. When $K = 0$ the system is linear, and inflow and outflow respond in the expected manner. These responses are shown in the right panel of Figure 5.13. Inflow exhibits an overshoot and decays exponentially to its new steady state. Outflow rises exponentially to the new steady state. The time constants for inflow and outflow are essentially the same and can be calculated by Equation [5.4].

The particular behavior of the nonlinear response becomes apparent when the

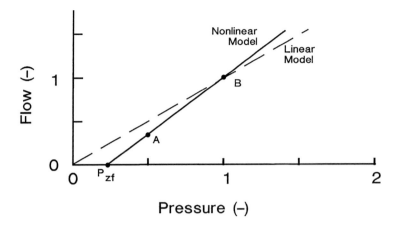

Figure 5.15: Steady state pressure–flow relations belonging to the linear and nonlinear versions of the model depicted in Figure 5.13. Points A and B correspond to the steady levels of pressure and flow shown in Figure 5.14. P_{zf} is the zero flow pressure intercept determined by linear extrapolation from the points A and B. The dashed curve is the curve corresponding to the linear simulations.

value of K is assumed to be different from zero in Equation [5.7]. The responses of inflow and outflow are illustrated in the left panel of Figure 5.14. The inflow exhibits an almost perfect step-shaped response. However, the outflow signal response is much slower, and resembles the shape of the outflow response in the linear system. The change of resistance with time is depicted in the right panel of Figure 5.14. Resistance decreases slowly with time and reaches a new steady state with a time course similar to that of the outflow. Because of the lower resistance value in the new steady state, inflow and outflow demonstrate more than a proportional increase with pressure. The problem with the interpretation of the inflow signal is that, when considered alone, the conclusion would be that the system is in a rapid equilibration, whereas the outflow seems to indicate a system with a slow response.

In Figure 5.15 the steady state pressure–flow curves for the linear and nonlinear model are presented. Points A and B correspond with the simulation example illustrated by Figure 5.14. Extrapolation to zero flow pressure from these two data points illustrates a zero flow pressure above the outlet pressure. The dashed curve is the pressure–flow relation holding for the linear example. It should be noted that the deviation between the nonlinear and linear pressure–flow relations is in fair agreement with diastolic pressure-flow relations which will be discussed in Chapter 7. Hence the effect discussed here is of realistic magnitude.

The capacitive flow in our model can simply be calculated as the rate by which the volume in the vascular compartment alters, dV/dt, and is the difference between inflow and outflow. The capacitive flow as a function of time behaves similarly in the linear and nonlinear system as can be concluded from the respective differences between the inflow and outflow signals. Capacitive flow, however, is distributed differently over the inflow and outflow signals. Application of a software package[2] to the input response of the pressure dependent resistance model provides a simple answer. Transfer functions are found and the system is judged to behave linearly. Hence, although the system is essentially nonlinear its input impedance can be described by linear theory. The problem is, obviously, with the interpretation of the parameters found. When the input impedance shows the behavior of a CR model one might conclude from a small RC-time that for a given value of resistance R the value of compliance C should be small. However, the time varying resistance reduces the compliance effect on inflow and hence the compliance, C, will be underestimated.

The simple model analysis of this section is highly relevant to the physiology of coronary circulation. In the past much emphasis has been on the analysis of the coronary arterial flow signal, while the venous outflow was overlooked for a long time. An important point of discussion pertains to time constants of arterial inflow and venous outflow. Measurement of arterial responses to step changes in pressure provide rapid responses, resulting in small estimates of compliance by RC interpretation. In contrast, response times of venous outflow to step changes in input pressure are slow, providing high estimates of RC constants and consequently high values of compliance.

5.6 Discussions of the linear models of coronary circulation

Linear system analysis is a strong tool enabling definition of the complexities of coronary pressure–flow relations. The strength of this method is its well-defined structure and the possibilities it provides of drawing analogies with nonbiological systems. In this chapter, the applications of linear system analysis were the load line analysis and input impedance. The dangers, however, related to the interpretation of linear models were also outlined by means of the same examples. It is therefore important to distinguish sharply between the quantification of systems behavior with a descriptive model and the interpretation in terms of physical properties of the structure under study. Both stages of analysis are relevant and have their own merits.

The contribution of the linear intramyocardial pump model to the understanding of coronary arterial pressure–flow relation is that it provides a description of

---

[2] AT-MatLab, from Mathworks, Inc., South Natick, Ma 01760.

pulsatility of phasic coronary flow in relation to pulsatility of arterial pressure. It shows that these properties are consistent with an explanation of flow pulsations on the basis of volume variations. In so far as systolic flow remains positive, these pulsations can be equally well explained by a time varying resistance, but the occurrence of retrograde systolic flow can be explained only by volume variations of the vascular bed. However, the model has no predictive power for the impediment of mean flow by cardiac contraction.

The coronary input impedance measurements resulted in a descriptive model relating to rapid variations in coronary flow and pressure. They are important to any other study where pressure and/or flow vary at a rate compatible with the frequency range over which the predictive model was tested. They have been useful in designing experiments on diastolic pressure–flow relations which will be discussed in Chapter 7. However, on the basis of the input impedance measurements alone it is impossible to predict mechanical behavior of the coronary circulation. For example, no distinction can be made between possible viscoelastic properties of coronary arteries and wave transmission in the epicardial arteries.

An important pitfall in linear analysis is that a nonlinear system may behave according to the linear rules and therefore induce an interpretation that may be in error. In the simple example of pressure dependent resistances, the behavior of the step response at the entrance is compatible with a linear system equipped with a small RC-time constant. However, since resistance changes in time, the rate of change of flow is not only determined by filling of compliance but also by the rate of change of resistance.

As will be discussed in the next two chapters, there is much evidence that the coronary circulation is a nonlinear system. We have illustrated that linear relations may be linearized around a working point. The linearized relationship, however, depends strongly on the working point chosen and great care must be exercised when extrapolating results obtained in one set of experimental conditions to a different set. For research in coronary circulation this seemingly trivial suggestion of caution is highly relevant. The interaction between coronary flow and heart contraction is often studied under conditions of pharmacological vasodilation. The question is whether such results can be extrapolated to the condition where vasomotor control is intact. One may expect that with vasomotor control intact, other working conditions will hold than at vasodilation. In general, flow rates are much higher at vasodilation and consequently microvascular pressures will be higher as well. As will be discussed in the next chapter, flow mechanics relates strongly to microvascular pressure.

5.7 Summary

Models are powerful tools in the analysis of the coronary circulation because this system cannot be studied directly at the level of the subendocardial microcirculation. A classification of models has been made, distinguishing between descriptive and predictive models. Moreover, models can be distinguished according to the way these are utilized. Physical models are concrete realizations while mathematical models are systems of constitutive mathematical relations. Linear system analysis is a well-developed field in engineering which can successfully be adopted for the analysis of biological systems.

The pulsatility of coronary flow was analyzed using the coronary load lines where the amplitude in pulse pressures was plotted versus the amplitude of flow pulsations. This relationship was obtained by applying a stenosis on the coronary perfusion line. The 'open clamp' pressure was found equal to half the systolic left ventricular pressure. Internal resistance varies with vasomotor tone altered by changing mean perfusion pressure. Collateral flow was also analyzed using load line analysis and resulted in a prediction of collateral flow from measurement of retrograde flow.

The input impedance of the coronary arterial system was analyzed applying three different models. Fits of these models to the measured modulus and phase as a function of frequency were reasonable in all three. However, during vasodilation, the predicted coronary compliance from a CR model may differ a factor of three from the compliance predicted by an RCR model.

Problems may arise with the interpretation of linear models providing a good fit to experimental data. The nonlinear nature of the coronary circulation and its linear behavior under certain circumstances make it difficult to distil physical properties from, e.g., measurements of input impedance.

References

[1] BASSINGTHWAIGHTE JB (1985) Using computer models to understand complex systems. *Physiol.* **28**: 439–442.
[2] CANTY JM JR, MATES RE (1982) A programmable pressure control system for coronary flow studies. *Am. J. Phys.* **243** (*Heart Circ. Pysiol.* **12**): H796–H802.
[3] CANTY JM JR, KLOCKE FJ, MATES RE (1985) Pressure and tone dependence of coronary diastolic input impedance and capacitance. *Am. J. Physiol.* **248** (*Heart Circ. Physiol.* **17**): H700–H711.
[4] ENG C, KIRK ES (1983) The arterial component of the coronary capacitance. In: *Mechanics of the coronary circulation.* Eds. MATES RE, NEREM RM, STEIN PD. New York: The American Society of Mechanical Engineers: 49–50.
[5] HARASAWA Y, SUNAGAWA K, HIYASHIDA K, NOSE Y, NAKAMURA M (1987) Frequency domain analysis of dynamic mechanical properties of the coronary arterial system and their roles in determining instantaneous coronary arterial flow studied in isolated canine heart. *Automedica Lond.* **9**: 170.

[6] HOFFMAN JIE (1989) The uses and abuses of models. In: *Modeling in biomedical research: An assessment of Current and Potential Approaches. Proceedings NIH Conference*: 17-21.
[7] KRAMS R (1988) *The effect of cardiac contraction on coronary flow. Introduction to a new concept.* PhD Thesis. Free University of Amsterdam. The Netherlands.
[8] LEE J, CHAMBERS DE, AKIZUKI S, DOWNEY JM (1984) The role of vascular capacitance in the coronary circulation. *Circ. Res.* **55**: 751-762.
[9] LJUNG L (1987) *System identification: Theory for the user.* Englewood Cliffs, Printice-Hall Inc., New Jersey.
[10] ROULEAU J, BOERBOOM LE, SURJADHANA A, HOFFMAN JIE (1979) The role of autoregulation and tissue diastolic pressures in the transmural distribution of left ventricular blood flow in anesthetized dogs. *Circ. Res.* **45**: 804-815.
[11] RUBIN SA (1987) *The principles of biomedical instrumentation. A beginner's guide.* Year Book Medical Publishers, Inc. Chicago, London.
[12] SAGAWA K (1972) The use of controle theory and systems analysis in cardivascular dynamics. *Cardiovascular fluid dynamics.* Ed. BERGEL DH, Academ. Press London-New York, Vol. **1**, chap **5**: 116-171.
[13] SAINT-FELIX D, DEMOMENT G (1982) Pressure-flow relationship in the canine left coronary artery: Study of linearity and stationarity using a time-domain representation and estimation methods. *Med. Biol. Eng. Compt.* **20** 231-239.
[14] SEELY S (1958) *Electronic tube circuits.* Mc GrawHill, New York: 61.
[15] SPAAN JAE, BREULS NPW, LAIRD JD (1981) Diastolic-systolic coronary flow differences are caused by intramyocardial pump action in the anesthetized dog. *Circ. Res.* **49**: 584-593.
[16] SPAAN JAE, BREULS NPW, LAIRD JD (1981) Forward coronary flow normally seen in systole is the result of both forward and concealed back flow. *Basic Res. Cardiol.* **76**: 582-586.
[17] TAYLOR MG (1966) The input impedance of assembly of randomly branching elastic tubes. *Biophysic. J.* **6**: 29-51.
[18] VANHUIS GA, SIPKEMA P, WESTERHOF N (1987) Coronary input impedance during cardiac cycle as determined by impulse response method. *Am. J. Physiol.* **253** (*Heart Circ. Physiol.* **22**): H317-H324.
[19] VERGROESEN I, NOBLE MIM, SPAAN JAE (1987) Intramyocardial blood volume change in first moments of cardiac arrest in anesthetized goats. *Am. J. Physiol.* **253** (*Heart Circ. Physiol.* **22**): H307-H316.
[20] WESTERHOF N, KRAMS R (1986) Comments on 'Pressure and tone dependence of coronary diastolic input impedance and capacitance.' *Am. J. Physiol.* **250** (*Heart Circ. Physiol.* **19**): H330-H331.
[21] WESTERHOF N (1990) Physiological hypotheses-Intramyocardial pressure.

A new concept, suggestions for measurement. *Basic Res. Cardiol.* **85**: 105–119.
[22] WYATT D, LEE J, DOWNEY JM (1982) Determination of coronary collateral flow by a load line analysis. *Circ. Res.* **50**: 663–670.

Chapter 6

Interaction between contraction and coronary flow: Theory

HEART CONTRACTION AFFECTS CORONARY PERFUSION in two experimentally distinguishable ways; the time averaged flow through the myocardium is reduced, depending on the depth in the heart muscle, and the flow is pulsatile. The relation between these two phenomena is not trivial and is hard to study because of technical difficulties. Up to now almost all experimental studies on the transmural distribution of flow during contraction were hampered by the fact that flow measurements are time averaged rather than instantaneous. On the other hand, information on the pulsatile nature of coronary flow is obtained from measurements on epicardial arteries or veins and hence provide a time varying flow signal per unit muscle mass which is the space average of the pulsatile flow over the different layers. As long as we are unable to measure time varying flow at different depths within the myocardium, the relation between space dependent time averaged flow and time dependent space averaged flow has to be determined by predictive models. These models postulate a mechanism for the effect of contraction on the coronary vasculature, resulting in mathematical predictions of, amongst others, coronary arterial or venous pressure–flow relations and microsphere distribution.

In this chapter the validation of the models will only be briefly discussed, and emphasis will be on the formulation and basic behavior of the different models presented in the literature. The different models will be analyzed in a general way for their ability to predict the relations between time averaged flow and pressure and phasic flow under conditions of constant pressure perfusion at pressures of 100 and 50 mm Hg and square wave left ventricular pressure. This latter wave form has been chosen to accentuate the characteristics of the models in predicting phasic flow. Moreover, only the situation without vasomotor control of the coronary circulation is considered. Validations of the different models will be discussed in more detail in Chapter 7. The linear intramyocardial pump model was discussed extensively in Chapter 5 because it fitted in the general approach of linear analysis. Hence, this model will not be discussed here. In Chapter 5 we concluded that the linear intramyocardial pump model adequately described pulsatile flow and pressure in the coronary artery when autoregulation is present but failed to explain the impeding effect of contraction on the time averaged flow.

The common denominator of the models discussed in this chapter is that they are nonlinear. The problems related to validation of nonlinear models were touched upon in Chapter 5, but will be discussed in the next chapter. However, it is worth noting at this point that a nonlinear model may be appropriate for describing signals obtained in a certain set of conditions but can fail to do so in other conditions. This specific point is not always recognized and often turns a complicated discussion into a controversy. Hence, it is worthwhile to compare the mechanical concepts within one chapter and to accentuate their assumptions. For this reason, this chapter is restricted to the models in their elementary form. In the literature, some modifications of the elementary models are presented in order to extend their possible applicability. Some of these modifications will be discussed in Chapter 7.

6.1 Systolic extravascular resistance model

In this model it is assumed that in diastole, especially at its end, contraction has no effect on the vascular bed. This concept was among those formulated and applied by Gregg and colleagues [10, 22]. The ratio between arterial pressure and flow at the end of diastole was called end-diastolic resistance and was regarded as reflecting the true resistance of the vascular bed. It was further assumed that in systole the resistance of the vascular bed was increased because of extravascular factors resulting in, e.g., deformation of vessels [21]. Hence, when the coronary artery is perfused at constant pressure, flow is low in systole because of the increased resistance.

A simple circuit symbolizing the extravascular resistance concept is illustrated in Figure 6.1. The circuit contains a switch which when 'activated' by the contraction of the heart brings an extra resistance in series with the diastolic resistance. This extra resistance represents extravascular resistance due to heart contraction. The diastolic resistance and the sum of diastolic and extravascular resistances can be calculated from the pressure–flow ratios in diastole and systole respectively. The extravascular resistance then follows from the difference between the total

6.1 Systolic extravascular resistance model

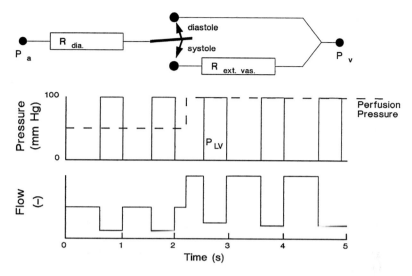

Figure 6.1: Schematic representation of the extravascular resistance model. The extravascular resistance is assumed to be present in the subendocardium and not in the subepicardial layer. Top: In systole an extra resistance ($R_{\text{ext.vas.}}$) is placed in series with the diastolic resistance (R_{dia}). Middle: Perfusion pressure (- - -) and left ventricular (—) pressure. Bottom: At constant perfusion pressure, flow is lower in systole than in diastole because of the extra resistance. Note that flow pulsations increase with perfusion pressure.

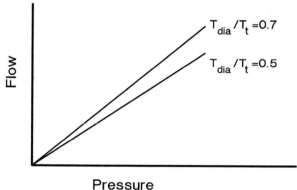

Figure 6.2: Mean pressure–mean flow relations predicted by the extravascular resistance model for two values of the diastolic time fraction. Note that the inverse of the slope has dimension of resistance. The lower slope indicates an increased time averaged resistance. However, the slope is not equal to the time averaged physical resistance.

resistances in systole and diastole.

6.1.1 Basic behavior of extravascular resistance model

According to the extravascular resistance model, systolic flow is low because coronary resistance is higher in systole than in diastole. A flow pattern predicted by the model for constant pressure perfusion has been calculated for an extravascular resistance three times higher than the diastolic resistance. This flow pattern is depicted in the bottom panel of Figure 6.1. Besides the perfusion pressure (dashed line), the middle panel also shows (solid line) the assumed square wave of the left ventricular pressure for the purpose of indicating the cardiac cycle. For the present analysis the left ventricular pressure is not of interest since it was assumed that heart contraction only activated the switch in the circuit and the value of the extravascular resistance was not related to the magnitude of left ventricular pressure.

An increase in heart rate at constant perfusion pressure will decrease mean flow simply by reduction of the fraction of time the heart is in diastole. The effect of heart rate on the mean pressure–mean flow relationship is caused by a rotation of the pressure–flow lines as illustrated in Figure 6.2. The ratio between the values of the diastolic and extravascular resistances were the same as in Figure 6.1. Mean pressure–mean flow relations were constructed for diastolic time fractions of 0.7 and 0.5 respectively.

6.1.2 Discussion of extravascular resistance model

It is impossible to stress sufficiently the fact that, although the inverse of a slope of a pressure–flow relation has the dimension of resistance, this does not imply that this slope represents a physical resistance. The curves were calculated with constant values of the diastolic and extravascular resistances. The pressure–flow line rotates clockwise with increasing heart rate because of a reduction of the diastolic time fraction and not because of an increasing physical resistance. An obvious step would seem to be to calculate a mean resistance from the inverse of the slope of the pressure–flow curve. However, a true time averaged resistance is not equal to the slope of the pressure–flow line either. If systolic flow would be zero at finite arterial pressure, systolic resistance would be infinite and hence the time averaged resistance would be infinite as well. This does not agree with the slope of the pressure–flow relation. Hence, the slope of a pressure–flow relation is only indirectly related to a physical resistance.

Obviously, it is possible to hypothesize that the extravascular resistance component is larger in the subendocardium than in the subepicardium. A more realistic model would then consist of different layers in parallel, each represented by the schematic of Figure 6.1. Since the model is linear within the two distinct phases of the heart beat, such a layer model can be represented by the single unit depicted in Figure 6.1 as long as all the switches are activated simultaneously. Hence, the description of phasic flow and mean pressure–mean flow relations would remain the same as discussed above. However, it would of course be impossible to calculate the distribution of the resistances over the layers from arterial pressure and flow patterns without additional a priori information on local resistance or, e.g., measurements of flow distribution obtained from microsphere distribution.

6.2 The waterfall model

The waterfall model postulates that the vascular bed is collapsible and that its fluid dynamic properties can be compared with a collapsible tube in a fluid environment as depicted in Figure 6.3, top panel. In such a vessel, the collapse occurs close to the outlet when the external pressure, P_{ext}, exceeds the blood pressure in the vessel at that point.

The model for the heart received its name from Downey and Kirk [7], but the mechanism was described by others studying vessel compression within the lung [20]. The name 'waterfall' has been given because of the analogy between the determinants of flow through a waterfall and the tube with collapse. In neither situation is flow influenced by the 'downstream pressure', i.e., the height of the fall in the former example.

The flow behavior of the 'waterfall vessel' can be distinguished at three different conditions of pressure, and can be mathematically expressed by Equation [6.1]. When external pressure is higher than inlet, P_{in}, and outlet pressure, P_{out}, of the vessel, the vessel is completely collapsed and flow through it is zero. Should the external pressure be lower than inlet and outlet pressure, the vessel is open and the flow through this is determined by the ratio between the pressure difference over the vessel and the vessel resistance, R_w. The third condition is when external pressure is higher than outlet pressure but smaller than inlet pressure. The vessel collapses near the end and the flow will be determined by the ratio between the pressure difference between inlet and external pressure and the resistance of the upstream part of the tube. The pressure distribution over the vessel in the latter example is depicted schematically in the middle panel of Figure 6.3.

The three-stage behavior of the waterfall was adequately described by Downey and Kirk [7] by the electrical analog depicted in the bottom panel of Figure 6.3. The model yields the following mathematical expressions.

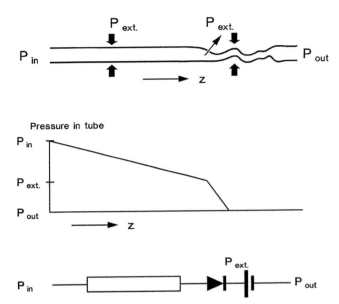

Figure 6.3: *Illustration of a tube with collapse as is assumed in the waterfall model. The top panel illustrates that collapse can occur at the tube outlet when surrounding pressure, P_{ext}, exceeds outflow pressure, P_{out}. The middle panel illustrates the pressure decay in the tube when surrounding pressure exceeds P_{out}. P_{in} is the pressure at the tube inlet. z is the distance along the tube from the inlet. The bottom panel gives the electrical equivalent of the waterfall model. The collapse is mimicked by a diode with a pressure source in series.*

$$\begin{cases} Q = 0 & \text{for } P_{ext} > P_{in} \text{ and } P_{ext} > P_{out} \\ Q = \dfrac{P_{in} - P_{out}}{R_w} & \text{for } P_{ext} < P_{in} \text{ and } P_{ext} < P_{out} \\ Q = \dfrac{P_{in} - P_{ext}}{R_w} & \text{for } P_{ext} < P_{in} \text{ and } P_{ext} > P_{out} \end{cases} \quad [6.1]$$

That relation [6.1] should hold can be rationalized by the following. Assuming that the vessel is collapsed at the outlet, flow through the tube and therefore the pressure drop over the proximal part of the tube will be zero. Because of this zero pressure drop, the pressure will be equal to inlet pressure everywhere in the tube and the collapse will thus be pushed open. As soon as flow is established there will be a pressure drop over the proximal part of the tube. If the flow becomes too high, this pressure drop will be too large and internal pressure at the collapse point would become lower than external pressure. The vessel will then collapse again. The only stable point is when the pressure drop over the proximal part of the vessel is balanced such that at a certain point, luminal and external pressures are equal.

The experimental results of Downey and Kirk [7] were compatible with the assumptions that tissue pressure equalled left ventricular pressure in the subendocardium, becoming atmospheric pressure in the subepicardium, and showing a linear decay between these two layers. This conclusion is in concordance with model calculations on the mechanics of heart contraction [2] and more recent measurements of tissue pressure with micropipettes [11].

The literature on vessel collapse has recently been reviewed extensively by Hoffman and Spaan [12].

6.2.1 Basic model behavior of the waterfall model

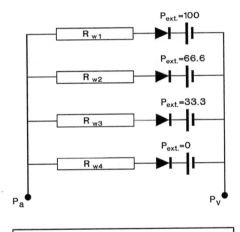

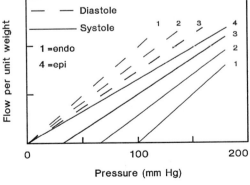

Figure 6.4: *Multilayer model for coronary perfusion based on the waterfall concept. Top: Illustration of a four-layer model for the left ventricular wall. The vascular bed in each layer is represented by resistance, diode and voltage source in series as shown in Figure 6.3. Bottom: Pressure-flow lines for the different layers in diastole (broken lines) and systole (solid lines). The subendocardial layer has a smaller resistance than the subepicardial layer ($R_{w1} < R_{w4}$) but in systole a higher back pressure.*

The waterfall model is elegant because it predicts in a simple way the pressure–flow relations in the different layers of the heart and as a result in the coronary artery. A four-layer waterfall model is illustrated in Figure 6.4. Each layer is represented by a resistance, diode and voltage source in series. In the original version of Downey and Kirk [7] it was assumed that the resistances over all layers were the same. Their model has been slightly modified here to account for the subendocardial resistance being lower than subepicardial resistance in the arrested heart (tissue pressure = 0). The subendocardial resistance was assumed to be 30% lower than subepicardial resistance to account for the microsphere distribution in the arrested heart as discussed in Chapters 1 and 7. The pressure–flow lines for the different layers of the arrested heart and the heart in permanent systole are illustrated in the lower panel of Figure 6.4. Note that the systolic curves are parallel to their respective diastolic curves within the same layer, but are not parallel for different layers because of resistance differences.

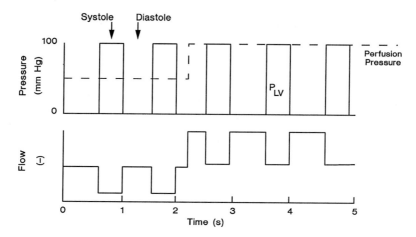

Figure 6.5: *Phasic flow in the coronary artery predicted by the waterfall model. Systolic flow is lower than diastolic flow because of an increase in back pressure over the different layers. In the top panel, the heavy line is left ventricular pressure, and the dashed line is arterial pressure.*

In the waterfall model, systolic flow in the coronary artery is low because of an increase in downstream pressure, also referred to as back pressure, which varies in magnitude over the different layers. Under normal circumstances, flow would not cease in any part of the ventricle because tissue pressure generated by left ventricular pressure can, according to the model, never exceed the systolic arterial pressure. However, when left ventricular pressure exceeds coronary arterial pressure, e.g., in a supravalvular stenosis, the model predicts that flow in the coronary artery would decrease in systole partly because of complete cessation of

6.2 The waterfall model

flow in subendocardial layers. Figure 6.5 illustrates the phasic flow predicted for the coronary artery with the square wave form of left ventricular pressure and coronary arterial pressures of 50 and 100 mm Hg.

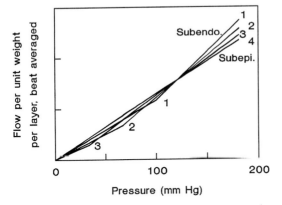

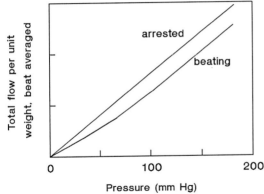

Figure 6.6: Pressure–flow lines in the beating heart predicted by the waterfall model. Top: Pressure-flow lines for the four different layers illustrated in Figure 6.4. Diastolic time fraction was as in Figure 6.5. Bottom: Coronary arterial pressure–flow line predicted for the beating heart compared to the one predicted for the arrested heart. Note the parallel shift of the curves for arterial pressure above maximal tissue pressure.

The waterfall model predicts a reduction in mean flow caused by the beating of the heart because of the reduction of perfusion time for the deeper layers and the increased systolic back pressure in these layers. The time averaged flow in each layer can readily be calculated from the predicted diastolic flow and systolic flow weighed by the time the heart spends in diastole and systole respectively. The pressure–flow lines for the four different layers of Figure 6.4 are depicted in Figure 6.6 upper panel. The curves merge, illustrating the compensatory mechanisms in the model, i.e., increased tissue pressure and reduced resistance for the subendocardial layer. The increased back pressure in each layer is counteracted by its lower resistance. Note that for each layer the pressure–flow line exhibits a corner point where arterial pressure exceeds the systolic tissue pressure of that layer. Also note that in the waterfall model, the inverse of the slope of the curve above this corner point equals the resistance of that layer.

The time and space averaged pressure–flow relation in the coronary artery is illustrated in the lower panel of Figure 6.6. Compared to the time and space averaged curve for the arrested heart and for pressure values above the highest tissue pressure, the curves run parallel, with pressure differences equal to the time and space averaged difference in tissue pressure between the arrested and beating state. This parallelism is essential to the model and is not influenced by the assumption that resistance is not equal in all layers. It is the direct result of the linear behavior of the model when arterial pressure is above the highest value of tissue pressure. In these circumstances the nonlinear elements in the circuit (the diodes) play no role and can be considered to be nonexistent.

Obviously, the waterfall model can be tuned by assuming pressure dependency of the resistances and by the addition of compliances [6, 17, 24]. These effects were studied by Westerhof et al. [5, 25] using a hydraulic model. The use of these additions will be discussed in Chapter 7.

6.3   Nonlinear intramyocardial pump model

In this model it is assumed that volume variations contribute transiently in a direct way to flow but also account for changes in resistance because of changes in vessel diameters. The conceptual agreement with the extravascular resistance model is that resistance changes due to extravascular effects on the vascular bed, and with the waterfall model that the vessels may collapse. The conceptual differences are, however, that in the pump model the variation in vessel diameters are greatly distributed over the different types of vessels as compared to the waterfall model and that time is needed to effect changes in diameter, whereas in the two other models, changes in extravascular resistance or collapse are regarded as being instantaneous.

Here, we will describe a model which was presented in its elementary form by Arts in his PhD thesis [1]. The model was evaluated quantitatively and slightly altered by Bruinsma et al. [4]. In the model, the ventricular wall is divided into a number of concentric layers. The vascular system in each layer is divided into three compartments: an arteriolar, capillary and venular compartment. The number of layers is arbitrary and depends on the purpose of the study. Because of the more complicated time dependent changes of vessel diameters, the description of the model is somewhat more extensive than that of the two former models. The running text is restricted to the description of the model behavior; a short description of the mathematical methods used is presented in Appendix B.

The compartmentalization of the model is depicted in the top half of Figure 6.7 while the physical behavior of the compartments is illustrated in the bottom half. The volume variation, distributed over the vessels of the three types represented by a compartment, is lumped into one element, 'the compliant bal-

6.3 Nonlinear intramyocardial pump model

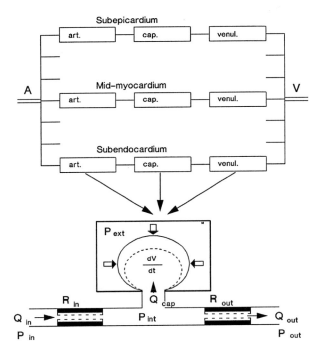

Figure 6.7: Distributed nonlinear intramyocardial pump model. Top: Illustration of the distribution of the compartments over different layers. A is artery, V is vein. Abbreviations: art., cap. and venul. stand for arteriolar, capillary and venular. Bottom: Illustration of the mechanisms determining the flow into and out of each compartment. The 'balloon' illustrates that the intramyocardial blood volume, V, can vary due to changes in external, P_{ext}, or luminal pressure, P_{int}. The time derivative of V equals capacitive flow, Q_{cap}. The total resistance of the compartment is lumped into an inflow, R_{in}, and outflow resistance R_{out}. Decreasing volume results in increasing resistances of the compartment.

loon'. The distributed resistance of each compartment is lumped into an inflow and outflow resistance both of which are taken as equal. As is suggested by the figure, a decrease in volume will result in a narrowing of the vessels and hence in an increase in resistance. The rate of volume variation equals the capacitive flow which in turn is related to the difference between inflow and outflow. A variation in blood volume can be caused by either a change in blood pressure inside the vessels, or by a change in tissue pressure. Actually, volume variations are thought to be brought about by a change in transmural pressure, $P_{in} - P_{ext}$. Hence, in this respect, the same assumptions are made as with the waterfall model. Tissue pressure equals left ventricular pressure in the subendocardium and is assumed equal to atmospheric pressure in the subepicardium.

In this chapter no interaction between the different layers is considered. The arterial pressures for all layers are assumed to be equal as are the venous pressures. As a result, the inflow and outflow of each layer can be calculated independently of the other layers. The total coronary arterial and venous flow can then be calculated by simply adding the values for the different layers. The different layers may account for the nonhomogeneous distribution of resistance and volume over the myocardial wall. This will be discussed later. We first will analyze the characteristical steady and transient behavior of the subendocardial model layer.

6.3.1 Pressure dependency of compartmental resistance

As was explained in the former paragraph, the basic assumption for the model is that resistance increases when the volume of the compartment decreases. However, although a relationship between vascular volume and resistance has been inferred [27], quantitative information is not available. We assumed a relationship in the form of

$$R = \frac{K}{V^2} \qquad [6.2]$$

where K is a constant.

The constant K of a compartment can be estimated from a single defined combination of volume and pressure drop.

A relation such as Equation [6.2] may be expected when the length of a vessel remains constant and the law of Poiseuille is applicable; then resistance is inversely proportional to the vessel diameter to the fourth power. Since volume is proportional to the diameter squared, Equation [6.2] is plausible. Although there is some rationale for Equation [6.2], the exact relation between resistance and volume is not of vital importance as long as the increase in resistance is more than the inverse of volume. The volume of the compartment is related to its transmural pressure. In general, the transmural pressure–volume curve of a biological compartment is sigmoid. This was assumed for all compartments. To simplify matters, one may assume that the pressure–volume curves are the same for all compartments except for the scaling of the volume axis. This is illustrated in the top panel of Figure 6.8. The characteristics of the pressure–volume curves are,

1. a finite volume at zero transmural pressure,

2. the possible collapse of the vessel if the external pressure is sufficiently higher than the inside pressure,

3. the compartments become less distensible at higher transmural pressures.

6.3 Nonlinear intramyocardial pump model

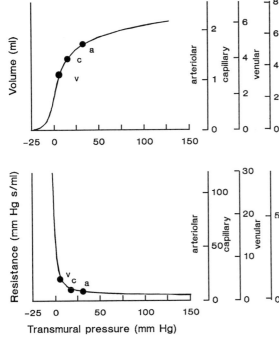

Figure 6.8: Dependency of volume (top panel) and resistance (bottom panel) of the compartments in the subendocardium on transmural pressure. The heavy dots indicate the reference condition at which pressure-drop over, flow through, and volume of the compartments are defined. a, c and v refer to the arteriolar, capillary and venular compartments. These points represent the diastolic extreme of the working range of the respective variables in the model for the beating heart.

After the shape of the pressure–volume relation has been decided, and the compartmental volume for a single value of transmural pressure is known, the volume axis can be scaled. The combination of values from which the scaling of the volume axis is derived is referred to as the reference condition for the pressure–volume relations.

The constant K for a compartment can be estimated from Equation [6.2] by the substitution of one combination of volume and resistance in Equation [6.2]. This combination, from which K is calculated, is referred to as reference condition for the scaling of volume-resistance relations. The reference conditions for the resistances of the three compartments can be calculated from the assumption of blood pressures within them at a given flow. When in addition the blood volumes of the three compartments are assumed, the K's for the three compartments can be calculated.

The reference conditions for the calculations below for the subendocardial layer were:

1. the arrested heart with tissue pressure zero,

2. flow = $4 \text{ ml} \cdot \text{s}^{-1} \cdot [100 \text{ g}]^{-1}$,

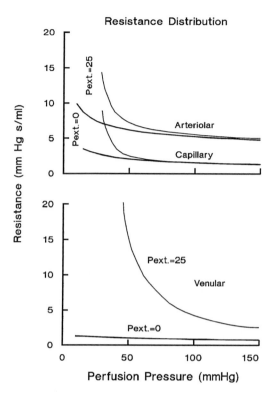

Figure 6.9: Resistance of the three subendocardial vessel compartments as a function of inlet pressure at two different tissue pressures. Top: Arteriolar and capillary compartments. Bottom: Venular compartment. Note that distribution of resistance is shifted to the venular compartment when tissue pressure is increased.

3. inlet pressure, $P_{in} = 50$ mm Hg, arteriolar pressure, $P_{art} = 35$ mm Hg, capillary pressure, $P_{cap} = 15$ mm Hg, venular pressure, $P_{ven} = 7.5$ mm Hg and outlet pressure, $P_{out} = 5$ mm Hg:

4. volumes of 1.8, 4.0 and 3.6 ml $\cdot$ $[100 \text{ g}]^{-1}$ for the arteriolar, capillary and venular compartments respectively.

The reference values for transmural pressures, resistances and volumes are indicated in Figure 6.8.

Obviously, the analysis of the dynamics of such a model requires some mathematics as described in Appendix B.

6.3.2 Steady state arterial pressure–flow relations during arrest

The hemodynamic behavior of three compartments in series and their interaction can be probed as follows. Assume a certain deviation of flow from the reference

6.3 Nonlinear intramyocardial pump model

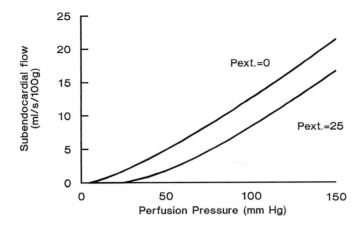

Figure 6.10: *Arterial pressure–flow relations at two different values of tissue pressure in the subendocardial model layer. The curvature is the result of the pressure dependency of the resistances. Note the almost parallel shift of the pressure–flow relation due to the increased tissue pressure. This shift is mainly determined by the increase in venular resistance.*

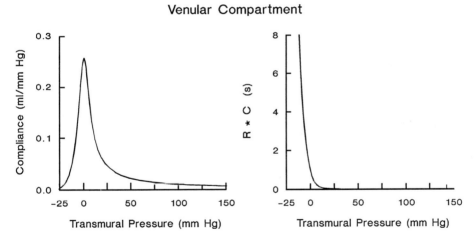

Figure 6.11: *Dependency on transmural pressure of compliance (left panel) and characteristic time, $R \times C$, for changing volume (right panel) of the venular compartment. The curves for the two other compartments exhibit similar courses.*

value due to an unknown increase in inlet pressure, but with fixed outlet pressure. The increasing flow over the last resistance will result in an increasing pressure within the venular compartment resulting in a decreasing resistance.

A new steady state will be reached if pressure in the venular compartment is higher than in the reference condition but not very much higher than would have occurred if the resistance had remained constant. The same reasoning applies consecutively for the capillary and arteriolar compartment, resulting in a new steady state with lower resistances and higher volumes of the compartments. It can be inferred from the steepness of the pressure–volume and pressure–resistance curves of Figure 6.8 that the effect on volume and resistance will be smallest in the arteriolar compartment and largest in the venular compartment. The resistance distributions over the three subendocardial compartments as a function of inlet pressure or perfusion pressure at two different values of external (tissue) pressure are presented in Figure 6.9. At zero external pressure the resistance distribution is virtually independent of perfusion pressure, especially at inlet pressures above 25 mm Hg, with the major resistance in the arteriolar compartment. However, at a tissue pressure of 25 mm Hg the venular resistance especially increases very sharply with perfusion pressure. The increase in venous resistance is so dramatic that it becomes the major site of coronary resistance. This is logical, because with an increase of external pressure the transmural pressure is reduced. This reduction of transmural pressure is less than the shift in external pressure since venular blood pressure will increase with the increased venous resistance.

Steady state subendocardial pressure–flow relations at the tissue pressures of 0 and 25 mm Hg are depicted in Figure 6.10. The pressure dependency of the resistances results in curved arterial pressure–flow relations especially at high tissue pressures. The pressure–flow relation shifts more or less parallel with tissue pressure.

6.3.3 Solutions for the subendocardial model layer of the contracting myocardium

Two quantities are important for the dynamic behavior of the model: compliance and the characteristic time for filling and emptying a compartment. The compliance is important since it determines the capacitive flow at a certain rate of change of transmural pressure. The compliance equals the slope of the pressure–volume relation and is therefore pressure dependent. This is depicted for the venular compartment in the left panel of Figure 6.11. Note that the compliance has a peak value at a low transmural pressure. The characteristic time for the venular compartment is depicted in the right panel of Figure 6.11. This has been calculated as the product between compliance and half of the compartmental resistance, e.g., Equation 5.4.

The characteristic time would be equal to the RC-time constant of the compartment if the compartment was studied in isolation. Hence, the RC-time must be regarded as an estimate of the characteristic time in view of the fact that in the model, the inlet and/or outlet of a compartment are connected to other compartments, affecting dynamic behavior. The characteristic time of the venular compartment is strongly transmural pressure dependent. For very low values of transmural pressure the characteristic time increases exponentially. Obviously, the time constants for the other compartments will also be transmural pressure dependent as well. However, since transmural pressure will be the lowest in the venular compartment, the time constant there will be the largest.

6.3.4 Compartmental volume variations

In the contracting myocardium tissue pressure rises and falls periodically. This causes the blood volumes of the compartments to vary during the heartbeat, rendering all the derived parameters time variant. As a result, the different interactions are very complex and difficult to predict. Model simulations can be of great help in assessing the implications of vascular volume variations for the coronary arterial and venous flow. Again, the contraction of the myocardium was simulated by a square wave form to emphasize the characteristic transient of the model and to ensure that these were not influenced by the time varying properties of the left ventricular pressure. The cycle duration of the square wave was 0.6 s and the diastolic time fraction 0.5. Tissue pressure was 90 mm Hg.

For two arterial pressures (50 and 100 mm Hg), the volumes and their resistances in the compartments are shown in Figure 6.12 as a function of time. The volume transients to a permanent diastole and permanent systole are presented as well.

Figure 6.12 contains a wealth of information that is too much to grasp in one glance. However, it is worth our while to understand the characteristic behavior of the model since it shows the complications of many experimental designs directed at elucidating the mechanics of coronary flow.

A first, general observation of the figure provides some obvious information on the beating state. The time averaged volumes of all three compartments are lower at the lower perfusion pressure. The relative volume variations in the arteriolar compartment are largest at the lower perfusion pressure. The maximum range over which arteriolar volume can vary is indicated by the permanent diastolic and systolic values respectively. Hence at 50 mm Hg inlet pressure and 90 mm Hg tissue pressure the compartments can be completely emptied, which is not so at 100 mm Hg inlet pressure. At 50 mm Hg perfusion pressure the volume variations in the venular compartment are much smaller than at 100 mm Hg. The cause of this difference is the large characteristic time of the venular compartment at the low volume under the former condition. At a perfusion pressure of 100 mm Hg the flow and therefore the transmural pressure in the venular compartment is higher and the characteristic times are lower.

It is important to notice that at a perfusion pressure of 50 mm Hg capillary volume remains high after 3 s of asystole. In theory, this volume can become as low as the venular and arteriolar volumes since tissue pressure is about 40 mm

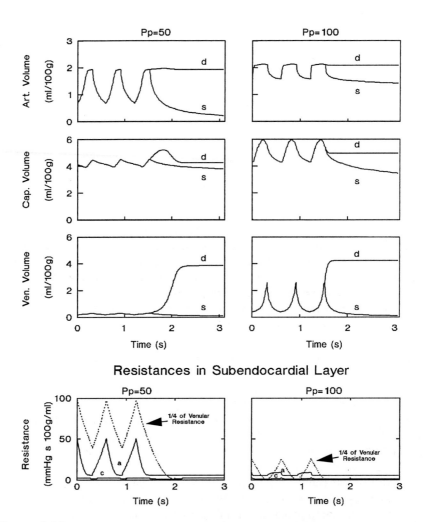

Figure 6.12: Volume and resistance variations of the different compartments in the subendocardial model layer with periodic varying tissue pressure and the transients to a permanent systole (s) and diastole (d) at two different arterial pressures. The left hand panels show the results for a perfusion pressure of 50 mm Hg and the right hand panels for 100 mm Hg. Note that the resistance of the venular compartment has been plotted applying an attenuation factor of 4 in order to show it on the same scale as the resistances of the arteriolar and capillary compartment.

Hg higher than pressure at the inlet and 85 mm Hg at the outlet of the vascular system. However, the venular and arteriolar compartments are emptied rather rapidly and prevent the capillary compartment from emptying as well. Hence, the model predicts that the collapse of the arteriolar and venular compartments will prevent the collapse of capillaries and keep them patent.

The model predicts that the major resistance will be located in the venular compartment in the dynamic situation. This was also true in the steady state at the high tissue pressure. Because of this the volume variations of the capillary compartment are relatively slight during the heart cycle and its resistance small compared to the other two compartments. Because the capillary volume is rather constant during the heart cycle, the contribution of the capillary compartment at a certain tissue pressure could be modelled by a constant resistance.

6.3.5 Flow simulations

Flow simulations for perfusion pressures of 50 and 100 mm Hg are shown in Figure 6.13. The inflow and outflow of the subendocardial arteriolar compartment are given in the top panels and for the subendocardial venular compartment in the middle panel. The added inflow and outflow of all layers represent the simulated total arterial and venous flows respectively. These are depicted in the bottom panel. Note that the arteriolar outflow and venular inflow equal the capillary inflow and outflow respectively.

In the first place, the model predicts that arteriolar inflow and venular outflow will be out of phase. The former is low or negative in systole and high in diastole while the latter is high in systole and low in diastole. The transients, especially from diastole to systole are fairly pronounced. This is due, of course, to the chosen square wave of tissue pressure. These spikes are attenuated in the flow signals summed over all the layers, as shown in the bottom panels, because the pulsatility of the flow signals decreases gradually to zero in the outer layers. Experimentally these spikes will never be measured, not only because tissue pressure will vary more gradually but also because the compliance of the epicardial arteries and veins will damp these flow variations. Moreover, in reality the inflow and outflow pressures of the different layers will be coupled, since some proximal and distal resistances respectively will be present, causing the compliance of the subepicardial layers to damp the pulses generated in the deeper layers.

The capacitive flow in a compartment is simply the difference between the inflow and the outflow and the magnitudes of capacitive flow for the arteriolar and venular compartment in the subendocardium can simply be estimated from Figure 6.13. The capacitive flow in the present simulation is due to the changing tissue pressure providing a pulsatile pumping action. Note that at 50 mm Hg perfusion pressure the pump action is higher at the inflow than at the outflow side of the subendocardial layer. At the perfusion pressure of 100 mm Hg the opposite is true. These differences can be understood from the levels of trans-

Subendocardial Layer

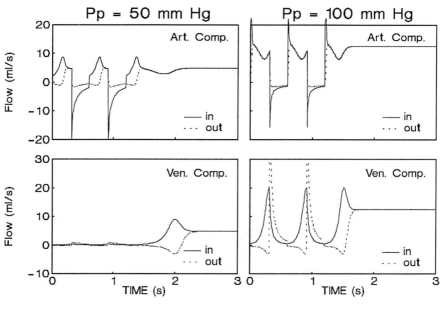

Summation Over 8 Layers

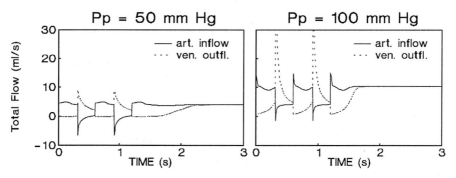

Figure 6.13: *Flow signals into and out of the different subendocardial compartments and of the total heart. The left panels are for a perfusion pressure of 50 mm Hg and the right panels for 100 mm Hg. The top panels depict the inflow and outflow for the subendocardial arteriolar compartment and the middle panels for the venular compartment. The difference between the inflow and outflow signals is the capacitive flow due to intramyocardial pumping. The bottom panels show the inflow and outflow signals for 8 layers in parallel.*

mural pressure relevant for the different compartments. At an inlet pressure of 100 mm Hg the arteriolar compartment has a higher transmural pressure and the vessels are stiff. The transmural pressure in the venular compartment is low and therefore the compliance is high; however, the transmural pressure is still high enough for the characteristic time to remain short. At the lower inlet pressure, flow and venular transmural pressure are low, and hence compliance is also low and the characteristic time large. Hence, the volume variations can occur only slowly.

6.4 Variable elastance model

6.4.1 Experimental support

Recently, Krams et al. [14, 15] reported on a series of experiments performed with an isolated cat heart perfused with blood. They illustrated that left ventricular pressure had almost no effect on coronary arterial flow but that the effect of contraction on coronary arterial flow was mainly mediated by contractility. A typical result of their experiments is illustrated in Figure 6.14.

The experimental results of Figure 6.14 strongly contradict the basic assumptions discussed with the waterfall model and the intramyocardial pump models with tissue pressure as generator. Only when an increase in left ventricular pressure is concomitant with an increase in contractility will the coronary arterial flow pattern alter. Obviously, in normal situations this often will be true (e.g. Figure 1.3) and hence experiments as performed by Krams et al. were needed to discover the relatively small importance of left ventricular pressure in itself.

6.4.2 Variable elastance concept

In order to explain their experimental results Westerhof and his colleagues introduced a new concept in coronary flow mechanics: the variable elastance model. This model is basically also an intramyocardial pump model; however, the driving force for the pump is different. It is assumed that the intramyocardial blood space is pressurized in the same way by surrounding muscle as is the left ventricular cavity. The concept of variable elastance as applied by Suga et al. [23] (see also Chapter 12) to describe the pump function of the left ventricle is then applied to the intramyocardial pump.

The similarity in the explanation of time varying elastance model for heart function and coronary flow mechanics is illustrated in Figure 6.15. In the varying elastance concept heart function at constant contractility is dictated by the diastolic and end-systolic pressure–volume relations on the one hand and end-diastolic filling and aortic pressure on the other hand. End-diastolic pressure is referred to as preload and aortic pressure as afterload. For a normal beating

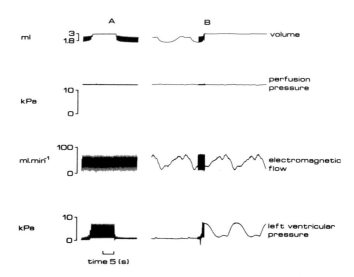

Figure 6.14: In the isolated blood perfused cat heart in a Langendorff preparation, left ventricular pressure barely affects the coronary flow pattern. Isobaric and isovolumetric beats result in almost identical coronary flow patterns. Volume was determined by a balloon in the left ventricle. Flow was measured in the cannulated root of the aorta. The panels on the left are at low paper speed and at the right at high paper speed. These experiments led to the formulation of the time varying elastance model. (From Krams et al. [13], with permission of authors and American Physiological Society.)

heart a pressure–volume loop generated by the left ventricle comprises an area equalling the external work performed by the ventricle during one beat. The elastance is defined as the slope of the pressure–volume relation defined by the fixed intercept on the volume axis and the time varying pressure and volume coordinates on the loop as time progresses during a beat. In the simplified model of Suga, this elastance varies with time in a fixed manner and predicts the course of other pressure–volume relations providing pre- and afterload are defined. Two extremes of contraction are the isovolumetric and isobaric contraction which in this figure are illustrated by the vertical and horizontal lines respectively.

According to Westerhof [26], the time varying elastance concept can be similarly applied to the mechanics of coronary circulation. A diastolic and end-systolic pressure–volume relation of the intramyocardial blood space is assumed to exist and the relation between pressure and volume to vary with time dictated by the same time varying elastance that dictates the pressure–volume relation of the left ventricle. This does not mean, however, that pressure and volume of the intramyocardial blood space necessarily follow the same loop as the left

6.4 Variable elastance model

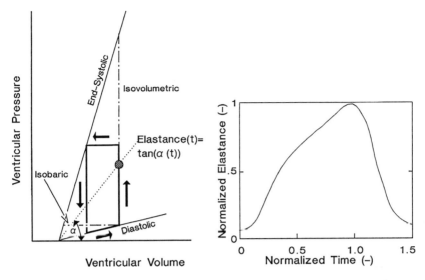

Figure 6.15: *Illustration of time varying elastance concept of Suga et al. [23] of left ventricular function. Left: The ranges over which pressure–volume relations of the left ventricle are limited to the area delineated by the diastolic and end-systolic pressure–volume relations. The well-known pressure–volume loop describing left ventricular function is illustrated in bold lines. The isovolumetric and isobaric beats at the same end-diastolic pressure–volume point are depicted with dash-dotted lines. The dotted line connects the reference point on the volume axis with the coordinates on the pressure–volume relation which vary with time as indicated by the arrows alongside the loop. The slope of this dotted curve, tan(α), is the elastance. Right panel: Time varying elastance during systole, reflecting the results from different interventions [23]. Elastance is normalized to its maximal value and time is normalized to the time between start of ventricular pressure and time of maximal elastance. (Redrawn from Suga et al. [23].)*

ventricle since the intramyocardial blood space does not possess valves dictating isovolumetric conditions. The time varying elastance model does explain in an elegant way some elementary observations which are illustrated in Figure 6.14.

When the coronary system is perfused at constant pressure one may assume that, up to a certain depth in the arterial system, blood pressure will be constant. Because of increasing elastance, intramyocardial blood volume has to decrease such that at the end of systole, its volume is dictated by the end-systolic pressure–volume relation. Since the volume difference between the diastolic and end-systolic pressure–volume relations increases with increasing perfusion pressure one may expect the diastolic-systolic flow difference to increase with in-

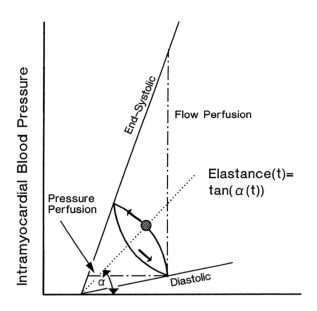

Figure 6.16: *Application of the Suga concept to coronary flow mechanics. Intramyocardial blood space is treated in the same way as left ventricular blood space in Figure 6.15. It is assumed that elastance of this volume equals that applying to the left ventricle. It may be assumed that at constant flow perfusion the volume will be fairly constant and coronary arterial pressure will vary with time. At constant pressure perfusion, blood volume varies and results in phasic coronary flow. Under more realistic circumstances, the pressure–volume relation of the coronary bed will form loops, where end-diastolic and end-systolic pressure–volume coordinates are defined by the diastolic and end-systolic pressure–volume relations.*

creasing perfusion pressure, which indeed happens in the vasodilated heart as Krams [16] demonstrated. When perfused at constant flow at least a part of the intramyocardial blood space is prevented from changing volume. Hence, the time varying elastance will cause intramyocardial blood pressure to vary isovolumetrically from the diastolic curve to the systolic curve. Moreover, it predicts that the pulsation in perfusion pressure will increase with the average perfusion pressure, which at vasodilation indeed takes place. In general, the coronary bed will neither be perfused at constant pressure nor at constant flow. Hence, the pressure–volume relation of the intramyocardial vascular space will form loops as illustrated by Figure 6.16.

Applying the time varying elastance concept to coronary flow mechanics can be considered a first step towards furthering an understanding of coronary flow mechanics. The concept is an elegant one since it provides simple explanations for basic characteristics of coronary flow. However, reaching a qualitative interpretation of experimental results obtained on the basis of this concept is complicated because of the distribution of resistance in the coronary circulation and because resistance will vary with vascular volume. A first attempt to model coronary arterial flow variations induced by time varying elastance is presented below.

6.4.3 A mathematical intramyocardial pump model with time varying elastance as pump generator

The time varying elastance concept can be quite simply incorporated into the nonlinear intramyocardial pump model by making the pressure–volume relations for the different compartments 'elastance' dependent. Once again, we will make an artificial distinction between diastolc and systole as was done when tissue pressure was the pump generator. However, now the distinction is made by assuming a diastolic and systolic pressure–volume relation. Hence, at the start of systole, a different relation between pressure and volume is suddenly forced and at the start of diastole, this relation is changed back to its diastolic shape. The important question, however, is which pressure–volume curves to assume. At present, studies are being performed in which the effect of barium contraction on blood distribution over the different vascular compartments is measured. Other studies have measured pressure–flow relations in hearts with barium contracture. The barium contracted heart is then considered as a steady state model for systole as was suggested by Munch *et al.* [19].

Levy *et al.* [18] demonstrated that intramyocardial blood volume can be reduced by about 50% by a permanent systole. Similar results were found by Goto *et al.* [8]. The reduction is more significant in the subendocardium than in the subepicardium. Pressure–flow relations in the barium contracted hearts were reported by Bellamy and O'Benar [3] and more recently by Goto *et al.* [9]. If pressure is reduced slowly enough, the pressure–flow relations show an intercept close to that of the diastolic hearts but their shape is much more curved and resembles the curve at high external pressure $P_{\text{ext}} = 25$ mm Hg, which is depicted in Figure 6.10. The scarce data that are now available may be summarized as follows: barium contracture does reduce vascular volume by a significant amount but vessels are not completely closed by contraction of the myocytes alone.

In order to assess the effect of time varying elastance on the coronary flow the nonlinear intramyocardial pump model was adapted. Only one layer was considered as basically the elastance variation should be similar at all depths in the myocardium. It was assumed that the pressure–volume relation, while maintaining its characteristic S-shape, suddenly switches from a diastolic course to a systolic course and vice versa. The difference between systolic and diastolic

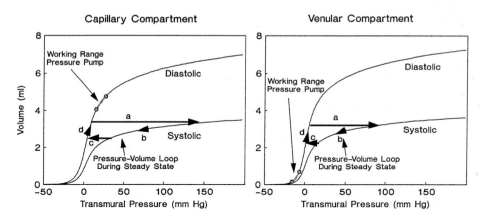

Figure 6.17: Pressure volume loops of capillary (left) and venular compartment (right) in the elastance intramyocardial pump model with diastolic and systolic pressure–volume relations. Perfusion pressure was taken as 50 mm Hg. At the onset of systole, the pressure–flow curve is suddenly changed. Because volume cannot change instantaneously, blood pressure in the compartment is increased according to the line segments denoted a. Because of the increased blood pressure blood will flow out of the compartment, reducing volume according to line segments b. At the onset of diastole blood pressure will suddenly decrease at constant volume (c) and increase to its original value (d). The working ranges for the 'tissue pressure pump' model are indicated on the diastolic pressure–volume curves.

pressure–volume curves is simply the volume scale. The volume scale of the systolic curve was attenuated by a factor of two compared to the diastolic curve for the capillary and venular compartments. This step-shaped alteration accentuates the effects of the time varying elastance. The pressure–volume relation of the arteriolar compartment was attenuated by only a factor 0.75 because of practical reasons. If the attenuation factor was larger, the computations became quite unstable when pressure–volume relations were suddenly switched. No attempt was made to solve these numerical problems since, as was illustrated above, the effects of the capillary and venular compartment dominate the mechanics of the coronary circulation in the beating heart.

At the end of diastole the pressure and volume of the capillary and venular compartments are defined by their respective diastolic pressure–volume relations. At the onset of systole the pressure–volume relations suddenly change to their systolic form. Since the volume of the compartments cannot alter instantaneously, blood pressure is generated in the compartments, as illustrated by the

6.4 Variable elastance model

line segments indicated by a in Figure 6.17. Because of the increased capillary and venular pressures, blood is driven out of these compartments and pressure will fall as dictated by the systolic pressure–volume relations and as indicated by line segments b. At the onset of diastole, the opposite occurs. Blood pressure in the compartments is suddenly reduced because of the switch in pressure–volume relations, as indicated by the line segments c in Figure 6.17. Since at this point of the contraction cycle volumes have decreased below their respective end-diastolic values, blood will be sucked into the compartments and volumes increase according to the diastolic pressure–flow relation. The rates by which volumes alter are obviously dictated by the resistances proximal and distal to the compartments.

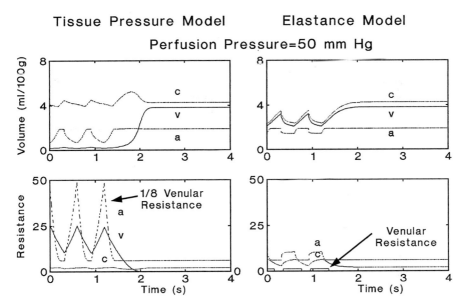

Figure 6.18: *Time dependency of compartmental volumes (top) and resistances (bottom) of a single layer of the elastance intramyocardial pump model compared to the simulations with the nonlinear intramyocardial pump or tissue pressure model (Figures 6.12 and 6.13). All volumes decrease in systole and increase in diastole. Since resistances are proportional to the inverse of volume squared they increase during systole and decrease during diastole. Note the rapid stabilization of the arteriolar compartment.*

These resistances are volume dependent just as in the tissue pressure pump model. The time dependency of volumes and resistances and the consequences of these for the flow into and out of the different compartments were simulated with the model depicted in Figure 6.7, but then for only one layer. Since all variations are induced by the changing pressure–volume relations reflecting the time varying elastance, we will refer to this model as the elastance pump model in contrast to the tissue pressure pump model. Model simulations were performed at a perfusion pressure of 50 mm Hg only. The simulation results will be interpreted in relation to the tissue pressure pump model, the results of which are shown in Figures 6.12 and 6.13 for a perfusion pressure of 50 mm Hg and systolic tissue pressure of 90 mm Hg. These predictions are reproduced in Figure 6.18 and 6.19.

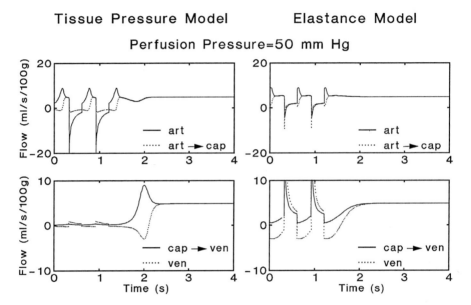

Figure 6.19: *Flow pattern into and out of the arteriolar compartment (top) and venular compartment (bottom) as predicted by the elastance pump model compared to the prediction of the nonlinear intramyocardial pump or tissue pressure model. Note that inflow and outflow of the capillary compartments equal the arteriolar outflow and venular inflow respectively.*

The predicted time varying volumes and compartmental resistances as a function of time for the elastance pump model are depicted in Figure 6.18. The transitions to a permanent diastole are also illustrated. The capillary and venular volumes in the beating condition vary between the values for permanent systole and diastole. However, in contrast to the tissue pump model, the systolic volumes will not decrease to zero merely as a result of a change in elastance. The most important difference between the two models is within the venular compartment. With the elastance pump model, the venular volume remains high and consequently, resistance is low. In the tissue pressure pump model, the venular resistance was high, which resulted in high blood pressure in the capillary compartment and hence in a high capillary volume. Since venular resistance remains low in the elastance pump model, the capillary volume decreased by about the same amount as that of the venular compartment. Hence, one might conclude that an important difference between the two pump models is related to the action of compression of the vascular bed. In the elastance pump model, this is more homogeneously distributed than in the tissue pressure pump model.

The effect of the varying volumes, which induce capacitive flows, and changes in resistance, which also induce time dependency of flow, on flows into and out of the different compartments are depicted in Figure 6.19. All flow patterns are pulsatile. As indicated by the observed signals, arterial flow is low in systole and high in diastole while the opposite holds true for the venous flow signal, which is high in systole and low in diastole. Figure 6.19 illustrates that the time varying elastance indeed causes a pulsatile pump action on coronary in- and outflow. The sharp transition in flow between the two different phases of the heart cycle is obviously due to the assumed on-off simulation of diastole and systole. With a smoother transition of elastance, these peaks will disappear. When comparing the predicted arterial and venous flow pattern with those in the tissue pressure pump model two distinctions become apparent. Arterial flow is less pulsatile and venous flow is more pulsatile in the elastance pump model than in the tissue pump model. These two characteristic differences are probably related. In the tissue pump model, venous flow was less pulsatile because of the high degree of compression of the venular compartment, increasing the venular resistance and damping pulsatile flow. The higher outflow resistance, however, amplifies the interaction between capillary and arteriolar compartment, making arterial flow more pulsatile. In the elastance pump model the effect of squeezing of the capillary compartment has a more evenly distributed effect over the arteriolar and venular compartment. Obviously, the predicted flow variations depend on boundary conditions and pressure–volume relations chosen.

It is important to note that with respect to time constants the behavior between the two pump models differs only slightly. The elastance pump model also predicts more rapid stabilization of arterial inflow than of venous outflow. Hence, as discussed before, a rapid stabilization of inflow may not be considered evidence for achieving steady state at the microvascular level.

6.5 Discussion

In the past 20 years, there has been a steady development in the quantitative models on the interaction between coronary circulation and myocardial mechanics. As long as a satisfying description of this effect is not available, new models will continue to be developed. This chapter was restricted to the presentation of models in their elementary form. Moreover, these were evaluated only in idealized conditions in order to accentuate the various characteristics.

It is difficult at this stage to conclude which model is the most appropriate. The systolic resistance model overaccentuates the importance of vascular resistance variations during the heart cycle, although such variations have to be considered. The waterfall model overaccentuates the possibility of intramyocardial vascular collapse that may occur under extreme circumstances. The intramyocardial pump models take into account the effect of volume variations, both in terms of capacitive flow and resistance variations. However, the driving force for the intramyocardial pump has yet to be defined. Tissue pressure as well as muscle elastance variations may contribute to the volume variations. In the next chapter the experimental support for the different models will be evaluated, which may be helpful in putting the different models in their physiological perspective.

6.6 Summary

In this chapter four elementary models were discussed which explained the interaction between cardiac contraction and coronary flow: the systolic extravascular resistance model, waterfall model, nonlinear intramyocardial pump model and varying elastance model. A first attempt to formulate the latter mentioned model in mathematical equations was presented.

In the systolic extravascular resistance model, systolic arterial flow is lower because of increased resistance. The reduction of time averaged coronary flow in the beating heart compared to the arrested heart is mainly due to the reduction in diastolic time fraction. The model is not predictive in the sense that the assumed interaction between contraction and coronary flow is not predicted quantitatively. In the waterfall model the reduced systolic flow is explained by an increased back pressure caused by an increased systolic tissue pressure varying in magnitude over the left ventricular wall. With constant systolic left ventricular pressure, the reduction of time averaged coronary flow by the beating of the heart is explained by the reduction in diastolic time fraction. In the nonlinear intramyocardial pump model the systolic–diastolic flow variations are caused by displacement of volume and varying resistance. Heart contraction reduces coronary flow at constant perfusion pressure because of reduction of diastolic flow fraction, although not necessarily linearly. This depends on the extent to which intramyocardial blood volume can vary through the cardiac cycle. The time varying elastance model predicts pulsatile coronary arterial and venous flow. The behavior is similar to the prediction of the tissue pressure intramyocardial pump model. It also predicts the rapid equilibration of diastolic flow while microvascular pressure and volumes continue to vary.

References

[1] ARTS MGJ[1] (1978) *A mathematical model of the dynamics of the left ventricle and the coronary circulation.* PhD Thesis. University of Limburg, Maastricht, The Netherlands.

[2] ARTS T, VEENSTRA PC, RENEMAN RS (1982) Epicardial deformation and left ventricular wall mechanics during ejection in the dog. *Am. J. Physiol.* **243** (*Heart Circ. Physiol.* **12**): H379–H390.

[3] BELLAMY RF, O'BENAR JD (1984) Cessation of arterial and venous flow at a finite driving pressure in porcine coronary circulation. *Am. J. Physiol.* **246** (*Heart Circ. Physiol.* **15**): H525–H531.

[4] BRUINSMA P, ARTS T, DANKELMAN J, SPAAN JAE (1988) Model of the coronary circulation based on pressure dependence of coronary resistance and compliance. *Basic Res. Cardiol.* **83**: 510–524.

[5] BURATTINI R, SIPKEMA P, VAN HUIS GA, WESTERHOF N (1985) Identification of canine coronary resistance and intramyocardial compliance on the basis of the waterfall model *Ann. Biomed. Eng.* **13**: 385–404.

[6] DANKELMAN J, STASSEN HG, SPAAN JAE (1990) Coronary circulation mechanics. In: *Coronary circulation. Basic mechanics and clinical relevance.* Eds. KAJIYA F, KLASSEN GA, SPAAN JAE, HOFFMAN JIE. Springer-Verlag Tokyo: 75–87.

[7] DOWNEY JM, KIRK ES (1975) Inhibition of coronary blood flow by a vascular waterfall mechanism. *Circ. Res.* **36**: 753–760.

[8] GOTO M, JANSEN CMA, STORK MM, FLYNN AE, COGGINS DL, HUSSEINI W, HOFFMAN JIE (1989) Effects of myocardial contraction on intramyocardial vessels. *Circulation* **80** *Suppl.* II: 212.

[9] GOTO M, FLYNN AE, DOUCETTE JW, MUEHRCKE D, JANSEN CMA, HUSSEINI W, HOFFMAN JIE (1990) Impeding effect of myocardial contraction on regional blood flow. *FASEB J*: **A404**.

[10] GREGG DE, GREEN HD (1940) Registration and interpretation of normal phasic inflow into a left coronary artery by an improved differential manometric method. *Am. J. Physiol.* **130**: 114–125.

[11] HEINEMAN FW, GRAYSON J (1985) Transmural distribution of intramyocardial pressure measured by micropipette technique. *Am. J. Physiol.* **249** (*Heart Circ. Physiol.* **18**): H1216–H1223.

[12] HOFFMAN JIE, SPAAN JAE (1990) Pressure-flow relations in the coronary circulation. *Physiol. Rev.* **70**: 331–390.

[13] KRAMS R, SIPKEMA P, WESTERHOF N (1989) Varying elastance concept may explain coronary systolic flow impediment. *Am. J. Physiol.* **257** (*Heart Circ. Physiol.* **26**): H1471–H1479.

---

[1] Arts MGJ is the same person as Arts T [2].

[14] KRAMS R, SIPKEMA P, WESTERHOF N (1989) Can coronary systolic-diastolic flow difference be predicted by left ventricular pressure or time-varying intramyocardial elastance. *Basic Res. Cardiol.* **84**: 149–159.
[15] KRAMS R, SIPKEMA P, ZEGERS J, WESTERHOF N (1989) Contractility is the main determinant of coronary systolic flow impediment. *Am. J. Physiol.* **257** (*Heart Circ. Physiol.* **26**): H1936–H1944.
[16] KRAMS R (1988) *The effects of cardiac contraction on coronary flow.* PhD Thesis. Free University of Amsterdam, The Netherlands.
[17] LEE J, CHAMBERS DE, AKIZUKI S, DOWNEY JM (1984) The role of vascular capacitance in the coronary arteries. *Circ. Res.* **55**: 751–762.
[18] LEVY BI, SAMUEL JL, TEDGUI A, KOTELIANSKI V, MAROTTE F, POITEVIN P, CHADWICK RS (1988) Intramyocardial blood volume in the left ventricle of rat arrested hearts. In: *Cardiovascular dynamics and models.* Eds. BRUN P, CHADWICK RS, LEVY BI. INSERM, Paris: 65–71.
[19] MUNCH DF, COMER HT, DOWNEY JM. (1980) Barium contracture: a model for systole. *Am. J. Physiol.* **239** (*Heart Circ. Physiol.* **8**): H438–H442.
[20] PERMUTT S, RILEY RL (1963) Hemodynamics of collapsible vessels with tone: the vascular waterfall. *J. Appl. Phys.* **18**: 924–932.
[21] RAFF WK, KOSCHE F, GOEBEL H, LOCHNER W (1972) Die extravasale Komponente des Coronarwiderstandes mit steigendem linksventrikulären Druck. *Pflügers Arch.* **333**: 352–361.
[22] SABISTON DC JR, GREGG DE (1957) Effect of cardiac contraction on coronary blood flow. *Circulation* **15**: 14–20.
[23] SUGA H, SAGAWA K, SHOUKAS AA (1973) Load independence of the instantaneous pressure-volume ratio of the canine left ventricle and effects of epinephrine and heart rate on the ratio. *Circ. Res.* **32**: 314–322.
[24] SUN Y, GEWIRTZ H (1987) Characterization of the coronary vascular capacitance, resistance and flow in endocardium and epicardium based on a nonlinear dynamic analog model. *IEEE Trans Biomed. Eng.* **34**: 817–825.
[25] WESTERHOF N, SIPKEMA P. VANHUIS GA (1983) Coronary pressure-flow relations and the vascular waterfall. *Cardiovasc. Res.* **17**: 162–169.
[26] WESTERHOF N (1990) Physiological hypotheses-Intramyocardial pressure. A new concept, suggestions for measurement. *Basic Res. Cardiol.* **85**: 105–119.
[27] WÜSTEN B, BUSS DD, DEIST H, SCHAPER W (1977) Dilatory capacity of the coronary circulation and its correlation to the arterial vasculature in the canine left ventricle. *Basic Res. Cardiol.* **72**: 636–650.

Chapter 7

Interaction between contraction and coronary flow: Experiment

It is clear from the preceding two chapters, that a universally accepted model of the coronary circulation has not yet been formulated. This implies that the mechanics of interaction between cardiac contraction and coronary flow are not yet properly understood.
This chapter attempts to serve two purposes:

1. emphasize key experimental observations on coronary flow mechanics,

2. evaluate existing models in relation to these observations.

Since existing models apparently fail, subjecting these to a quantitative evaluation would appear to have only limited value. However, an evaluation of the merits and shortcomings of the existing models might provide a stimulus for further thinking and formulation of new hypotheses. The quantitative evaluation of models will focus on the waterfall model and the tissue pressure driven intramyocardial pump model, because at present they are formulated in a testable way.

It is not too hard to formulate the shortcomings of the various models, at least in their original forms. The extravascular resistance model is too simple since it does not explain why the phasic wave form of the venous flow is out of phase with the arterial wave form at constant pressure perfusion. The waterfall model makes also no prediction of venous flow wave form. Moreover, the waterfall model in its original form can not explain retrograde coronary arterial flow. The linear intramyocardial pump model is not able to predict a decreased endocardial flow due to heart contraction. Both the waterfall model and nonlinear pump model are able to relate the effects of cardiac contraction on coronary flow to tissue pressure. The models fall short when tissue pressure is related to left ventricular pressure [21], since coronary flow remains pulsatile in an empty beating heart, which, according to these models, should not occur. It is somewhat more difficult to point to elementary shortcomings of the elastance model since its predictions are not yet well-formulated. However, as will be discussed below, experiments show that time averaged subepicardial flow is not a function of heart rate, which seems hard to explain with the elastance model. One would expect tissue elastance to vary in the subepicardium as well. Moreover, the finding that right coronary arterial flow is less pulsatile than left coronary flow favors the concept that ventricular pressure rather than time varying elastance is responsible for these flow variations.

The mechanics of the coronary circulation are most certainly nonlinear. A property of a nonlinear system is that its behavior is dependent on the working point. Freely translated, this may imply that the assumptions underlying the different models could be true under one operational condition but not under another one. For example, the test of pulsatile flow in an empty beating heart could be too severe for a waterfall or intramyocardial pump model since the deformations of intramyocardial vessels involved are much more extreme than in a normal beating heart. The effect of these large deformations may not be relevant for the normal beating heart.

In the literature, attempts have been made to combine the strong point of different models. For example, several models combining the waterfall concept and intramyocardial pump have been presented. Some of these models will be discussed below.

7.1 Parallel shift of pressure–flow relations

A classic experimental finding is the parallel course of the coronary arterial pressure–flow lines measured during cardiac arrest and during beating [16]. The experiment was performed in an open chest anesthetized dog with a cannulated left anterior descending artery. The perfused vascular bed was fully dilated with adenosine. The vessel was perfused at constant flow and mean arterial pressure was measured as function of flow; thus changes in mean pressure are proportional to changes in beat averaged resistance. When the heart was arrested by vagal stimulation the coronary pressure at constant flow decreased, showing the impeding effect of heart contraction. At a perfusion pressure above systolic left ventricular pressure, the pressure–flow curves are parallel. The parallel shift of the pressure–flow relation was interpreted as evidence for the waterfall hypothesis. The prediction of the parallel shift by the waterfall model was demonstrated

7.1 Parallel shift of pressure–flow relations

in Figure 6.6. However, Figure 6.10 illustrated that pressure–flow curves in a model of the non-beating subendocardium based on pressure dependent resistances may shift in parallel when tissue pressure is raised.

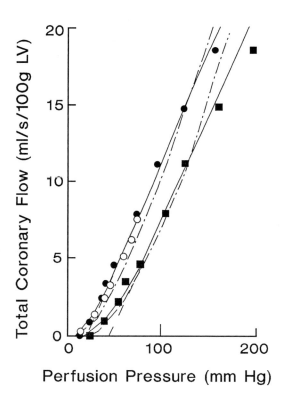

Figure 7.1: Predicted and experimental pressure–flow relations for the beating and arrested heart. Heavy lines are as predicted by the nonlinear intramyocardial pump model as described in Chapter 6. The closed symbols are from Figure 7 of Downey and Kirk [16], the open circles from [27]. The pressure values of these data were scaled such that the datum at arterial pressure of 100 mm Hg for the arrested heart from [16] coincided with the appropriate curve and the datum from [27] at 80 mm Hg. Obviously, the data can also be fitted by the waterfall model. The dash-dotted curves are obtained with a different pressure–volume curve for the arteriolar compartment (see Section 7.2).

A typical result of an experiment from Downey and Kirk [16] is depicted in Figure 7.1 with the flow axis scaled to allow comparison with the intramyocardial pump model. In Figure 7.1, the measuring points provided in Figure 7 of the Downey and Kirk paper [16] are compared with theoretical pressure–flow lines predicted by the tissue pressure nonlinear intramyocardial pump model (heavy lines). This model consisted of 8 layers. Tissue pressure was assumed to vary linearly over these layers between left ventricular pressure and atmospheric pressure. The pressure–volume curves for the different compartments are discussed in Chapter 6. It appears that the experimental data are described quite well by the nonlinear intramyocardial pump model allowing scaling on the basis of a single data point. Hence, the parallel courses of pressure–flow lines observed cannot be taken as exclusive evidence for the waterfall model. Obviously, the shape of the pressure–flow relations predicted by the intramyocardial pump model depend on the pressure–volume relations which have been assumed for different compartments. This point will be discussed in the next section, where the relation between pressure–volume curves and pressure dependency of resistance will be discussed.

According to the time varying elastance model, the reduction in flow by the beating of the heart should not be related to the left ventricular pressure, but to the stiffening of the wall during contraction. However, it is not yet clear whether this should predict a parallel shift of pressure–flow relations at higher perfusion pressure.

7.2 Pressure dependency of coronary resistance

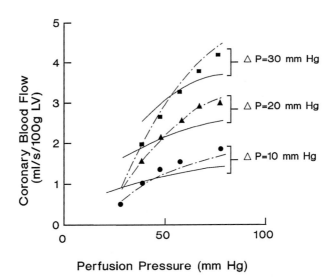

Figure 7.2: Coronary flow in an arrested heart at constant driving pressure but varying venous pressure. Data are from Hanley et al. [20]. The heavy lines are the predictions from a one-layer, three-compartmental intramyocardial pump model. The dash-dotted lines are also a prediction by the nonlinear pump model but now an alternative pressure–volume relation for the arteriolar compartment has been used as is illustrated in Figure 7.3. This pressure dependency of resistance resulted in the dash-dotted pressure–flow relations of Figure 7.1. It was concluded that the experimental data illustrated an extreme example of pressure dependency of resistance.

Pressure dependency of coronary resistance in the arrested heart was demonstrated by Hanley et al. [20] in a right heart bypass preparation. The left main coronary artery was cannulated. The difference in coronary arterial and coronary venous pressure was kept constant but the level of pressure was increased.

Only the data of the figure compiled by them are reproduced in Figure 7.2. If the coronary vasculature was indistensible its resistance would be constant and flow would only depend on pressure difference and not on the level of pressure. However, flow increases with the level of pressure which is evidence for a decrease of resistance. The experiment was simulated by the intramyocardial pump model with the standard pressure–volume relations of Figure 7.3. The result is depicted by the heavy lines. It seems that these standard pressure–volume curves result in a lower dependency of resistance on pressure, as was also found experimentally. However, it seems that the data shown in Figure 7.2 from Hanley et al. [20], are from the experiment exhibiting the largest pressure dependency of resistance in their series of experiments. Nevertheless, we attempted to fit these extreme data to our model by changing the pressure–volume curve of the arteriolar compartment. The arteriolar compartment was selected since, according to Figure 6.9, the arteriolar resistance is dominant when the heart is not beating. The new arteriolar pressure–volume relation is depicted in Figure 7.3, where it is compared with the standard curve. The simulation of the protocol of Hanley et al. [20] is depicted in Figure 7.2 by the dash-dotted curves.

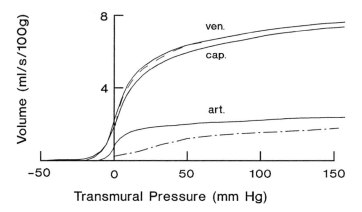

Figure 7.3: *Pressure–volume relations for the arteriolar and venular compartments of the nonlinear intramyocardial pump model based on tissue pressure. The heavy lines are the standard curves and close to the ones defined in Figure 6.8. The dash-dotted curve is an alternative for the arteriolar compartment such that the pressure dependency of flow at constant driving pressure in the arrested heart is predicted as shown in Figure 7.2. The dash-dotted pressure–flow relations in Figure 7.1 were calculated using this relationship. The dashed curve is an alternative venular pressure–volume relation, describing collapse at zero transmural pressure, used below and in Chapter 10.*

The alternative pressure–volume relation for the arteriolar compartment results also in different pressure–flow relations for the arrested and beating heart.

These results are provided by the thin lines in Figure 7.1. The curvature of the pressure–flow relations for the arrested heart now is much stronger due to the higher sensitivity of arteriolar resistance to pressure. One should note that this difference is not introduced by the structure of the model. The dynamic behavior of the model does not play any role in this comparison since the steady state is under discussion. Probably the data shown in Figure 7.2 are from the experiment exhibiting the strongest pressure dependency of resistance in the experimental series.

Of course, the prediction of the effect of cardiac contraction on the alternative arteriolar pressure–volume relation is dependent on the dynamic characteristic of the model. The interesting point is that the predicted curve for the beating heart again runs parallel to that of the arrested heart and is calculated with the same pressure–volume relations. This can be explained by the role of the venous compartment. The pressure–volume relation in the arrested state is determined by the arteriolar compartment, but the shift from this curve due to heart contraction is caused by the venous compartment. Since this compartment was not changed, the shift remained in the same order of magnitude as for the standard venous pressure–volume curve.

The elastance model as elaborated on in Chapter 6 will predict essentially the same pressure–flow relation as the tissue pump model. The effect of heart contraction on the pressure–flow relation depends strongly on the systolic pressure–volume relations to be assumed for the elastance model. These relationships might be obtained from hearts in permanent systole, as can be obtained by barium contracture.

7.3 Effect of heart rate on microsphere distribution

An important test for models on the coronary circulation is the distribution of microspheres over the left ventricular free wall. In Figure 1.10 it was shown that endocardial–epicardial flow ratio decreases as heart rate increases. The data from this figure are also shown in Figure 7.5 and compared with model results. However, before discussing the different model predictions some data of Bache and Cobb [4] will be discussed in more detail.

Bache and Cobb [4] injected microspheres in a fully dilated coronary vascular bed at different heart rates. Average systemic arterial pressure was fairly constant at about 100 mm Hg. The mean values for subepicardial flow at different heart rates were 5.27 ± 0.18 (SE), 5.09 ± 0.54 (SE), 6.07 ± 0.57 (SE) and 6.19 ± 0.63 (SE) ml $\cdot$ min^{-1} $\cdot$ g^{-1} at 100, 150, 200 and 250 beats $\cdot$ min^{-1}, respectively. Hence, subepicardial flow was essentially constant, or even showed a slight increase with heart rate. Such an increase might have been more pronounced in the

7.3 Effect of heart rate on microsphere distribution

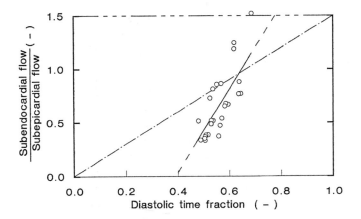

Figure 7.4: *Subendocardial-subepicardial flow ratio as function of diastolic time fraction. The data are from Bache and Cobb [4]. The top horizontal line represents the ratio expected without influence of heart contraction on coronary flow and equals the endo/epi ratio obtained in the arrested heart (e.g., Figure 7.5). The dash-dotted line (-.-.-) represents the theoretical prediction if endocardial flow is linearly related to the relative duration of diastole.*

outermost subepicardial layer since in the experiments of Bache and Cobb [4], the free wall was only cut into four layers. An increase in flow at the very subepicardium might have been masked by the flow decrease in the inner part of this layer. In the early days, an increase in flow due to contraction was believed to be made possible by the massaging effect of contracting muscle on the intramyocardial vessels. An increase in subepicardial flow has recently also been reported by Flynn et al. [18], who performed experiments at a constant time averaged perfusion pressure. However, even accepting that cardiac contraction increases subepicardial flow, more detailed information on the coronary arterial pressure variations during the interventions should be made available to exclude the possibility of an increased driving pressure, either systolic or diastolic. However, none of the models formulated up to now has the potential to predict a beneficial effect of contraction on subepicardial perfusion. For now it will be assumed that subepicardial flow is constant. Hence, endocardial/epicardial flow ratios at constant perfusion pressure essentially reflect the behavior of subendocardial flow.

In Figure 7.4 the endocardial/epicardial flow ratio as found by Bache and Cobb [4], (their Figure 1) is presented as a function of the diastolic time fraction. Diastole was defined by the period during which the aortic valve was closed and its duration deduced from the aortic pressure signal. A diastolic time fraction of one represents an arrested heart and of zero, a permanent systole. The data show an increase of endo/epi flow ratio with the diastolic time fraction. An interesting conclusion follows from this figure. From other experiments (see Figure 7.5) we know that the endo/epi flow ratio in an arrested heart at a perfusion pressure of 100 mm Hg is about 1.5. This ratio is indicated in Figure 7.4 by the top horizontal dashed line. If the endocardial flow were purely diastolic and independent of systole, we would expect a linear relation between endo/epi flow ratio and the diastolic time fraction as indicated by the dash-dotted line: ratio equals 1.5 at diastolic time fraction one and zero at diastolic time fraction zero. As is clear from Figure 7.4 the experimental data do not support the concept of pure diastolic perfusion independent of systole. The regression curve shows a slope that differs substantially from the theoretical line. This deviation can be explained, however, with models allowing for interaction between systole and diastole. The repetition rate of systole at a very low heart rate is slow such that intermediate diastoles are long enough to refill the small vessels, cancelling the squeezing effect of systole. However, at higher heart rates, diastole becomes too short to allow refilling and hence microvascular resistance in diastole remains higher than the value found at cardiac arrest. Consequently, in the range of diastolic time fractions where endocardial flow falls, this fall is not only due to reduction of diastolic time but also to an increased diastolic resistance. This increased resistance is then due to the repetition of systoles.

Figure 7.4 also explains why so much experimental support could be found for the waterfall model. Most of the data in the literature have been collected at heart rates above 100 beats · min^{-1}. In that range, the theoretical curve based on the idea of undisturbed diastolic perfusion crosses the scattered data. Hence, there is reasonable agreement between theory and experiment. However, the models should be tested especially at low heart rates with a large diastolic time fraction. These experiments have not been performed yet.

The crossing of the regression curve with the horizontal curve, representing the absence of systolic effect, could indicate the diastolic time fraction above which systole has no effect. In the figure, the two curves cross each other at a diastolic time fraction close to 0.75 which would be obtained at a heart rate of about 80 beats · min^{-1}. Diastolic and systolic times are then in the order of 0.56 and 0.19 s respectively. This diastolic time value would indicate the recovery time of microvascular resistance from compression by systole. Obviously, this time does not necessarily mark the point at which volume displacements no longer occur. These volume variations may take longer, as was discussed in Chapter 1.

The nonlinear intramyocardial pump model predicts systolic–diastolic interaction. It is therefore worthwhile to compare predictions on endo/epi flow ratio with experimental results. This comparison is presented in Figure 7.5. The data in this figure are the same as in Figure 1.10 and were selected for standard conditions of vasodilation and coronary arterial pressure. The tissue pump model was evaluated for two different pressure–volume relations for the venous compart-

7.3 Effect of heart rate on microsphere distribution

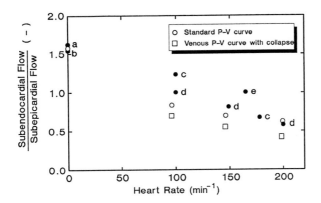

Figure 7.5: Comparison of experimental data (●), (see Figure 1.10) on ratio between endocardial and epicardial flow with prediction of the nonlinear tissue pressure pump model. The open circles, ○, and boxes, □, were calculated with the nonlinear intramyocardial pump model using the standard and alternative pressure–volume relations, P–V, for the venous compartment (Figure 7.3).

ments; the standard curve and the curve drawn as a broken line in Figure 7.3. As is clear from the figure, the model predicts a more rapid decrease of subendocardial flow with heart rate than experimentally found but predicts the endo/epi ratio well at the heart rate of 200 beats · min^{-1}. It should be noted that the discrepancy between model and experiment in this figure might partly be explained by the uncertainty in assumed left ventricular pressure curves used for the model calculations. However, we will not focus on this point in our analysis but on the systolic–diastolic interaction.

When the alternative curve is used, the model predicts a larger effect of heart contraction on subendocardial flow than with the standard curve. The effect of the alternative curve was evaluated since it exhibits a collapse at transmural pressures higher than zero and hence a waterfall behavior might be expected. However, as was discussed in Chapter 6 (see Figures 6.12 and 6.13), a collapse in steady state does not necessarily imply that collapse will occur in systole, as assumed in the waterfall model, since the period of compression is too short. Although the model does not predict a complete systolic collapse of the venular compartment it does predict a strong impediment of the time averaged subendocardial flow because of the predicted relative slow recovery of the venular volume in diastole. The impediment is stronger with the alternative curve since the vessels are more easily compressed delaying diastolic recovery. Too strong a predicted interaction between systole and diastole may also be the reason for the discrepancy between model and experiment at a heart rate around 100 beats · min^{-1}. In this respect it is worth noting that the elastance model predicts a more moderate interaction between systole and diastole (e.g., Figures 6.18 and 6.19).

It may be concluded from this section that the possibilities of validating models and discriminating between them by studying flow distribution over the left ventricular wall as functions of heart rate at a variety of perfusion conditions have not yet been exhausted.

7.4 Contractility and microsphere distribution

Before the varying elastance concept was formulated, Marzilli et al. [35] produced evidence for a direct effect of contractility on coronary flow. These results deserve some emphasis in this chapter because of the recently postulated varying elastance concept. Marzilli et al. cannulated the LAD and perfused this artery with a perfusion system. Microspheres were injected to measure subendocardial and subepicardial flows. The microsphere injection was done under control conditions and after two interventions, i.e.,

1. infusion of lidocaine which depressed contractility, and

2. infusion of isoproterenol which increased contractility.

Contractility changes were confirmed by local measurement of wall thickening. The coronary bed was fully dilated by infusion of adenosine into the perfusion line. Their results on flow distribution as function of wall thickening are summarized in Figure 7.6 left panel. Mean aortic pressure and mean LAD perfusion pressure were about 100 mm Hg which are similar to the experimental conditions of Bache and Cobb [4]. As is clear from Figure 7.6, lidocaine decreased wall thickening and increased both subepicardial and subendocardial flows, whereas isoproterenol caused opposite effects. It should be noted that the left ventricular pressure was similar under all conditions.

The experimental outcome is in agreement with the predictions of the time varying elastance concept. With constant ventricular cavity pressure, flow increased when contractility was decreased and decreased when contractility was increased. The effects are the largest at the subendocardium, suggesting that contractility effects are stronger in the subendocardium than in the subepicardium. This would contradict the microsphere data presented by Bache and Cobb, which showed that subepicardial flow is independent of heart rate. If subepicardial flow is independent of heart rate it should not be affected by contraction. In what way, then, can lidocaine and isoproterenol influence subepicardial flow? A possible explanation is the division in layers for microsphere counting. The ventricular wall in the study by Marzilli et al. [35] was only cut into three while Bache and Cobb divided the ventricular wall into four layers. The thicker the subepicardial layer is cut, the more will it exhibit effects similar to the subendocardial wall. Hence, it might well be possible that the epicardial effect of contractility

7.4 Contractility and microsphere distribution

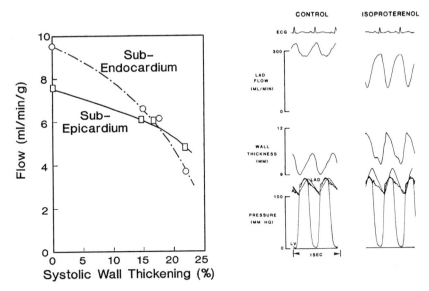

Figure 7.6: *Effect of selective contractility alterations on microsphere distribution and coronary arterial flow in the fully dilated bed as estimated by Marzilli et al. [35]. LAD was perfused artificially and contractility in its distribution area altered by either lidocaine or isoproterenol. Left: Effect on subepi- and subendocardial flow. Flow, calculated from microsphere distribution, is plotted versus local wall thickening. Right: Effect of lidocaine infusion on flow pulsatility in cannulated coronary artery. Note the absence of any effect here. (From Marzilli et al. [35], by permission of authors and American Heart Association Inc..)*

was absent. However, according to the same reasoning the effect at the very subendocardium will be more pronounced than found in the inner third of the ventricular wall. Hence the increase in subendocardial flow induced by the injection of lidocaine is at least 50%, similar to the increase to be expected when arresting the heart. This would indicate that left ventricular pressure does not contribute to the impediment of subendocardial flow at all. Recently VanWinkle et al. [45] reported results on microsphere distribution in the empty beating heart showing that subendocardial flow is reduced as much in an empty beating heart compared to arrest as in the beating heart generating pressure. These results confirm that left ventricular pressure, at least in the extreme circumstance of an empty beating heart, is not the dominating factor in impeding subendocardial flow.

Because the conclusions of the Marzilli et al. [35] study are so damaging to the tissue pressure hypothesis, their results must be considered critically. In the right panel of Figure 7.6, the typical phasic recording of a lidocaine injection measurement is reproduced. The increase in mean flow due to the infusion of lidocaine is evident. However, the pulsations in flow remain of the same order as those obtained under control and must be caused by the left ventricular pressure. This would appear to be in contradiction with the conclusion that flow is only affected by contractility. Moreover, Krams et al. [31, 32] in an isolated cat heart preparation, showed diminished pulsations when contractility was lowered. On the other hand, the flow pulsatility could be caused by factors different from those causing the reduction in mean flow perfusion. Arterial flow may be pulsatile because of compression of the proximal side of the intramyocardial vasculature, but this would not affect mean flow as it results from interaction between compression and coronary circulation at the venular part.

The phasic recordings in Figure 7.6 illustrate the effect of the impedance of the perfusion system on the coronary flow signal. At constant pressure perfusion, the systolic coronary flow normally can become negative. Thus perfusion system impedance has reduced the swing in diastolic-systolic flow in Marzilli's experiment and might have had an effect on the microsphere distribution. However, it seems unlikely that such an effect could be completely responsible for the findings on microsphere distribution discussed above.

A similar experiment was performed by Klassen and Zborowska-Sluis [26], but these authors came to an opposite conclusion. In this experiment the circumflex artery was perfused at constant flow. Calcium chloride was infused into a segment of the left coronary artery, increasing force generation as measured locally by a strain gauge. When vasomotor tone was abolished, force could be increased by 12% without affecting perfusion pressure or left ventricular pressure. Endo/epi flow ratios were equally unaffected by this degree of force increase. This finding suggests that contractility affects coronary flow when pushed to the extreme but not in the range of normal operation. Experiments like those of Klassen should be performed, but then with small alterations in left ventricular pressure.

7.5 Intramyocardial compliance

Intramyocardial blood volume is not constant but depends on several factors. As was shown in Figure 1.4, coronary venous outflow continues after coronary arterial occlusion and then decays to zero in a few seconds. The decay of outflow after coronary occlusion is direct proof of a compliant intramyocardial vasculature. This compliance is the result of the distensibility of the microvessels as discussed in Chapters 1, 2 and 3. Intramyocardial blood volume is also affected by contraction of the heart muscle. This is illustrated by Figure 7.7 which indicates that when the heart is arrested, intramyocardial blood volume increases. When inflow stops after a significant increase in blood volume, outflow decays to zero, reflecting the emptying of a windkessel. The increase in intramyocardial blood volume induced by cardiac arrest was about 2 ml per 100 g tissue [46] and did not differ much with vasodilation. The time constant for the increase in blood volume induced by cardiac rest was about 1.8 s with autoregulation intact and 1.2 s after vasodilation. From a recent study applying near-infrared spectroscopy an even larger time constant for volume variations following an arterial occlusion may be derived [38].

Similar experiments were performed by Kajiya et al. [24]. However, before arresting the heart the coronary arterial line was clamped. Hence, intramyocardial volume was decreased by an extra amount due to cessation of inflow. Venous outflow was measured using a laser Doppler technique. A typical result of their experiments is provided in Figure 7.8. Venous outflow was restored after a delay, which, although dependent on the magnitude of flow, was about one second. Then venous outflow increased exponentially, indicating the filling of a windkessel. The unstressed volume was estimated from the period of zero outflow after restoration of inflow and the intramyocardial compliance was estimated from the exponential rise of venous flow by applying an RC model. The unstressed volume was of the order of 4 ml $\cdot$ [100 g]$^{-1}$, and compliance of the order of 0.07 ml $\cdot$ mm Hg^{-1} $\cdot$ [100 g]$^{-1}$.

It has been shown by Goto et al. [19] that diastolic pressure–flow relations measured in the period of filling of the unstressed volume are different from those measured after filling. The difference corresponds with a lower resistance when the unstressed volume is not yet filled. This is not what one would expect since resistance should be higher at lower intramyocardial volumes. However, in the period of filling of the unstressed volume restoring forces are active and tend to increase intramyocardial volume. These restoring forces may overcompensate for the effect of increased resistance due to the low absolute level of intramyocardial volume.

The compliance value found from the increase in venous outflow after restoration of flow, the decay of venous outflow in a long diastole after cessation of inflow (see next section), and measurements from venous outflow after arterial occlusion in a normal beating heart all result in an estimate of compliance in the range between 0.07 and 0.11 ml $\cdot$ mm Hg^{-1} $\cdot$ [100 g]$^{-1}$. When Vergroesen et al. [46] divided their measured increase of intramyocardial blood volume by the decrease in half averaged left ventricular pressure they arrived at a compliance value of 0.1 and 0.14 ml $\cdot$ mm Hg^{-1} $\cdot$ [100 g]$^{-1}$ for the conditions of autoregulation and vasodilation respectively, which is in the range of compliance values measured by other methods. This agreement was seen as evidence that tissue pressure related to left ventricular pressure was the external loading pressure of the intramyocardial compliance.

Obviously, the tissue pressure driven intramyocardial pump model fits well with the cited studies on intramyocardial compliance. The out-of-phase relation between inflow and outflow signals predicted by their model was illustrated in Figure 6.13. These phase relations were studied in more detail by Chadwick

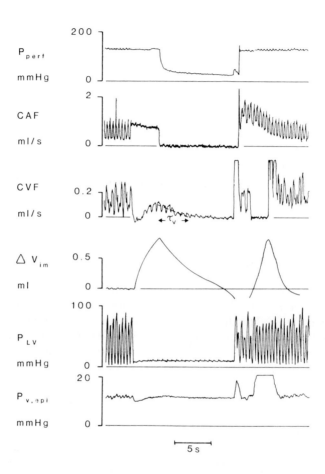

Figure 7.7: Illustration of intramyocardial compliance and effect of cardiac contraction on intramyocardial blood volume. When the ventricular pacemaker is turned off and perfusion pressure (P_{perf}) maintained, intramyocardial blood volume (V_{im}) increases, demonstrating that this is reduced by contraction. When coronary arterial flow (CAF) is stopped during the long diastole, venous flow (CVF) falls, demonstrating the windkessel effect of intramyocardial vessels during diastole as was true after arterial occlusion in the beating heart (Figure 1.4). Note that the time constant for decay, τ_v, is longer than the duration of a heart beat. Note also the decrease in epicardial venous pressure at the onset of arrest, indicating a possible reflow of venous blood into the intramyocardial vessels. (From [39], by permission of the American Heart Association, Inc..)

7.5 Intramyocardial compliance

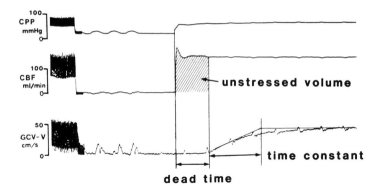

Figure 7.8: Illustration of compliance and unstressed volume of the intramyocardial circulation [24]. The perfusion line was first clamped for several seconds, after which the heart was arrested. Unstressed volume is the volume stored before venous outflow becomes measurable. (From Tsujioka et al. [42], by permission of the authors and Springer Verlag.)

et al. [11]. Apart from a small correction needed for wave transmission in the epicardial veins this study confirms the conclusion of our analysis above. There is, however, also a clear compatibility when the time varying elastance is considered as the cause for interaction between cardiac contraction and coronary flow. Such a model also describes compression of the intramyocardial space resulting in volume variations. It may very well be that a more detailed and quantitative analysis of induced volume alterations, theoretically and experimentally, might discriminate between the two forms of pump generators.

An experiment that clearly supports the concept of varying elastance is demonstrated in Figure 7.9. The experimental animal was the dog and the preparation was similar to the one used in the experiment of Figure 7.7. The additional signal measured was pressure in a small cannulated epicardial vein. Obviously, flow was stopped in the vein, although this does not imply that drainage of a part of the tissue is significantly impaired as the coronary venous system has numerous anastomoses. The pressure measured in this vein may be considered a reflection of the pressure proximal to the level of venular anastomoses and hence to reflect intramyocardial blood pressure.

In the period before the long diastole was induced the venous pressure variations are about half the left ventricular pressure variations. This obviously fits nicely with the concept of left ventricular pressure transmitted through the myocardial tissue and tissue pressure varying from left ventricular pressure at the endocardium to atmospheric at the epicardium. During the period of arrest, coronary arterial flow decreased due to vasoconstriction but inflow persisted. The rise in venular pressure, therefore, reflects the increase in volume of the intramy-

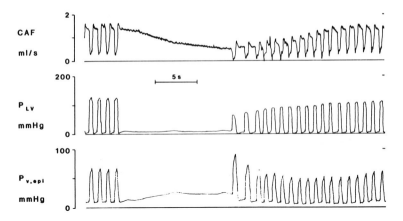

Figure 7.9: Pressure in a small occluded epicardial vein during beating and arrest. Top panel: Coronary blood flow. Middle panel: Left ventricular pressure. Bottom panel: Venous pressure. Note the constriction during cardiac arrest and the augmented venous pressure pulse after the end of arrest. Perfusion pressure was maintained at 100 mm Hg.

ocardial vessels. In the first beat after arrest, small venous pressure is twice as high as left ventricular pressure. It is unlikely that this venous pressure pulse is generated by the left ventricular pressure. However, this increased pressure pulse is in agreement with the elastance concept. Since intramyocardial blood volume has increased, the pressure generated in the intramyocardial blood space will be higher. The subsequent decrease in venular pressure, with increasing systolic left ventricular pressure, would then be the result of decreasing intramyocardial blood volume.

7.6 Pulsations in coronary pressure at constant flow perfusion

It has been recognized by Lee *et al.* [33] that in the waterfall model an intramyocardial compliance proximal to the waterfall element is needed to explain the phasic characteristics of coronary flow. They introduced a model that combined intramyocardial compliance and a vascular waterfall. Their studies showed that the magnitude of pulsations of coronary pressure at constant flow perfusion are pressure dependent, which was interpreted as proof for the existence of waterfalls. The idea was that at lower perfusion pressures, a larger subendocardial layer was without flow in systole and that therefore the arterial pressure pulsations are reduced. On the basis of the waterfall model, this reasoning makes

7.6 Pulsations in coronary pressure at constant flow perfusion

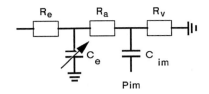

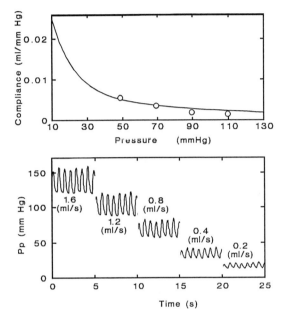

Figure 7.10: Effect of mean perfusion pressure on the magnitude of pressure pulsations at constant flow perfusion. Top: A simple linear intramyocardial pump model extended with a proximal pressure dependent compliance C_e and a small resistance R_e. Middle: Pressure dependency of this proximal compliance. Data points in this panel are from Canty et al. [9]. Bottom: Simulation results, exhibiting the decreasing magnitude of pressure pulsations at decreasing pressure.

sense. However, an alternative explanation is readily at hand. As was discussed in Chapter 5, Canty et al. [9] demonstrated that input compliance of the coronary system is pressure dependent (see Figure 5.12); compliance increases with decreasing pressure. Hence, assuming that the pressure pulsations are generated by intramyocardial pressures, these pulsations are more damped with decreasing perfusion pressure. We verified this possibility [14] by simulating the protocol of Lee et al. [33] with a very simple model illustrated in Figure 7.10. The linear intramyocardial pump model was extended with a proximal pressure dependent compliance in accordance with the findings of Canty et al. [9]. This pressure dependency is illustrated in the middle panel of Figure 7.10. The bottom panel presents the results of these simulations which show virtually the same behavior as found experimentally.

The decreasing pressure pulsation at decreasing perfusion pressure can also be explained with the varying elastance model of Krams et al. [30], as was discussed in Chapter 6. According to their theory, the intramyocardial blood space fills less at lower perfusion pressure and the pressure that can be built up in this space is less than would occur at lower left ventricular preload. It should be noted that when autoregulation is present, the pulsations of perfusion pressure at constant flow perfusion are independent of coronary arterial pressure. This is evident from Figure 5.5. The independence of perfusion pressure pulsations was understood at the time to be caused by tissue pressure dominance of interaction between contraction and coronary flow. In the varying elastance concept this will be interpreted differently. Since flow is quite independent of perfusion pressure when autoregulation is intact, it may be expected that intramyocardial vascular volume is unaltered by arterial pressure and that the variation of elastance would have an effect independent of coronary arteriolar pressure.

7.7 Diastolic pressure–flow lines

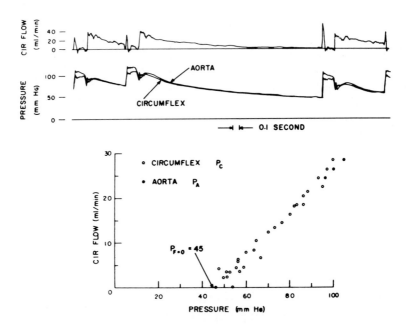

Figure 7.11: Coronary circumflex, CIR, flow and aortic pressure in a chronic instrumented awake dog. Top: Time varying signals. Bottom: Flow plotted versus pressure. Note the cessation of flow at high aortic pressure. (From Bellamy [5], by permission of the author and the American Heart Association, Inc..)

During the last 15 years, there has been much emphasis on the relation between pressure and flow during diastole. This field of research was stimulated by Bellamy [5] who observed in chronically instrumented dogs that coronary arterial flow could become zero while aortic pressure was still substantially above right atrial pressure. One of his observations is reproduced in Figure 7.11. This figure also depicts in the bottom panel the pressure–flow relation constructed from the pressure and flow tracings. Bellamy suggested that the cessation of flow was caused by the collapse of arterioles, similar to vessels with waterfall behavior. The collapse would then be caused by both the tissue pressure and smooth muscle tone in the arteriolar walls. This assumption was supported by the finding that the diastolic pressure–flow curves altered during the reactive hyperemic response. The intercepts of the extrapolated pressure–flow lines and their slopes were lower at decreased tone. This is consistent with the idea that tone affects both resistance and a collapse pressure. However, such an interpretation of pressure–flow curves during reactive hyperemia by a steady state model is dangerous. It implicitly assumes that tone will be constant during individual diastoles and hence can only change during systole [41]. Moreover, an extra problem with the interpretation involves the extrapolation of the pressure–flow curves to obtain zero flow pressure since the curves are nonlinear [29]. However, the experiment was repeated in open chest anesthetized dogs [15] and tone was changed to different levels via the autoregulation mechanism by altering perfusion pressure before letting this pressure decay in order to measure pressure–flow lines. The long diastoles in which these pressure–flow lines were obtained were induced by vagal stimulation (Figure 7.12). Positive zero flow intercepts were found, confirming the finding of Bellamy. With lower tone, the slope of the pressure–flow curves changed according to a lowered resistance and decreased zero flow pressure. These observations supported the idea that coronary flow was controlled by the interplay of alteration in resistance and collapse pressure due to smooth muscle activation in the arteriolar walls by changing perfusion pressure.

The linearity of the diastolic pressure–flow line has been seen as evidence for the interpretation that the inverse of the slope equalled resistance. However, this concept was weakened by the finding of others that diastolic pressure–flow lines can be curvilinear, especially at pressures close to zero flow pressure [27]. Moreover, although the inverse of a slope of a diastolic pressure–flow relation has the dimension or units of a resistance, this does not necessarily mean that it represents a vascular resistance. A simple example is shown by the long diastole experiment shown in Figure 7.9. Perfusion pressure was kept constant at 100 mm Hg during this experiment. The diastolic pressure–flow line that can be constructed from this measurement is a vertical line and the extrapolation of this curve intercepts the pressure axis at a value equal to perfusion pressure. The infinite tangent would suggest zero coronary resistance. We can be sure that with a decreasing pressure, flow would have decreased as well and we would have found a finite slope, and hence finite resistance.

An important limitation related to diastolic pressure–flow lines and their interpretation was reported by Eng et al. [17] and is demonstrated in Figure 7.13.

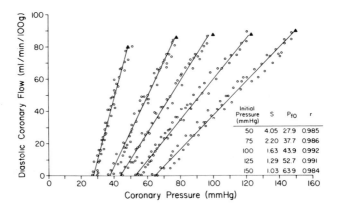

Figure 7.12: *Diastolic pressure–flow relations at 5 different values of initial coronary arterial pressure in a perfused circumflex coronary artery. Autoregulation was intact. Perfusion pressure decayed exponentially until P_{zf} (P_{f0}) was reached. S = slope of pressure–flow lines, r = correlation coefficient. Pressure decay started appr. 1 second after the beginning of a long diastole, allowing the intramyocardial compliance to fill. (From Dole and Bishop [15], by permission of authors and American Heart Asssociation Inc..)*

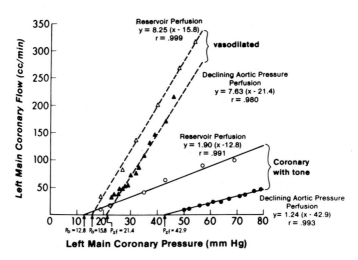

Figure 7.13: *The effect of changing perfusion pressure on the diastolic pressure–flow lines obtained during vasodilation and with tone intact. The closed symbols show results obtained by exponential decay of perfusion pressure. The open symbols show results obtained by rapid switching of the perfusion line to a source with adjustable pressure at the same time as the long diastole began. (From Eng et al. [17], by permission of authors and American Heart Association Inc..)*

7.7 Diastolic pressure–flow lines

Diastolic pressure–flow lines were obtained using two different approaches. In the first approach the cannulated coronary artery was connected to a perfusion source in which the pressure decayed exponentially. This method resulted in pressure–flow relations with higher intercept pressures when regulation was intact than during vasodilation. The second approach consisted of connecting the coronary perfusion line to a perfusion source with constant pressure, at the same moment as the pacer was switched off, inducing a long diastole. This was performed several times in succession but with varying pressures in the reservoir. Hence a pressure–flow relation could be constructed at further constant conditions of vasomotor tone or vasodilation. This procedure resulted in pressure–flow curves parallel to those obtained by decaying pressure, but with a much lower pressure intercept.

As has been discussed above, the intramyocardial blood space has a compliance and time is needed to change the volume stored in it. Hence, it is quite possible that the arterial pressure at zero flow is caused by the windkessel action of the intramyocardial compliance. In fact, Chilian and Marcus [13] showed a continuation of venous outflow at cessation of arterial inflow which is evidence for the discharge of the intramyocardial compliance via the veins.

The effect of intramyocardial compliance on P_{zf} is of special relevance to the experiments of Dole and Bishop [15] depicted in Figure 7.12. Decay of pressure started after allowing approximately 1 second for stabilization. Figure 7.7, however, showed that during such a period, intramyocardial blood volume and consequently microvascular pressure increases.

An additional evaluation of diastolic pressure–flow lines comes from Tomonaga et al. [44]. These authors continued to decrease arterial pressure during a long diastole and did not halt when flow reached zero but continued to determine pressure–flow relations during retrograde flow. Their results are illustrated in Figure 7.14. Clearly, retrograde flow can only be explained by the discharge of distal compliance. As is clear from Figure 7.14, the pressure–flow relation for positive values of flow depends on the speed of reduction of pressure. If reduction of pressure had halted when the flow became zero, the resulting limited portion of the pressure–flow curve could have been interpreted as arteriolar collapse.

The experimental evidence collected in this section is worthwhile analyzing in a broader context. The experiment of Eng et al. [17] reproduced in Figure 7.13 is clear evidence that there is no such mechanism as an arteriolar waterfall. When perfusion pressure is switched to a pressure below the zero flow pressure obtained with the pressure decaying method, a fair amount of antegrade flow seems to be possible. This makes collapse of arterioles in end-diastole unlikely. Eng et al. suggested that the shift in pressure–flow relation obtained by applying an exponential pressure decay was due to an input compliance. When pressure has decayed, an additional capacitive flow has to be subtracted from the actual flow obtained which should amount to $C_{in}\,dP/dt$; this is the rate of change by which

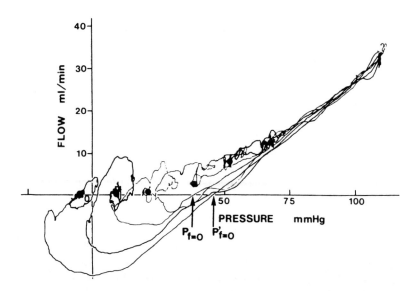

Figure 7.14: Diastolic pressure–flow relations with arterial pressure decreased below P_{zf} ($P_{f=0}$). The curves are continuous in the negative flow range, depending on the rate of change of pressure. Retrograde flow can be explained only by compliance. Since no sudden changes in course of the curves are observed at P_{zf} it is unlikely that compliance does not affect diastolic pressure–flow relations for pressures higher than P_{zf}. (From Tomonaga et al. [44], by permission of authors and Steinkoff Verlag.)

the volume in the compliance alters. However, the C'_{in} needed to explain the shift of curves obtained is much larger than the input compliance that was derived in Chapter 6. An alternative explanation for the observations reported in the figures is based on intramyocardial compliance. As was discussed by Tomonaga et al. [44], intramyocardial compliance is the only mechanism that can explain the retrograde flow when pressure is reduced below zero flow pressure.

Under the assumption that the shift in pressure–flow line by Eng et al. [17] was induced by input compliance a 'capacitance free' method of measuring diastolic pressure–flow lines was developed. By first decreasing and then increasing perfusion pressure at the same rate [2, 8, 36] and averaging the flows at the same pressure obtained during the downward and upward slope of the protocol a pressure–flow relation was obtained. Since the capacitive flows are the same but of opposite signs the capacitive effects should average out. However, this method only compensates for input compliance effects but not for intramyocardial compliance effects. The mathematical expressions for capacitive flow are more complicated for intramyocardial compliance and do not cancel out when averaging flows obtained with decreasing and increasing pressures.

7.7 Diastolic pressure–flow lines

The diastolic pressure–flow relations of Dole and Bishop [15] were obtained by decreasing pressure. Pressure decay started some time after the induction of long diastole. Their experimental results show a high degree of consistency with the load line analysis of pulsatile coronary flow and pressure shown in Figure 5.5 and can be described by the linear intramyocardial pump model. In the model, the pressure intercept is interpreted as the pressure in the intramyocardial blood compartment and the slopes of the pressure–flow lines reflect the inlet resistance of the compartment. The decreasing slope of the load line with decreasing perfusion pressure was related to arteriolar tone reduction. This corresponds with the increasing slope of the diastolic pressure–flow line at decreasing pressure.

The correlation found between intercept pressure and perfusion pressure as measured by Dole fits well with the ratio between inlet resistance and total resistance as found from the load line analysis. The above provides strong support for the theory that zero flow pressure as estimated from coronary arterial pressure–flow relations is caused by intramyocardial compliance and does not reflect a collapse pressure in the arterioles. One should, however, appreciate that in an attempt to explain zero flow pressure with a compliance based model the pressure dependency of intramyocardial compliance and resistance [34] should be taken into account. On theoretical grounds, collapse should not be expected when the vessels are fully dilated [3]. Kanatsuka et al. [25], applying an intravital microscopic technique with floating objective, studied the change of inner diameters of microvessels while obtaining diastolic pressure–flow relations in the fully dilated coronary bed. As to be expected, the arteriolar diameters did decrease with decreasing pressure but collapse could not be observed. A pressure difference of 10 mm Hg remained between coronary arteries and right atrium when red blood cells came to rest in arterioles, capillaries and venules. These observations are in agreement with the study of muscle circulation studied in a closed box [43]; in these experiments too, microvascular flow came to rest at a finite driving pressure. Hence, it seems possible that flow stagnates notwithstanding a small arterial–venous pressure difference which may be due to rheological properties of the blood. On the other hand, in the coronary circulation, the observations of Kanatsuka et al. [25] are consistent with a waterfall mechanism in the coronary epicardial veins as has been discussed in Chapter 4. Diastolic left ventricular pressure was 8 mm Hg in their experiments and close to the arterial zero flow pressure measured. The effect of diastolic ventricular pressure [2] is higher when the pericardium is present [47] which stresses the possible importance of compression of the epicardial veins in the magnitude of the coronary arterial zero flow pressure.

The absence of evidence of collapse by direct observations does not mean that arterioles cannot collapse due to severe vasoconstriction. Such constrictions have been observed under the stimulus of pharmacological agents [23]. Also, tetanic contraction of the left ventricular wall induced by barium contracture may lead to a severe reduction of coronary flow at a high arterial pressure [6]. However, these observations of collapse under extreme conditions do not imply that collapse is a mechanism active under normal working conditions of the heart.

However, as pointed out by Klocke *et al.* [27, 28] it is very difficult to prove from arterial and coronary venous flow alone that there is no collapse. Most of the observations on these flow signals are consistent with a point of zero flow somewhere in the microcirculation. Flow directions proximal and distal of such a point would then be opposite. However, such a hypothesis would imply that the point of collapse would vary its anatomical location continuously as judged from the ratio between zero flow pressure and the arterial–venous pressure difference. This ratio alters with vasodilation indicating the movement of the collapse point to the venous side [40]. A different factor that may have contributed to the high zero flow pressure found in preparations with a single cannulated coronary artery is collateral flow [37] as was discussed in Chapter 5. For a recent review of diastolic pressure–flow curves, the reader is referred to [22].

7.8 Discussion

The conclusion of the chapter is that, unfortunately, no model describes coronary flow mechanics over the whole range of working conditions. However, from the experimental observations discussed, some conclusions as to the relevance of a number of required ingredients for models on the coronary circulation may be drawn. Without doubt, the intramyocardial space is compliant, as otherwise the large intramyocardial volume variations could not be explained. However, this compliance need not be constant, but very probably varies throughout the cardiac cycle as well as being pressure dependent. Coronary resistance is almost certainly pressure dependent and a model of the coronary circulation should account for this. Another important observation, which a model should be able to account for, is the effect of cardiac contraction on microsphere distribution in the heart; as rate changes subepicardial flow is only slightly affected but subendocardial flow is changed very strongly. Because subepicardial flow is independent of heart rate, it is most likely that, at least in this part of the myocardium, coronary flow is not affected directly by the contracting myocytes. This is supported by the observation of Ashikawa [1] that red cell velocity signals in subepicardial arterioles, capillaries and venules are very similar. However, on the other hand, Ashikawa shows retrograde flow in epicardial arterioles during a short period at the beginning of systole. This would point in the direction of at least a transient effect of direct interaction. Such a direct effect was also inferred from observation of systolic decrease of flow in the septal artery prior to that in epicardial arteries [10]. However, the compliance of the epicardial arteries may have introduced a delay between flow signals in the penetrating coronary arteries and the epicardial ones [12].

A combination of the nonlinear intramyocardial pump model [7] and time varying elastance model [48] is the most promising for explaining both phasic coronary arterial and venous flow and time averaged flow. Both models focus on the intramyocardial blood space as being compliant and pressurized by systole. In the nonlinear pump model this is assumed to happen via tissue pressure which may either be related to ventricular pressure or to contraction of the myocytes. In the varying elastance model, this pressurization is caused by changing wall elastance. For the beating heart, the waterfall model provides little future. The rate of change of the intramyocardial blood volume is too slow to justify the assumption of complete local collapse.

An important factor that deserves much more study is the effect of venous pressure on coronary flow. Epicardial venous pressure could very well act as the mechanism which prevents intramyocardial blood vessels from collapsing. As was discussed in Chapter 4, coronary venous pressure is kept close to diastolic left ventricular pressure. If ventricular pressure increases, the increase of pressure in the interstitium might be compensated for by increasing venous pressure, keeping transmural vascular pressure within the myocardium constant.

An important point is that models should be validated in a physiological or pathophysiological working range. One may wonder whether the study of a fully vasodilated coronary bed at a perfusion pressure of 100 mm Hg can contribute to our knowledge of the coronary bed distal of a stenosis with a much lower perfusion pressure and where vasomotor tone is only locally absent. This does not imply that studies performed under artificial circumstances are unable to shed light on certain mechanisms. However, validation under realistic conditions always should be attempted.

7.9 Summary

At present there is no model that can describe all the phenomena observed in relation to coronary flow mechanics. This may partly be attributed to inconsistent and unrealistic experimental conditions. However, because of the nonlinear behavior of the coronary circulation, some assumptions may be true in one set of circumstances but not in others. The dispute at the moment especially concerns the extent to which coronary flow is affected by left ventricular pressure and contractility.

Curvature of pressure–flow lines and the effect of cardiac contraction on these can be explained equally well by a waterfall model or a model with pressure dependent resistances and compliances. Models on the coronary circulation should account for a considerable intramyocardial compliance, for the absence of effect of cardiac contraction in the subepicardium and a strong effect in the subendocardium.

Diastolic pressure–flow lines cross the pressure axis when coronary arterial pressure is reduced to below the zero flow pressure. This can be explained only by a significant intramyocardial compliance. It is unlikely that zero flow pressure is caused by tone induced collapse of arterioles during normal control of coronary flow.

References

[1] ASHIKAWA K, KANATSUKA H, SUZUKI T, TAKISHIMA T (1984) A new microscope system for the continuous observation of the coronary microcirculation in the beating canine left ventricle. *Microvasc. Res.* **28**: 387–394.
[2] AVERSANO T, KLOCKE FJ, MATES RE, CANTY JM JR (1984) Preload-induced alterations in capacitance-free diastolic pressure-flow relationships. *Am. J. Physiol.* **246** (*Heart Circ. Physiol.* **15**): H410–H417.
[3] AZUMA T, OKA S (1971) Mechanical equilibrium of blood vessel walls. *Am. J. Physiol.* **221**: 1310–1321.
[4] BACHE RJ, COBB FR (1977) Effect of maximal coronary vasodilation on transmural myocardial perfusion during tachycardia in the awake dog. *Circ. Res.* **41**: 648–653.
[5] BELLAMY RF (1978) Diastolic coronary pressure-flow relations in the dog. *Circ. Res.* **43**: 92–101.
[6] BELLAMY RF, O'BENAR JD (1984) Cessation of arterial and venous flow at a finite driving pressure in porcine coronary circulation. *Am. J. Physiol.* **246** (*Heart Circ. Physiol.* **15**): H525–H531.
[7] BRUINSMA P, ARTS T, DANKELMAN J, SPAAN JAE (1988) Model of the coronary circulation based on pressure dependence of coronary resistance and compliance. *Basic Res. Cardiol.* **83**: 510–524.
[8] CANTY JM JR, KLOCKE FJ, MATES RE (1987) Characterization of capacitance-free pressure–flow relations during single diastoles in dogs using an RC model with pressure-dependent parameters. *Circ. Res.* **60**: 273-282.
[9] CANTY JM JR, KLOCKE FJ, MATES RE (1985) Pressure and tone dependence of coronary diastolic input impedance and capacitance. *Am. J. Physiol.* **248** (*Heart Circ. Physiol.* **17**): H700–H711.
[10] CAREW TE, COVELL JW (1979) Effect of intramyocardial pressure on the phasic flow in the intraventricular septal artery. *Cardiovasc. Res.* **10**: 56–64.
[11] CHADWICK RS, TEDGUI A, MICHEL JB, OHAYON J, LEVY BI (1990) Phasic regional myocardial inflow and outflow: comparison of theory and experiments. *Am. J. Physiol.* **258** (*Heart Circ. Physiol.* **27**): H1687–H1698.
[12] CHILIAN WM, MARCUS ML (1982) Phasic coronary flow velocity in intramural and epicardial coronary arteries. *Circ. Res.* **50**: 775–781.
[13] CHILIAN WM, MARCUS ML (1984) Coronary venous outflow persists after cessation of coronary arterial inflow. *Am. J. Physiol.* **247** (*Heart Circ. Physiol.* **16**): H984–H990.

[14] DANKELMAN J, STASSEN HG, SPAAN JAE (1990) Coronary circulation mechanics. In: *Coronary circulation. Basic mechanism and clinical relevance.* Eds. KAJIYA F, KLASSEN GA, SPAAN JAE, HOFFMAN JIE. Springer-Verlag Tokyo: 75–87.
[15] DOLE WP, BISHOP VS (1982) Influence of autoregulation and capacitance on diastolic coronary artery pressure-flow relationships in the dog. *Circ. Res.* **51**: 261–270.
[16] DOWNEY JM, KIRK ES (1975) Inhibition of coronary blood flow by a vascular waterfall mechanism. *Circ. Res.* **36**: 753–760.
[17] ENG C, JENTZER JH, KIRK ES (1982) The effects of the coronary capacitance on the interpretation of diastolic pressure-flow relationships. *Circ. Res.* **50**: 334–341.
[18] FLYNN AE, COGGINS DL, ALDEA GS, AUSTIN RE, GOTO M, HUSSEINI W, HOFFMAN JIE (1989) Ventricular contraction increases subepicardial blood flow: evidence for a deep myocardial pump. *FASEB J.* **3**: A1305.
[19] GOTO M, TSUJIOKA K, OGASAWARA Y, WADA Y, TADAOKA S, HIRAMATSU O, YANAKA M, KAJIYA F (1990) Effect of blood filling in intramyocardial vessels on coronary arterial inflow. *Am. J. Physiol.* **258** (*Heart Circ. Physiol.* **27**): H1042–H1048.
[20] HANLEY FL, MESSINA LM, GRATTAN MT, HOFFMAN JIE (1984) The effect of coronary inflow pressure on coronary vascular resistance in the isolated dog heart. *Circ. Res.* **54**: 760–772.
[21] HEINEMAN FW, GRAYSON J (1985) Transmural distribution of intramyocardial pressure measured by micropipette technique. *Am. J. Physiol.* **249** (*Heart Circ. Physiol.* **18**): H1216–H1223.
[22] HOFFMAN JIE, SPAAN JAE (1990) Pressure-flow relations in coronary circulation. *Physiol. Rev.* **70**: 331–390.
[23] ITO Y, KITAMURA K, KURIYAMA H (1979) Effect of acetylcholine and catecholamines on the smooth muscle cell of the porcine coronary artery. *J. Physiol. Lond.* **294**: 595–612.
[24] KAJIYA F, TSUJIOKA K, GOTO M, WADA Y, CHEN XL, NAKAI M, TADAOKA S, HIRAMATSU O, OGASAWARA Y, MITO K, TOMONAGA G (1986) Functional characteristics of intramyocardial capacitance vessels during diastole in the dog. *Circ. Res.* **58**: 476–485.
[25] KANATSUKA H, ASHIKAWA K, KOMARU T, SUZUKI T, TAKISHIMA T (1990) Diameter change and pressure-red blood cell velocity relations in coronary microvessels during long diastoles in the canine left ventricle. *Circ. Res.* **66**: 503–510.
[26] KLASSEN GA, ZBOROWSKA-SLUIS DT (1979) The effect of myocardial force on coronary transmural flow distribution. *Cardiovasc. Res.* **13**: 365–369.
[27] KLOCKE FJ, MATES RE, CANTY JM JR, ECLIT AK (1985) Coronary pressure-flow relationships. Controversial issues and probable implications.

Circ. Res. **56**: 310–323.
[28] KLOCKE FJ, MATES RE, CANTY JM JR, ECLIT AK (1985) Response to the article by Spaan on 'Coronary diastolic pressure-flow relation and zero flow pressure explained on the basis of intramyocardial compliance' (*Circ. Res.* **56**: 293–309, 1985). *Circ. Res.* **56**: 791–792.
[29] KLOCKE FJ, WEINSTEIN IR, KLOCKE JF, ECLIT AK, KRAUS DR, MATES RE, CANTY JM, ANBAR RD, ROMANOWSKI RR, WALLMEYER KW, ECHT MP (1981) Zero-flow pressures and pressure-flow relationships during single long diastoles in the canine coronary bed before and during maximum vasodilation. *J. Clin. Invest.* **68**: 970–980.
[30] KRAMS R, SIPKEMA P, WESTERHOF N (1989) Can coronary systolic-diastolic flow difference be predicted by left ventricular pressure of time varying intramyocardial elastance? *Basic Res. Cardiol.* **84**: 149–159.
[31] KRAMS R (1988) *The effect of cardiac contraction on coronary flow. Introduction to a new concept.* PhD Thesis. Free University of Amsterdam, The Netherlands.
[32] KRAMS R, SIPKEMA P, ZEGERS J, WESTERHOF N (1989) Contractility is the main determinant of coronary systolic flow impediment. *Am. J. Physiol.* **257** (*Heart Circ. Physiol.* **26**): H1936–H1944.
[33] LEE J, CHAMBERS DE, AKIZUKI S, DOWNEY JM (1984) The role of vascular capacitance in the coronary arteries. *Circ. Res.* **55**: 751–762.
[34] MAGDER S (1990) Starling resistor versus compliance which explains the zero-flow pressure of a dynamic arterial pressure-flow relation?. *Circ. Res.* **67**: 209–220.
[35] MARZILLI M, GOLDSTEIN S, SABBAH HN, LEE T, STEIN PD (1979) Modulating effect of regional myocardial performance on local myocardial perfusion in the dog. *Circ. Res.* **45**: 634–640.
[36] MATES RE, KLOCKE FJ, CANTY JM JR (1987) Impedance to coronary flow. In: *Activation, Metabolism and Perfusion of the Heart.* Eds. SIDEMAN S, BEYAR R. Martinus Nijhoff, Dordrecht, The Netherlands: 409–419.
[37] MESSINA LM, HANLEY FL, UHLIG PN, BAER RW, GRATTAN MT, HOFFMAN JIE (1985) Effects of pressure gradients between branches of the left coronary artery on the pressure axis intercept and the shape of steady state circumflex pressure-flow relations in dogs. *Circ. Res.* **56**: 11–19.
[38] PARSONS WJ, REMBERT JC, BAUMAN RP, GREENFIELD JR JC, PAINTADOSI CA (1990) Dynamic mechanisms of cardiac oxygenation during brief ischemia and reperfusion. *Am. J. Physiol.* **259** (*Heart Circ. Physiol.* **28**): H1477–H1485.
[39] SPAAN JAE (1985) Coronary diastolic pressure-flow relation and zero flow pressure explained on the basis of intramyocardial compliance. *Circ. Res.* **56**: 293–309.
[40] SPAAN JAE (1985) Response to the article by Klocke *et al.*on 'Coronary

pressure-flow relationships: controversial issues and probable implications'. (*Circ. Res.* **56**: 310-323, 1985). *Circ. Res.* **56**: 789-791.

[41] SPAAN JAE (1979) Does coronary resistance change only during systole? *Circ. Res.* **45**: 838-839.

[42] TSUJIOKA K, GOTO M, HIRAMATSU O, WADA Y, OGASAWARE Y, KAJIYA F (1990) Functional characteristics of intramyocardial capacitance vessels and their effects on coronary arterial inflow and venous outflow. In: *Coronary circulation. Basic mechanism and clinical relevance.* Springer-Verlag Tokyo.

[43] TANGELDER GJ, SLAAF DW, RENEMAN RS Skeletal muscle microcirculation and changes in transmural and perfusion pressures. *Prog. Appl. Microcirc.* **5**: 93-108.

[44] TOMONAGA G, TSUJIOKA K, OGASAWARA Y, NAKAI M, MITO K, HIRAMATSU O, KAJIYA F (1984) Dynamic characteristics of diastolic pressure-flow relation in the canine coronary artery. In: *The Coronary Sinus.* Eds. MOHL W, WOLNER E, GLOGAR D. Steinkoff Verlag Darmstadt, Springer-Verlag New York: 79-85.

[45] VANWINKLE DM, SWAFFORD AN, DOWNEY JM (1990) The subendocardial extravascular resistance in dog hearts is independent of ventricular lumenal pressure. *FASEB J.* **4**: A946.

[46] VERGROESEN I, NOBLE MIM, SPAAN JAE (1987) Intramyocardial blood volume change in first moments of cardiac arrest in anesthetized goats. *Am. J. Physiol.* **253** *(Heart Circ. Physiol.* **22**): H307-H316.

[47] WATANABE J, MARUYAMA Y, SATOH S, KEITOKU M, TAKASHIMA T (1987) Effects of the pericardium on the diastolic left coronary pressure-flow relationship in the isolated dog heart. *Circulation* **75**: 670-675.

[48] WESTERHOF N (1990) Physiological hypotheses–Intramyocardial pressure. A new concept, suggestions for measurement. *Basic Res. Cardiol.* **85**: 105-119.

Chapter 8

Arteriolar mechanics and control of flow

ED VAN BAVEL, MAURICE JMM GIEZEMAN and JOS AE SPAAN

ARTERIOLES ARE THE SITE OF CORONARY FLOW CONTROL, and their tone dependent mechanical properties determine an important part of the input impedance of the coronary system. Understanding the behavior of the coronary system as a whole would be much easier if the basic mechanics of the arteriolar wall were understood. However, the mechanics of smooth muscle in general is a field much less developed than the mechanics of striated muscle and heart muscle. The interaction between the smooth muscle cells and endothelial cells is far from being clarified. Only recently have experiments been performed on isolated coronary arterioles which allow their behavior to be studied without interference from the surrounding tissue.

In Chapters 6 and 7, pressure–volume relationships of the various blood compartments were used based on hypothetical mechanical properties of individual vessels. In this chapter, the mechanical properties of arterioles will be discussed and some data on isolated vessels will be presented. Furthermore, the relation between the mechanical properties of individual vessels and the pressure dependency of both arterial volume and resistance is discussed.

Arterioles are intrinsically capable of controlling flow by the so-called myogenic mechanism. This is the tendency of the arterioles to increase their level of contraction upon an increase in pressure. However, the most important determinant of coronary flow is the oxygen requirement of the heart, which means that a metabolic signal overrules the myogenic response. This myogenic response of the arterioles must be defined at the isolated arteriolar level to provide a sensible hypothesis about its role in the coronary circulation.

8.1 Morphology of the arteriolar wall

The wall of each type of blood vessel can be subdivided into three layers. The layer closest to the lumen is the intima which, in general, consists of one continuous layer of endothelial cells. These cells are usually very elongated, and are orientated in the longitudinal direction. The middle layer, the media, is the layer in which the smooth muscle cells are positioned. In large vessels, these cells can be orientated in any direction between longitudinal and transverse; however, in the arterioles the orientation is close to transverse. Depending on the size of the arterioles and species, the smooth muscle layer is one to three cells thick. The smooth muscle cells are embedded in a matrix of connective fibers, consisting of collagen and elastin. The part of the medial volume which is occupied by smooth muscle cells is larger in arterioles than it is in conductance vessels [17]. A large elastic lamina is present at the inner border of the media, and sometimes a less developed elastic lamina is also present between media and the outer layer, the adventitia. This adventitia contains mostly collagen fibers as well as some specialized cell types and nerve fibers.

The force for contraction is generated by actin and myosin filaments in the smooth muscle cells. However, in contrast to striated and heart muscle, these filaments are not ordered in sarcomeres. The filaments may be orientated in all directions relative to the smooth muscle cell axis [17]. Furthermore, the orientation of the filament as well as the orientation of the smooth muscle cells themselves is dependent on the state of contraction. This dependency of wall structure on arteriolar constriction is evident from Figure 8.1 which was taken from Greensmith and Duling [7]. The four panels show cross sections of vessels fixed at four different levels of smooth muscle tone. As is to be expected from geometrical considerations, the thickness of the different layers increases with vasoconstriction. The inner layers of the wall are folded by the constriction.

During constriction, some of the filaments are no longer orientated in a circumferential direction, and it is suggested by Greensmith and Duling that these filaments no longer participate in the development of active tangential tension. From the observations that orientation of the filaments is variable, and strongly influenced by diameter changes, it is clear that relating arteriolar resistance to the force generated by the filaments is practically impossible [7]. The seemingly poor organization of the filaments within the smooth muscle cells complicates the relation between their generated force and tangential wall stress.

The resistance of a vessel is, according to Poiseuille's law, inversely proportional to the fourth power of the inner radius. For a vessel with an irregular wall, such as the constricted arteriole, a hydraulic diameter may be introduced. This is the equivalent diameter of a cylindrical tube with the same Poiseuille resistance. If the folds in the inner wall of the arteriole are not sharp, as for example in panel B of Figure 8.1, the luminal cross-sectional area of this equivalent tube will be close to that of the arteriole. However, when the folds are large,

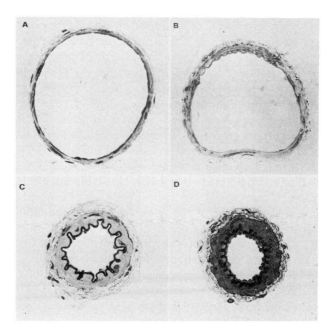

Figure 8.1: Dependency of the structure of arteriolar wall on the state of vasoconstriction. The diameters of the lumen were altered to 125% (A), 111% (B), 72% (C) and 34% (D) of their approximate diameter at zero transmural pressure. Note the different layers of the arteriolar wall which are especially clear in panel C. The inner layers of the wall exhibit folds due to the contraction. (From Greensmith and Duling [7], by permission of authors and American Physiological Society.)

forming small slits as in panels C and D of Figure 8.1, the cross-sectional area of the equivalent tube will be close to that of the area determined by the inner tops of the ridges. Hence, the resistance in the folds could be considered to be infinite. Consequently, there is an uncertainty about the diameter to be used in calculating the resistance which corresponds to the depth of the folds. Because of the power nature of Poiseuille's law, the resulting uncertainty in resistance may easily be in the order of 50%.

8.2 Myogenic response

The myogenic response is defined as an increase in active force production of smooth muscle cells induced by raising transmural pressure. Actually, an arteriolar diameter decreases instead of increasing when transmural pressure is raised, as would occur when the material properties of the arteriolar wall remain unaltered. The myogenic response is also referred to as a Bayliss response, because he was the first to describe this mechanism [2]. In 1902, Bayliss observed that arteries *'appeared to writhe like a worm'* when arterial pressure was raised. He recognized the importance of the myogenic response for the regulation of organ flow when he wrote: *'the peripheral powers of reaction possessed by the arteries is of such a nature as to provide as far as possible for the maintenance of a constant flow of blood through the tissues supplied by them, whatever may be the height of the general blood pressure'*. Myogenic responses have been reviewed by Johnson [10] and for their possible role in coronary control by McHale et al. [12].

Although myogenic responses were first recognized nearly a century ago, surprisingly little effort has been made to quantify these responses in isolated vessels. The quantification of mechanical and control behavior of isolated arterioles is of importance to avoid interaction of the arterioles with surrounding tissue, either directly or indirectly by circulating blood.

The concept of *myogenic response* should be distinguished from the concept of *myogenic tone*. The latter is a synonym for spontaneous tone in the arteriolar walls. An arteriole may exhibit spontaneous tone independent of its surrounding tissue but not show a myogenic response, as was demonstrated by Uchida and Bohr [18] in constant flow perfused segments of resistance vessels in skeletal muscle from around which tissue was removed.

During the past few years, we have studied the mechanics of isolated arterioles from mesentery and myocardium. Arterioles were dissected from surrounding tissue and mounted between two microcannulas [20], allowing constant perfusion of the vessel. Vessels were allowed to stabilize for 30 minutes after cannulation at a transmural pressure of 80 mm Hg before any intervention started. The perfusate contained a fluorescing dye to allow the continuous measurement of the volume of the arteriole over some length from the intensity of fluorescence light. This signal was calibrated so as to represent the average cross-sectional area of the vessel segment observed. Not all the arterioles showed spontaneous tone. However, in those, tone could be induced by norepinephrine.

An example of myogenic responses measured on an isolated mesenteric arteriole exhibiting spontaneous tone after isolation is illustrated in Figure 8.2. The cross-sectional area was studied in response to stepwise alterations in luminal pressure before and after the administration of acetylcholine. This latter intervention removed all smooth muscle tone.

The reduction of pressure from 80 to 40 mm Hg reduced the cross-sectional area, as is to be expected in a vessel with an elastic wall. The myogenic response is obvious from the subsequent vasodilation. The cross-sectional area returned to approximately its initial value. The reverse reaction of the cross-sectional area occurred when pressure was once again increased to 80 mm Hg: initially, the cross-sectional area increased because of elastic effects but then decreased

8.3 Myogenic response

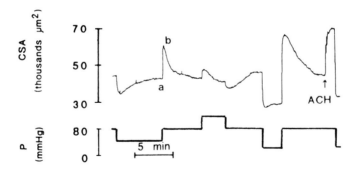

Figure 8.2: Myogenic response of an isolated mesenteric arteriole exhibiting spontaneous tone, measured by fluorescence technique using FITC. Note that the steady state cross-sectional areas of the vessel at 40, 80 and 120 mm Hg are quite similar. A reduction of pressure to a very low value eliminated smooth muscle tone almost completely as is clear from the peak cross-sectional area after restoration of pressure to 80 mm Hg. This peak is almost similar to the cross-sectional area at this pressure after relaxation by acetylcholine, ACH. The difference between cross-sectional areas indicated by a and b, divided by the pressure step, is a measure of compliance at the tone and pressure at the start of the pressure step (see Figure 8.12). This will be discussed further in Section 8.6. (From VanBavel [19].)

back to its initial value due to the increase in smooth muscle tone. Due to the myogenic response, the cross-sectional area at pressures of 40, 80 and 120 mm Hg is virtually the same. The vessel could almost completely be dilated by a reduction of pressure to 20 mm Hg. The peak cross-sectional area, after restoration of pressure from 20 to 80 mm Hg, almost equals the cross-sectional area at this higher pressure after acetylcholine administration.

Myogenic responses have also been observed in coronary arterioles by Kuo et al. [11]. The steady relation between pressure and diameter of a coronary arteriole obtained by these authors is illustrated in Figure 8.3. They also reported that there was some difference in myogenic response between subendocardial and subepicardial arterioles.

As is clear from Figure 8.2 and 8.3, the myogenic response provides the arterioles with an intrinsic ability to autoregulate flow and to show a reactive hyperemic response of flow without any feedback from an ischemic stimulus from the tissue. Obviously, when surrounded by tissue, the myogenic response has to function in concert with the metabolic stimuli for the control of flow. An important discrepancy between the myogenic response observed in our isolated arterioles and organ flow regulation concerns the rate of the responses. As will be elucidated in our next chapter, the rate of change of coronary resistance is much higher than the rate of change of diameter due to myogenic response in isolated vessels.

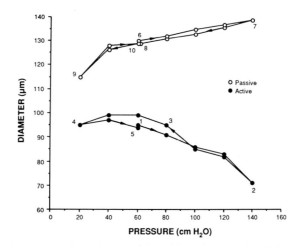

Figure 8.3: Relation between pressure and diameter in a coronary arteriole during steady state. The relatively flat portion of the relations illustrates the myogenic control of this vessel diameter. (From Kuo et al. [11], by permission of the authors and the American Physiological Society.)

8.3 Arteriolar vasomotion

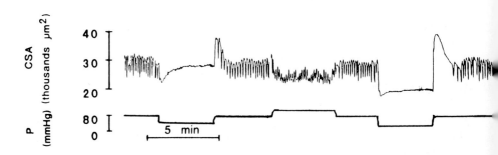

Figure 8.4: Example of vasomotion of an isolated, cannulated mesenteric arteriole. Note the superimposed myogenic responses and the pressure dependency of vasomotion. (From VanBavel et al. [20].)

In vivo microcirculatory observations have revealed the existence of cyclic diameter variations of arterioles and venules in a number of organs. This property is called vasomotion. It has been demonstrated in only a few isolated vessels, the most famous of which is the portal vein [9]. Due to its size, this vein is easy to handle and it is often considered to be a useful model for the study of vasomotion. However, the smooth muscle in this vein may be more related to visceral smooth muscle tissue than to smooth muscle in other blood vessels. Therefore, the process of vasomotion in the portal vein may be more comparable to intestinal peristaltic motion than to resistance vessel vasomotion.

In vitro observations of vasomotion on resistance sized isolated arterial vessels are limited to a few preparations like the mesenteric arterial arcade of the rat [19, 21], and the cerebral arteries of spontaneously hypertensive rats [16]. Figure 8.4 shows an example of spontaneous vasomotion in a mesenteric arcade vessel. During the first period of pressurization to 80 mm Hg, slow vasomotion is present. When pressure is lowered to 40 mm Hg, a myogenic response appears which resembles those discussed in the previous section. Vasomotion is no longer present. Restoration of the pressure to 80 mm Hg leads to another myogenic response, and at the same time vasomotion reappears. Increasing pressure even further induces a change in vasomotion: the amplitude decreases, while the frequency increases. This pressure dependency of vasomotion has also been established *in vivo* preparations [3].

Although vasomotion has been the subject of many studies, most of them on *in vivo* models, little is known about its physiological importance. It has been suggested that the flow alterations induced by vasomotion might be useful for the removal of plugged white blood cells. Intaglietta suggested a positive effect of vasomotion on capillary fluid exchange [8]. Vasomotion might also have a positive effect on the ability of the arterioles to control resistance. Resistance of a vessel is related to the inverse of the radius to the power of four. Hence, when the flow needs to be controlled within 4% by controlling the vessel radius, this radius has to be controlled to within 1%. With vasomotion, the inaccuracy which occurs when the flow is maintained constant by controlling vessel radius can be compensated for by varying the resistance in time, thereby controlling time averaged flow.

One should be cautious in calculating a resistance from a time averaged diameter of an arteriole when it exhibits vasomotion. Compare for instance, in a nonrealistic but easy example, a vessel which has a square wave type of vasomotion between 0 and 100 μm, and a vessel with a steady diameter of 50 μm. Both vessels have the same time averaged diameter, but the first has a conductance which is 8 times higher in the open period, resulting in a mean conductance which is 4 times higher.

Vasomotion has not yet been seen in isolated coronary arterioles. The reason for this is not clear. This may be merely due to the difference in the contractile apparatus between the two types of vessels. However, research on isolated coronary arterioles is just starting. Vasomotion may very well be able to be observed under conditions not yet examined. The observations which show that vasomotion is dependent on local transmural pressure suggest that its mechanism may be related to the mechanism of myogenic responses.

8.4 Strain and stress in the arteriolar wall

With respect to the hemodynamic implications of arteriolar mechanics, the relation between pressure and cross-sectional area is most relevant. However, the mechanical properties of the vascular wall must be considered in terms of strain and stress. By disregarding the direct effect of curvature on wall properties, the circumference may be related to radius of the arteriole by the simple geometrical consideration,

$$L_\text{w} = 2\pi[r + \frac{1}{2}d_\text{w}] \qquad [8.1]$$

where:

L_w is the circumference,
r is radius,
d_w is wall thickness.

The circumferential stress in the arteriolar wall can be related to pressure and radius by the law of LaPlace:

$$S_\text{w} = \frac{P_\text{tr} r}{d_\text{w}} \qquad [8.2]$$

where:

S_w is the wall stress,
P_tr is transmural pressure.

Equation [8.2] is a simplified form of the more general expression which should be considered when it becomes important to introduce wall mechanics [1, 15]. Since we may assume that the stress within the vessel wall is carried by fibers which remain constant in number and only vessel geometry changes, it is useful to apply the notion of tension, which can be written as $T = S_\text{w} d_\text{w}$, to our problem. This tension may be assumed to be related to the force per fiber in the wall. For the relation between tension and pressure this yields the law of LaPlace for wall tension:

$$T = Pr \qquad [8.3]$$

Within the arterial wall, three different tissue types can be identified which are able to carry force: elastin, collagen and smooth muscle. In a simplified assumption one might consider these structures to be independent in their mechanical behavior according to Equation [8.3]. The total wall tension can then be obtained

8.4 Strain and stress in the arteriolar wall

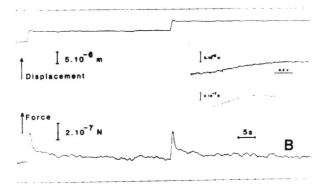

Figure 8.5: Stress relaxation of smooth muscle cells enzymatically isolated from rat aorta. The recordings are from an experiment with an initial cell length of 20.1 μm. There was no calcium in the superfusate. However, the same behavior was observed in the presence of calcium. The insert gives the second pressure step with the accompanying force at a faster scale. (From VanDijk et al. [22], by permission of authors and American Physiological Society.)

by adding the tension in the three different structures since they are anatomically parallel. Different radii may be applied to calculate the tension in relation to transmural pressure.

It is unlikely that smooth muscle contributes to the static passive properties of the arteriolar wall. This can be concluded from a study by VanDijk et al. [22] on isolated smooth muscle cells from rat aorta and bovine circumflex arteries. In this study single smooth muscle cells could be folded over the tip of a micropipette and the two cell ends could be clamped to the bottom of a glass dish on a microscope. The micropipette was connected to a force transducer and could put tension on the cell. Displacement was measured through the microscope. A typical result of that study is illustrated in Figure 8.5. Cells could easily be extended over twice their original length without any force left to be measured by the transducer. The force increase at the start of the response died away over some seconds.

The mechanical properties of elastin and collagen in the wall become apparent when studying the cross-sectional area as a function of pressure after dilation of the smooth muscle by acetylcholine. With our preparation and using the fluorescence technique, the pressure was changed up and down according to a ramp function while cross-sectional area was continuously measured. Tension could be calculated from pressure and cross-sectional area according to Equation [8.2] as a function of diameter over a wide range of pressures. A typical result from a mesenteric arcade artery is illustrated in Figure 8.6. Note the linearity of the relationship over a wide range of radii. The vessel became very stiff when the radius was 150% of its unloaded value obtained by extrapolation. It is very prob-

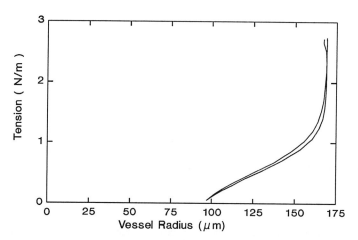

Figure 8.6: *Relation between tension and radius of passive small mesenteric arcade vessel obtained continuously by varying the pressure in ramp fashion. The slope of the curve at given diameter reflects the stiffness of the wall. Note the strong increase in stiffness after a considerable extension of the vessel.*

able that the distensible part is dominated by the elastin fibers and the stiffer region by the collagen.

The tension that can be generated spontaneously by the smooth muscle cells becomes apparent when comparing the pressure–cross-sectional area relationships of vessels with and without tone. The results of a series of experiments obtained by a protocol illustrated in Figures 8.2 and 8.4. are provided in the left panel of Figure 8.7. The curve related to the active vessels increased when pressure was raised from 20 to 40 mm Hg, as occurred with the coronary vessel shown in Figure 8.3. However, cross-sectional area decreases myogenically when pressure is raised from 60 to 100 mm Hg. Note that at a pressure of 20 mm Hg, the active curve coincides with the passive curve, which agrees with the finding that smooth muscle cells in the arteriolar wall can be completely relaxed by a reduction in transmural pressure.

The total tension within the wall can be calculated from the active curve depicted in the left panel of Figure 8.7. It can be considered to be the resulting tension developed by two parallel tension bearing structures, the elastic fibers and the activated smooth muscle cell layer. Assuming that the relation between tension and radius for the passive fibers is not affected by smooth muscle contraction, the actively developed tension can be calculated by taking the difference between total and passive tension. As is clear from these calculations, the smooth muscle activity keeps vessel diameter at around 75% of its value at maximal dilatation and a distending pressure of 80 mm Hg.

8.4 Strain and stress in the arteriolar wall

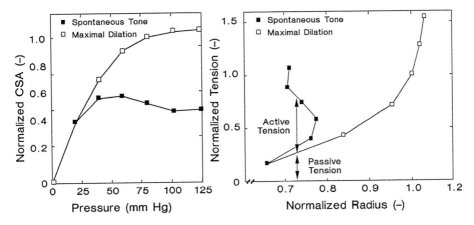

Figure 8.7: Active and passive tension in the arteriolar wall. Left: Pressure–cross-sectional area relations before (myogenic response) and after vasodilation. Right: Relations between vessel diameter and wall tension calculated from the curves depicted in the left panel. Tension is normalized to passive tension of pressure of 80 mm Hg. Forces pulling at the same object may be added. Hence, total wall tension is the sum of the tension of passive elastic and active tensions. Assuming that the relation between tension and radius for the passive fibers remains unaltered during contraction, the actively developed tension can be obtained by subtracting passive tension from total tension.

Because of technical difficulties, measurements on arterioles with diameters smaller than 50 µm are not yet available. It is tempting to extrapolate from the results obtained on larger vessels to these smaller ones. Let us try to do so for the passive vessels. To simplify matters, we will assume that the wall of passive vessels consists of parallel arrangements of single fibers, each having the combined properties of collagen and elastin. We shall first examine the possibility that the number of parallel elastic fibers in the wall is simply proportional to the unloaded radius, r_0, of the vessel, with proportionality constant k. The tension in each single fiber, T_{sf}, will be a function of the relative lengthening of that fiber, and therefore of the relative increase in radius of the vessel:

$$T_{sf} = f\left(\frac{r}{r_0}\right) \qquad [8.4]$$

We will assume this function to be unrelated to the vessel size. The shape of this function will resemble that of Figure 8.6, thus at higher values of r/r_0 the function increases rapidly. The number of parallel fibers equals kr_0. These parallel fibers carry the total tension in the wall:

$$T = kr_0 f\left(\frac{r}{r_0}\right) \qquad [8.5]$$

Applying the Laplace relationship leads to

$$P_{\text{tr}} = T/r \text{ or } P_{\text{tr}} = k\frac{f(r/r_0)}{(r/r_0)} \qquad [8.6]$$

Thus, under the above conditions the pressure needed to distend passive vessels by a certain fraction is constant along the vascular bed. That is, pressure–radius relationships are invariant apart from a scaling of the radius axis. Since pressure in the arterioles is lower than in the arteries, the above analysis would suggest that the arterioles are less distended with respect to their unloaded radius. Therefore, distensibility of these vessels at their *in vivo* pressure would be higher than that of the arteries.

The assumptions made above may not be very realistic. However, they may serve as a starting point for the analysis of mechanical properties of vessels of various sizes. The number of parallel fibers in the above model is proportional to both the fraction of the wall occupied by these fibers, and the wall thickness. Some information on these quantities is available from anatomical studies [17, 23]. In general, wall thickness to lumen ratio increases along the arterial bed, while the fraction of the wall occupied by elastic fibers decreases. The effects of these heterogeneities on the pressure–radius relation are opposing and the net outcome is therefore hard to predict. Hence a direct measurement of this relation in vessels along the bed remains relevant.

Figure 8.8 compares pressure–diameter relations of cannulated porcine coronary vessels of various sizes. Since information on the unloaded diameter was not available for all three vessels, the diameters have been normalized to the value at 80 mm Hg, rather than to the value at zero pressure. As can be seen, the three relationships are markedly similar, despite the 20-fold difference in diameter, and despite the normal difference in *in vivo* intravascular pressure. The comparison suggests that the passive properties of coronary vessels may be rather constant along the bed. Therefore the increasing wall thickness to lumen ratio will probably be accounted for by smooth muscle cells, rather than by elastic fibers. Figure 8.8 also depicts the average passive results of our mesenteric study. The passive properties of these vessels differ significantly from the coronary vessels. They are less stiff in the pressure range between 20–50 mm Hg than are the coronary vessels.

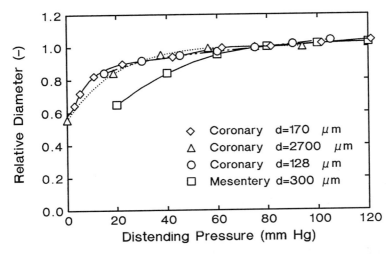

Figure 8.8: *Pressure-diameter relations of porcine coronary arteries of various sizes and mesenteric small arteries. The diameters are inner diameters. Circles: from Kuo et al. [11] diameter at 80 mm Hg was 128 μm. Diamonds: unpublished observations from our own laboratory, diameter was 170 μm. Triangles: from Nagata et al. [14], right coronary artery with a diameter of 2.7 mm. Nagata et al. published outer diameters including the ones for potassium constricted vessels. Based on our experience this vessel must have been almost fully closed, and we calculated inner diameter using the outer diameter of the closed vessel as an estimate of wall cross-sectional area. Squares: data on mesenteric vessels from our laboratory.*

8.5 Myogenic responses in relation to autoregulation of flow

Above, the myogenic response was quantified by the relation between arteriolar diameter and transmural pressure. We concluded that myogenic tone may play a role in coronary autoregulation since it causes the resistance vessels to constrict when distending pressure is elevated. However, a more quantitative prediction of the effect of spontaneous tone on pressure–flow relations requires the use of a model approach. Two very simplified models will be considered, both of which are illustrated in Figure 8.9. The first model consists of one resistance. One could say that a direct extrapolation of myogenic change in diameter of an arteriole to autoregulation of a whole organ is based on the implicit assumption of such a model. The second model consists of three resistances and is meant to evaluate the possible interaction between arterioles in series, all of which exhibit myogenic responses. Such a model would be more realistic since control of coronary resistance is distributed over arteriolar and arterial vessels with different diameters.

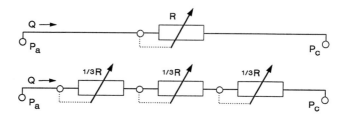

Figure 8.9: *Models for the evaluation of the role of myogenic response in the autoregulatory properties of an arterial tree. Top: Single resistance model. Bottom: Model of three resistances in series. It is assumed that the resistances, R, are related to the pressure at their inlet as can be calculated from the pressure–diameter relationships obtained from isolated arterioles. Q = flow, P_a = arterial pressure, P_c = capillary pressure.*

In this three-compartmental model each resistance is assumed to be related to the pressure at its inlet. A downstream pressure of 20 mm Hg is assumed for both models as an estimate of capillary pressure. The possible effect of flow on this pressure is ignored.

8.5.1 Relation between pressure and resistance with and without myogenic tone

The resistance of a compartment was calculated by applying the law of Poiseuille. This resistance has been normalized to its value at vasodilation and a distending pressure of 80 mm Hg. The effect of pressure on the resistance was then calculated, assuming the pressure–cross-sectional area relationship of the mesenteric arterioles as they were presented in Figure 8.7. The resulting pressure–resistance relationships are depicted in the left panel of Figure 8.10. Note that resistance increases with pressures in the range between 60 and 100 mm Hg. Such an increase in resistance is a prerequisite for the vascular bed to exhibit autoregulation. The range in which resistance increases with pressure will be referred to as the myogenic working range. When vascular tone is abolished, the resistance is strongly dependent on pressure, which is in agreement with the models on coronary flow mechanics discussed in Chapters 6 and 7. In the passive vessel, resistance becomes fairly constant at higher pressures. This is due to the stiffening of these vessels.

8.5.2 Width of the autoregulatory plateau

Pressure–flow relations for the fully dilated and autoregulated state according to the one- and three-compartmental model are depicted in Figure 8.10. The

8.5 Myogenic responses in relation to autoregulation of flow

passive pressure–flow relations of the two models exhibit a course quite similar to the experimental ones discussed in Chapter 7. There is curvature at the low pressure side of the curve which disappears when pressure is increasing.

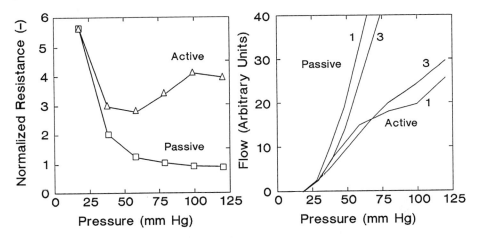

Figure 8.10: *Pressure dependency of arteriolar resistance and pressure–flow relations. Left: Resistance of a vessel with and without tone as a function of pressure. The pressure–cross-sectional area relationships for the mesenteric bed presented in Figure 8.7 are used to calculate these relations, assuming Poiseuille's law. The resistance of the vasodilated vessel at a distending pressure of 80 mm Hg was taken as unity. Note the increase of resistance when the vessels are spontaneously active between 60 and 100 mm Hg, the myogenic working range. Right: Pressure–flow relation calculated by the one-(1) and three-(3)compartmental models, assuming for each compartment the pressure–resistance relation as depicted in the left panel. Note that in the one compartment model, the pressure–flow relation for myogenic activity indeed exhibits an autoregulatory plateau. This plateau, however, disappears when more than one compartment in series is considered. Note that the pressure–flow relations for the fully dilated bed exhibit a course quite similar to the experimental and theoretical ones discussed in Chapters 5–7.*

The interpretation of the active curves is more complicated. Let us first discuss the results, taking only one compartment into consideration. The active pressure–flow relation exhibits a plateau which corresponds to the plateau in pressure–flow relations of an organ with autoregulation. However, the pressure range over which the regulation is effective seems small compared to what has been measured in physiological experiments (e.g., Chapters 1 and 9). The upper pressure limit is obviously due to the limited range over which the smooth muscles are responsive to an increase in pressure and the amount of tension that can be developed. The lower pressure limit of the autoregulatory range may be determined by two phenomena: the mechanical properties of the passive tissue in the arteriolar wall and the strength of the myogenic tone of the smooth muscle cells. This can be understood as follows. If the passive pressure–cross-sectional area curves are steeper, as a result of which the resistance of the passive vessels will fall faster with pressure, the myogenic activity can be expected to occur at lower pressures. As discussed above, the passive pressure–cross-sectional area relationships of the coronary small arteries are steeper than those of the mesentery shown here. Hence, indeed, we may look for a wider myogenic working range and hence autoregulatory plateau for the coronary vascular bed. This is also suggested by the data on coronary arterioles illustrated in Figure 8.3. On the other hand, if the myogenic tone which has developed is stronger, this may also result in a lower limit for the myogenic working range, because the active tension in the arterial wall will become zero at lower pressures.

The autoregulation predicted by the three-compartmental model is much less than with the one-compartmental model. This is due to the fact that the stimulus for myogenic constriction of the distal compartments is reduced by the pressure drop over the proximal compartments. Moreover, because of the limited myogenic working range the most distal compartment is brought into the pressure range where myogenic tone can no longer be developed. Since we know from experimental observations that flow is controlled over many arteriolar segments in series, the role of myogenic tone in autoregulation is not trivial, despite its prediction on the basis at a single arteriolar segment.

8.5.3 The optimal strength of myogenic tone

In the section above, an experimental pressure–cross-sectional area curve was taken to evaluate its predictive power for autoregulation. In this section we will evaluate some hypothesized relationships. This analysis is illustrated in Figure 8.11. In the left hand panel two hypothesized pressure–resistance relationships are depicted. The myogenic working ranges of these curves are limited only by zero cross-sectional area. Curve 1 fits the experimental data on the pressure–resistance relation depicted in Figure 8.10 when tone is present. The predicted pressure–flow relations for the one- and three-compartmental models are illustrated in the right panel of the figure. Obviously, the predicted curve for the one-compartmental model coincides with the pressure–flow relations depicted in the right panel of Figure 8.10 in the range of 60 to 100 mm Hg. The predicted pressure–flow relation shows that even when the myogenic working range is extended, the increase in resistance induced by increasing pressure via the myogenic mechanism is not strong enough to predict a wide plateau in the autoregulation curves. Moreover, the conclusion that regulation by the myogenic mechanism is diminished by having compartments in series remains a problem with this pressure–resistance relationship.

As a next step in the analysis, perfect autoregulation for the one-compartmental model was assumed as illustrated by curve 2 in the right panel in Figure 8.11. The pressure–resistance relation needed to predict perfect autoregulation was calculated. This is curve 2 in the left panel of the figure. As a next step, this pressure–resistance relation was then applied to all compartments in the three compartmental model and the pressure–flow relation was predicted. This relation coincided with the curve of the one-compartmental model and hence also exhibits perfect autoregulation. It therefore may be concluded that the attenuation of the myogenic tone by resistance vessels in series is less when myogenic tone responds more strongly to pressure.

The outcome of our analysis suggests that if autoregulation is completely caused by myogenic tone there will be a narrow range of the sensitivity of resistance to pressure. Pressure–resistance relations with a slope equal to that of curve 1 barely predict autoregulation. However, the pressure–flow relation with a slope steeper than that of curve 2 in the left panel of Figure 8.11 relation would exhibit a negative slope in the autoregulation range. Such a negative slope seems unrealistic. Collectively, it would appear both from models and experimental data that the myogenic mechanism cannot completely explain autoregulation but will play roles partly dictated by other factors.

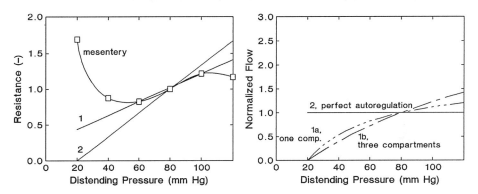

Figure 8.11: Left panel: Pressure–resistance relationships. The open squares are the same data points for the vessels with tone as were depicted in Figure 8.10. Curve 1 is the extrapolation of the myogenic working range over a wider range of pressure. Curve 2 is derived assuming perfect autoregulation with one compartment. Right panel: Pressure–flow relationships. Curves 1a and 1b refer to curve 1 in the left panel. 1a is the result of one compartment and 1b with three compartments in series. Note that autoregulation diminishes when the compartments are in series. Curve 2 exhibits perfect autoregulation and was used to calculate curve 2 in the left panel. This pressure–resistance relation was then applied to the one- and three-compartmental model. Hence, when one compartment predicts perfect autoregulation, several compartments in series will do so as well.

8.6 Compliance of arterioles

The compliance of a vessel is defined as the ratio between a change of volume and the change in distending pressure causing this volume alteration. In the experimental preparation described above, the cross-sectional area of arterioles was measured. The ratio between a change in cross-sectional area and the change in distending pressure causing the cross-sectional area change is the compliance per unit length. In our experiments on isolated vessels cross-sectional area is usually normalized to the cross-sectional area measured at a distending pressure of 80 mm Hg. In this section we will refer to the relative compliance as the ratio between the change in absolute cross-sectional area divided by the cross-sectional area at 80 mm Hg of the dilated vessel and the change in distending pressure. Relative compliance can easily be transformed into real compliance by multiplication by the volume at 80 mm Hg and at maximal vasodilation.

Distensibility equals the ratio between the relative changes in cross-sectional area and pressure. The definition of distensibility resembles that of the relative compliance defined above, except for the fact that the cross-sectional area change is related to the actual cross-sectional area in the former and to a fixed cross-sectional area in the latter definition.

Compliance is obviously determined by the stiffness of the vessel wall. The relation between these two quantities is provided by

$$E = \frac{2\pi r^3}{Cd} \qquad [8.7]$$

where:

- E is Hooke's elasticity modulus,
- C is compliance per unit length,
- r is radius,
- d_w is wall thickness.

The compliance of the vascular bed is an important determinant of the arterial pressure–flow relations. In Chapter 5 the input compliance for the coronary circulation was derived from input impedance measurements and the effect of tone on this quantity studied. Obviously, the input compliance is made up from the compliances of the total vascular bed. It is therefore important to gain insight into the compliance of single vessels in order to interpret data obtained on the vascular system as a whole.

8.6.1 Effect of tone on static compliance

The effect of tone on the distensibility and on the relative compliance of isolated small mesenteric arteries is illustrated in Figure 8.12. The data were obtained from the averaged data on small mesenteric arteries reported on in Figure 8.7. The data on vasodilation were obtained from the slope of the curve drawn

8.6 Compliance of arterioles

smoothly through the vasodilated data points provided in this figure. The data on vessels with intact tone were obtained from the average peak change in the relative cross-sectional area induced by a pressure step. Note that no steady state compliance in vessels with tone can be defined because of the myogenic response induced by the pressure step. The data from the vessels with tone in Figure 8.12 not only reflect the effect of pressure on the relative compliance but also the effect of tone as determined by the pressure level. The level of constriction at the pressures indicated can be derived from the reduction in cross-sectional area as defined in Figure 8.7.

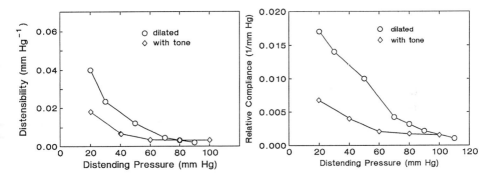

Figure 8.12: *Effect of tone on distensibility (left) and relative static compliance (right) of isolated mesenteric small arteries. The data are from the same set of experiments as depicted in Figure 8.7, top panel. Values for dilated vessels were obtained from the slope of a smooth curve drawn through the data. Relative compliances for the vessels with tone were obtained from the peak changes in cross-sectional area induced by a sudden pressure step as illustrated in Figures 8.2 and 8.4. Note that a steady state compliance with intact tone cannot be obtained since the change in pressure will alter tone.*

With vasodilation, compliance increases with decreasing pressure because the stiffness of the wall is reduced (e.g., Figure 8.6). When tone is present, compliance is lower than with vasodilation (right panel of Figure 8.12). Note that at higher pressures, the compliance of the vessel with tone is about the same as that of a vessel without tone. At 80 mm Hg, the vessels are constricted for about 50% and hence the passive elements of the vessel wall are unstretched. Compliance at pressures above 80 mm Hg is therefore determined by the smooth muscle cells. Since at 100 mm Hg relative compliance is equal for vessels with and without tone, but cross-sectional area is smaller when tone is present, one may conclude that the constricted vascular wall is less stiff than when distended at maximal vasodilation.

The compliance of the vessels with tone will approach the compliance of the dilated vessels at a pressure of around 20 mm Hg, since tone will disappear if pressure is reduced to this level, as was illustrated in Figures 8.2 and 8.7. That this is not the case in Figure 8.12 is probably due to too large a pressure step, from 20–80 mm Hg, and the rapid development of tone.

8.6.2 Quasi–static distensibility of dilated coronary arteries

Measurements of distensibility and compliance by steady state changes of pressure in cross-sectional area are not well reproduced because of the slow changes in tissue properties often referred to as creep. Therefore, a series of experiments were performed in the experimental preparation described above in which distending pressure continuously changed in ramp fashion between about 0 and 120 mm Hg. Cross-sectional area was measured continuously and distensibility was calculated as a function of pressure calculated. A typical result for a small coronary artery is illustrated in Figure 8.13.

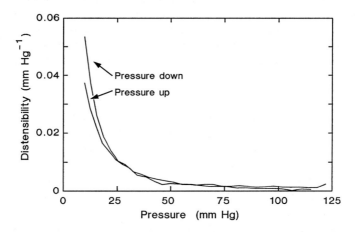

Figure 8.13: Static distensibility of a cannulated small coronary artery. Pressure was varied continuously in ramp fashion from 5 to 120 mm Hg and back in recurring cycles of about 10 minutes duration. The result shown in this figure was obtained after conditioning by 5 runs. Distensibility increases at low pressures [6].

8.6.3 Frequency dependency of distensibility of active and passive small coronary arteries

Because of the viscoelasticity of the vessel walls, the distensibility and compliance of the arterioles will be frequency dependent. This was assessed in our laboratory

8.6 Compliance of arterioles

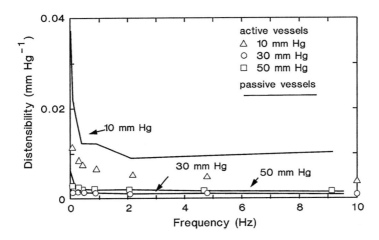

Figure 8.14: *Dynamic distensibility of a cannulated small coronary artery (diam 190 μm at 80 mm Hg and vasodilation) at vasodilation (solid curves) and at spontaneous tone (markers). These curves have been constructed by measuring the cross-sectional area variations induced by small cyclic pressure variations, superimposed on a steady state level of 10, 30 or 50 mm Hg. At a pressure of 80 mm Hg this tone resulted in a cross-sectional area reduction of 40%. The points at the ordinate represent 'static' measurements.*

by inducing very small pressure oscillations, with an amplitude of 2 mm Hg about the mean distending pressure. Relative changes in amplitudes of cross-sectional area variation divided by the amplitude of pressure variation resulted in the distensibility. The distensibility as a function of frequency of small coronary arteries is depicted for three mean distending pressures in Figure 8.14.

The lowest frequency at which distensibility was estimated was 0.1 Hz. Note that both with and without tone, distensibility at this frequency is reduced by factors of 2 to 3 with respect to the steady distensibilities at the same distending pressures. The distensibility is then practically constant over the frequency range between 1 and 10 Hz. Note that the distensibilities are only slightly affected by the presence of tone in this frequency range.

The frequency dependency of distensibility can be described by models taking into account the damping effect of the viscoelastic elements. Such models have been described for the vascular wall by, e.g., Dobrin *et al.* [4, 5] and Murphy [13].

8.7 Discussion

Understanding the mechanics of single arterioles is important to both the interpretation of coronary arterial pressure–flow lines and the control of coronary blood flow. It most certainly is too simplistic to assume that, if the properties of every single vessel are understood, the behavior of the complete system will be understood as well. The interaction between the several subsystems in the circulation adds a dimension to the problem which should not be underestimated. However, information on the properties of single vessels, functioning without interaction with their surroundings, remain an important basis for the understanding of the system as a whole.

In this chapter, data on mesenteric and coronary small arteries were mixed when assessing the role of small arteries in the coronary circulation. Moreover, it was assumed that the very small arterioles behave in a fashion similar to the larger isolated vessels. Such extrapolations are always dangerous, not so much with respect to the general properties of vessel walls but with regard to their quantification. However, caution should be exercised even when extrapolating results from arterioles obtained from the epicardium and endocardium. Kuo et al. [11] showed different myogenic behavior for the subepicardial and subendocardial small arteries. No studies have as yet been conducted on the small arteries in the mid-myocardium.

8.7.1 Vasodilation

An impressive amount of research is being done on the interpretation of coronary pressure–flow relations and flow distribution in the myocardium after complete vasodilation of the arterioles. This is being performed because the variation in arteriolar tone is an unpredictable event which considerably hampers the interpretation of coronary arterial pressure–flow signals in terms of compression by extravascular forces or elastic wall properties. The mechanics of the arteriolar wall after pharmacologically induced dilation are obviously highly relevant to these type of studies.

There is quite a difference between the passive pressure–cross-sectional area relationships of the coronary arterioles and those of the mesenteric arterioles. This is illustrated in Figure 8.8 where the data available on these two types of small arteries are reviewed. The obvious reason for this difference must be looked for in the properties of the wall and it is reasonable to assume that the cause lies in the difference in amount of elastin and collagen tissue contained in the wall. The pressure–volume relations used for model purposes in Chapters 6 and 7 coincide very well with the passive pressure–cross-sectional area relation of the coronary arteries. At the time this relationship was deduced from data on distensibilities of several vessels in the literature. The shape of this relationship is of importance since it determines the course of the pressure–flow relations in the vasodilated bed in the arrested heart (see Figure 7.1).

The experiments reported in this chapter showed, apart from the pressure dependency, a clear effect of frequency on the distensibility of passive small arteries. Such a dependency is consistent with a viscoelastic behavior of the vascular wall. In Chapter 5, we saw that to interpret input impedance relations during long diastoles, the model had to take viscoelasticity into account. We have not yet performed model fits to our data to evaluate whether the factor describing viscoelasticity in our results would be consistent with the factor derived from input impedance measurements.

The frequency dependency of compliance was not accounted for by the models discussed in Chapters 6 and 7. Hence, one might conclude that the compliance component in the description of time varying flow signals was overestimated. However, the time dependency of resistance is a major factor in the dynamic predictions of these models. Hence the conclusions of these model studies are not seriously affected by the frequency dependence of the passive properties of the wall.

The shape of the pressure–cross-sectional area relation emphasized that care should be taken in extrapolating data obtained in one set of conditions to the other. A very important parameter is the capillary blood pressure, as the downstream pressure of the arterial tree. The cross-sectional area of small arteries and arterioles is most sensitive to vascular transmural pressure in the range of 30 mm Hg and lower. This is the normal pressure range for capillary blood pressure. The probability is high that capillary pressure will rise with increasing flow rate. Apart from the effect this may have on the mechanics of myocardial perfusion, it will elevate the downstream pressure of the arterial tree, widening and stiffening the smallest vessels from this tree and thereby lowering their resistance and compliance.

8.7.2 Arterioles and regulation of flow

The slope of the pressure–cross-sectional area ratio is of importance for the ability of the arterioles to contribute to a plateau in the autoregulation curve. Such a plateau requires vasoconstriction to occur following an increase in perfusion pressure. The analysis of the potential of the myogenic response for determining autoregulation behavior in an organ showed that this can only be effective with a negative slope of the pressure–cross-sectional area relation which has been shown to be the case with the isolated mesenteric small arteries as well as with the subepicardial arterioles. If myogenic tone were the sole mechanism responsible for autoregulation, subendocardial flow would lack such a flow regulation. It is known that, although the reserve may be exhausted at higher coronary arterial pressure in the subendocardium than in the subepicardium, there is definitely subendocardial autoregulation. The possible interactions between myogenic control and metabolic control are discussed in Chapter 9.

When smooth muscle in the arteriolar wall contracts, the distensibility of the passive elements is increased because these are shortened. The dynamic mechanical wall properties become dominant at higher levels of contraction. Decreasing distending pressure affects the arteriolar compliance via a reduction in vascular volume and via a change in vascular elastic properties. The former reduces the compliance of the vessel. The latter increases compliance by means of a reduction in tone. At very low distending pressures the passive and active pressure–compliance curves come together, and around 20 mm Hg tone in the vascular wall will have decreased completely.

8.8 Summary

Arterioles and small arteries are the 'instruments' of flow control. They function by alteration of their diameter, induced smooth muscle contraction and relaxation. The relation between wall stress and distending pressure is not unique as this is also determined by the vessel radius. The relation between stress, pressure and vessel radius is described by the law of LaPlace. Especially at high levels of contraction, the arteriolar wall is as thick as the lumen, and wall thickness must be taken into account when calculating wall stress. However, for a first order approximation the more simple thin wall formula may be used. Moreover, since the forces in the wall are carried by fiber structures, the concept of tension is appropriate.

Isolated small arteries exhibit myogenic tone and a myogenic response. The response is defined as constriction following a distending pressure increase or dilation following pressure decrease. The concept of myogenic tone refers to the arteries' ability to maintain a stable tone at a stable distending pressure. Tone may increase so much that steady state arterial diameter is actually smaller at higher pressures than at lower pressures. Such a pressure range is referred to as the myogenic working range. The potential of myogenic tone to contribute to the plateau found in autoregulation curves was evaluated. It is shown that when the slope of the pressure–cross-sectional area relation is insufficiently steep, proximal vessels exhibiting myogenic tone will reduce the stimulus for tone development in the more distal vessels. Hence, autoregulation is less likely to occur with myogenic vessels in series.

The distensibility of passive vessels increases with decreasing pressure. Coronary arteries of different resting diameter show the same dependency of normalized cross-sectional area on pressure. Passive small arteries from the mesenteric bed show a different course and are less rigid below 60 mm Hg. The small arteries all show viscoelastic behavior. Their distensibility decreases with increasing frequency. However, the largest change is in the frequency range between 0 and 0.5 Hz.

References

[1] AZUMA T, OKA S (1971) Mechanical equilibrium of blood vessel walls. *Am. J. Physiol.* **221**: 1310–1321.
[2] BAYLISS WM (1902) On the local reactions of the arterial wall to changes in internal pressure. *J. Physiol. Lond.* **28**: 220-231.
[3] BURROWS ME, JOHNSON PC (1981) Diameter, wall tension, and flow in mesenteric arterioles during autoregulation. *Am. J. Physiol.* **241** (*Heart Circ. Physiol.* **10**): H829–H837.
[4] DOBRIN PB, CANFIELD TR (1977) Identification of smooth muscle series elastic component in intact carotid artery. *Am. J. Physiol.* **232** (*Heart Circ. Physiol.* **1**): H122–H130.
[5] DOBRIN PB (1978) Mechanical properties of arteries. *Physiol. Rev.* **58**: 397–460.
[6] GIEZEMAN MJMM, VANBAVEL E, MOOIJ T, SPAAN JAE (1990) Distensibility of isolated small rat mesenteric arteries without tone. *FASEB J.*: 4(3): A587.
[7] GREENSMITH JE, DULING BR (1984) Morphology of the constricted arteriolar wall: physiological implications. *Am. J. Physiol.* **247** (*Heart Circ. Physiol.* **16**): H687–H698
[8] INTAGLIETTA M (1981) Vasomotor activity, time-dependent fluid exchange and tissue pressure. *Microvasc. Res.* **21**: 153–164.
[9] JOHANSSON B, MELLANDER S (1975) Static and dynamic components in the vascular myogenic response to passive changes in length as revealed by electrical and mechanical recordings from the rat portal vein. *Circ. Res.* **36**: 76–83.
[10] JOHNSON PC (1980) The myogenic response. In: *Handbook of Physiology. The cardiovascular system. Vascular smooth muscle.* Eds. BOHR DF, SOMLYO AP, SPARKS HV JR. Am. Physiol. Soc., Bethesda, **2 (II)** chapter 15: 409–442.
[11] KUO L, DAVIS MJ, CHILIAN WM (1988) Myogenic activity in isolated subepicardial and subendocardial coronary arterioles. *Am. J. Physiol.* **255** (*Heart Circ. Physiol.* **24**): H1558–H1562.
[12] MCHALE PA, DUBÉ GP, GREENFIELD JC JR (1987) Evidence for myogenic vasomotor activity in the coronary circulation. *Prog. Cardiovasc. Dis.* **30**: 139–146.
[13] MURPHY RA (1980) Mechanics of vascular smooth muscle. In: *Handbook of Physiology. The cardiovascular system. Vascular smooth muscle.* Eds. BOHR DF, SOMLYO AP, SPARKS HV JR. Am. Physiol. Soc., Bethesda, **2 (11)** chapter 13: 325–351.
[14] NAGATA Y, ARAKI H, TOMOIKE H, NAKAMURA M (1985) Vasoconstrictor agents correlatively alter diameter and tension development in isolated pig coronary arteries. *Basic Res. Cardiol.* **80**: 210–217.

[15] OKA S, AZUMA T (1970) Physical theory of tension in thick-walled blood vessels in equilibrium. *Biorheology* **7**: 109–117.
[16] OSOL G, HALPERN W (1988) Spontaneous vasomotion in pressurized cerebral arteries from genetically hypertensive rats. *Am. J. Physiol.* **254** (*Heart Circ. Physiol.* **23**): H28–H33.
[17] RHODIN JAG (1980) Architecture of the vessel wall. In: *Handbook of Physiology. The cardiovascular system. Vascular smooth muscle.* Eds. BOHR DF, SOMLYO AP, SPARKS HV JR. American Physiological Society, Bethesda, **2 (II)** chapter 1: 1–29.
[18] UCHIDA E, BOHR DF (1969) Myogenic tone in isolated perfused resistance vessels from rats. *Am. J. Physiol.* **216**: 1343–1350.
[19] VANBAVEL E (1989) *Metabolic and myogenic control of blood flow studied on isolated small arteries.* PhD Thesis. University of Amsterdam, The Netherlands.
[20] VANBAVEL E, MOOIJ T, GIEZEMAN MJMM, SPAAN JAE (1990) Cannulation and continuous cross-sectional area measurement of small blood vessels. *J. Pharmacol. Meth.* **24**: 219-227.
[21] VANBAVEL E, GIEZEMAN MJMM, MOOIJ T, SPAAN JAE (1991) Influence of pressure alterations on tone and vasomotion of isolated mesenteric small arteries of the rat. *J. Physiol.* in press.
[22] VANDIJK AM, WIERINGA PA, VANDERMEER M, LAIRD JD (1984) Mechanics of resting isolated single vascular smooth muscle cells from bovine coronary artery. *Am. J. Physiol.* **246** (*Cell Physiol.* **15**): C277–C287.
[23] ZWEIFACH BW (1961) The structural basis of the microcirculation. In: *Development and structure of the microcirculation.* Ed. LUISADA AA. McGraw-Hill, New-York: 198–205.

Chapter 9

Static and dynamic analysis of local control of coronary flow

JENNY DANKELMAN, ISABELLE VERGROESEN and JOS AE SPAAN

9.1 Introduction

CORONARY FLOW IS CONTROLLED by the myocardium at the tissue level. This local control can be characterized by two manifestations: the adaptation of blood flow to the level of oxygen consumption and the relative independence of blood flow from coronary arterial pressure. The former manifestation is referred to as flow adaptation to metabolism, the latter one as autoregulation. Alternative terms for flow adaptation to metabolism found in the literature are metabolic regulation and functional hyperemia. However, autoregulation may also be mediated by metabolic processes and therefore metabolic regulation is an ambiguous term. Hyperemia means 'increased blood flow' and consequently hyperemia implies the definition of a standard control value of flow. The term flow adaptation to metabolism, or simply flow adaptation, expresses the ability of the coronary system to adapt flow to metabolic needs of the heart, and is the term further used here.

An important question is whether or not flow adaptation and autoregulation are manifestations of the same control loop or different ones. One could argue, for example, that autoregulation is the result of a myogenic mechanism (Chapter 8) and flow adaptation due to a vasodilator (or constrictor), related to metabolism.

Hence, the two manifestations of flow control would then be the result of two independent processes. A major argument against this is the apparently well-defined relation between flow, pressure and oxygen consumption. In view of this relation, it is unlikely that these two manifestations of coronary control are unrelated. Also, the two processes could be countereffective to one other as illustrated in the example below.

If oxygen consumption is increased by cardiac work, resulting in an increase of arterial pressure, the metabolic signal would cause vasodilation; however, the concomitant increase in pressure would result in a signal to attempt to maintain flow constant by vasoconstriction. Hence, there must be a balance between the two submechanisms otherwise the net effect could either be a vasodilation or a vasoconstriction.

The notion of flow control implies that flow itself is a controlled variable, meaning that it is somehow measured and that action is taken to adjust the flow when it deviates from a preset value. Some basic problems are related to this concept. In the first place, as it is clear from above, flow is coupled to oxygen consumption and hence the preset value of flow must be related to this variable. Secondly, a mechanism must be present that is flow sensitive and able to alter smooth muscle tone. There are mechanisms in the arteriolar wall that affect arteriolar smooth muscle [36], and are flow sensitive. However, flow induces vasodilation and results in positive feedback whereas a negative feedback is needed. Careful scrutiny of the problem reveals that there is no reason why flow should be the controlled variable. Many other variables are involved such as tissue oxygen tension, tissue adenosine concentration, tissue pH, and diameters of arterioles.

Each of the variables involved can be viewed as the potential controlled variable and flow would then be the result of this process. Hence, if tissue oxygen tension is the controlled variable – a serious possibility which will be considered below – one should speak of local control of tissue oxygen tension. The reason for referring to control of flow is because it is a variable which is easily measured and also because of the fact that the actual controlled variable has not yet been identified.

This chapter will first characterize the control of coronary flow by some typical experimental results. Then it will be shown that a majority of these static and dynamic characteristics can be explained on the basis of a model based on the assumption that tissue P_{O_2} is the controlled variable. The same model approach will be used to evaluate the potency of adenosine to control flow. Finally, the experimental evidence for the involvement of the myogenic mechanism will be evaluated.

9.2 Steady state behavior of flow control

Experimentally, the effects of oxygen consumption and perfusion pressure are best studied in a preparation with a cannulated coronary artery. This is because interventions to alter oxygen consumption by stimulating cardiac action often alter arterial pressure. Moreover, altering coronary perfusion pressure affects the mechanical performance of the heart such that it alters its oxygen consumption, an effect referred to as Gregg effect [27]. This coupling between oxygen consumption and coronary arterial pressure makes it imperative that the study of regulation of coronary flow should be done under well-controlled conditions in respect of both oxygen consumption and perfusion pressure.

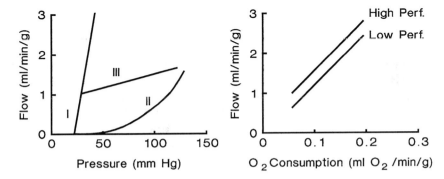

Figure 9.1: Schematic illustration of the static behavior of local coronary control. Left: Illustration of pressure–flow relations. III is the pressure–flow relation at a hypothetical constant oxygen consumption. Note the pressure–flow relations at maximal vasodilation (I) and maximal vasoconstriction (II). These two curves mark the pressure–flow area in which arteriolar smooth muscle tone can change to affect flow. See text for a further explanation. Right: Illustration of the relation between oxygen consumption and coronary flow with perfusion pressure as a parameter. Note that flow is linearly but not proportionally related to oxygen consumption.

Perfusion of the heart is tightly coupled to its oxygen needs and is only weakly determined by perfusion pressure. These basic characteristics of coronary flow control, however, only hold true within a limited range of perfusion pressures. Some typical experimental results on steady state flow control were presented in Chapter 1. Here the basic characteristics are schematically presented in Figure 9.1.

If, at a hypothetically fixed level of oxygen consumption, the coronary arterial pressure should change from venous pressure to a value of, for example, 160 mm Hg, three trajectories I, II and III could be recognized. Trajectory I reflects the range where the arterioles are maximally dilated because of hypoxic vasodilation. The curve for maximal vasodilation is discussed in Chapters 7 and 8. In trajectory II, the vasomotor tone is maximally stimulated and flow is dependent on pressure. Not much data is available on the curve of maximal vasoconstriction, making this curve highly speculative in the lower pressure range. The curves for maximal vasodilation and maximal vasoconstriction define the area where flow can be truly controlled by altering vasomotor tone. The effect of control of vasomotor tone is indicated by trajectory III. This trajectory is called the autoregulatory plateau of the coronary pressure–flow relation. If oxygen consumption is brought to a new, but higher level the plateau will be above, but parallel, to the one at control oxygen consumption and be limited by the pressure–flow relations of the maximally dilated and maximally constricted vascular bed.

If oxygen consumption is altered at constant perfusion pressure, the relation between flow and oxygen consumption will be linear. These relations will shift in parallel if perfusion pressure is altered, as is illustrated in the right hand panel of Figure 9.1.

In experiments with a cannulated left main coronary artery the following correlation formula was found to describe trajectory III in the coronary pressure–flow relation

$$\mathrm{CBF} = a\mathrm{MVO}_2 + bP_p + c \qquad [9.1]$$

The numeric values of the constants a, b and c are critically analyzed in the discussion to this chapter (Section 9.10.1) and summed up in Table 9.1.

9.3 Characteristics of dynamic coronary flow control

In accordance with the static analysis of coronary flow control presented above, two very different basic dynamic responses may be distinguished:

1. the response to a sudden change in oxygen consumption and

2. the response to a sudden change in the perfusion of the heart, either by change in flow at constant pressure or change in pressure at constant flow.

The former constitutes the dynamic characterization of flow adaptation and the latter that of autoregulation. Experiments according to these protocols have been systematically performed in our laboratory using an open chest anesthetized goat preparation with a cannulated left main coronary artery. The dynamic responses were measured at either constant pressure or at constant flow. We decided to compare these two different perfusion conditions, since the tissue P_{O_2} model discussed below predicted that there would be a difference. This expectation of a difference in rate of response is based on the knowledge that when flow is kept constant, the feedback loop of flow control is cut open. The dynamic responses were also measured at different levels of either perfusion pressure or flow since nonlinearities in the control system were expected. This nonlinear behavior would be evidenced by the dependency of the response on the magnitude of either perfusion or oxygen consumption. The alterations in pressure, flow and heart rate were moderate. Pressure and flow underwent changes in the order of 20%. Heart rate changes were in the order of 30 beats · min^{-1}.

A comparison of the rate of change of all these responses requires the definition of a dependent variable which can be determined from the experimental signals. Preferably, a variable reflecting the time varying resistance effective in controlling flow should be used, hence arteriolar resistance. However, for a system with compliances it is not possible to deduce the resistance component of the circuit from arterial pressure and flow signals alone. In order to allow comparison of the dynamic responses of the coronary system to different perturbations, we resorted to the application of an index. This index was the relative change in the ratio between pressure and flow measured in the coronary artery. We calculated the response of this index to a perturbation in two steps. First, the beat averaged values of pressure and flow and the ratio between the two were calculated for the response in which a control period before the perturbation, and a control period after the effect of the perturbation had faded away, were included. This ratio reflects the coronary resistance in the steady state. The index per beat was subsequently calculated by

$$\mathrm{BCI} = \frac{\overline{P(t)/Q(t)} - \overline{P_i/Q_i}}{\overline{P_e/Q_e} - \overline{P_i/Q_i}} \qquad [9.2]$$

where $\overline{P(t)/Q(t)}$ is the ratio between arterial pressure and flow both averaged per beat. $\overline{P_i/Q_i}$ and $\overline{P_e/Q_e}$ are the pressure/flow ratios measured in the control conditions before and at the end of the interventions (e.g., Equation [1.2]).

The practical advantage of this dimensionless index is that the rate of change of the different perturbations can easily be compared, since this always starts at zero and always ends at unity. An increase in heart rate will result in a vasodilation, leading to a decrease in the pressure–flow ratio. A reduction in heart rate will result in a vasoconstriction and hence an increase in pressure–flow ratio. The index, however, increases from zero to unity in both conditions, enabling the time responses to be superimposed. This makes slight differences between the responses to different interventions visible. An extra advantage of the index is that it masks variations in experimental conditions which would make a comparison of nonnormalized data complicated.

The strength of the index approach for the dynamic response of coronary flow control has been shown by Belloni and Sparks [3]. These authors showed that the BCI–time response was slightly different if this resulted from an increase in heart rate or a decrease in heart rate. This difference points to a directional sensitivity in the response of the coronary system, a sensitivity not expected to be found in linear control systems in which these responses would have been found to be identical.

The introduction of a dimensionless index for the evaluation of time dependent processes is not exclusive to the field of coronary research. In engineering it has found general application, not only in control engineering but also in problems of heat and mass transfer.

9.3.1 Rate of change in flow adaptation

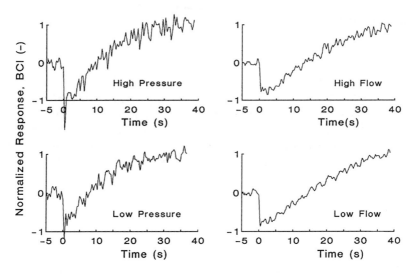

Figure 9.2: Summary of the dynamic change in normalized pressure/flow ratios, BCI, as a result of heart rate changes. BCI is defined by Equation [9.2]. Left panels are results obtained with constant pressure perfusion and right panels with constant flow perfusion. Upper panels show the average results of all experiments with high pressure and high flow and bottom panels show average results obtained with low pressure and low flow. (Redrawn from Dankelman et al. [8].)

The dynamic changes of normalized pressure–flow relations in response to the heart rate change in 7 goats with 156 interventions are grouped in Figure 9.2 [8]. The basic characteristic of the four averaged responses are similar. After the change in heart rate, there is a sudden initial reversed response. With an increase in heart rate, an increasing index reflects a decreasing resistance if no compliance effects are involved. The initial reversed response can be explained by a sudden increase in resistance due to the increased heart rate. This increased resistance is plausible and can be explained by the theories discussed in Chapters 6 and 7 for the fully dilated vascular bed. The extravascular resistance and waterfall model would explain this increase of time averaged pressure/flow ratio by a reduced diastolic time fraction. This would also partly be the explanation of the nonlinear intramyocardial pump model based on tissue pressure as well as elastance. However, part of the initial reversed response is certainly also due to capacitive effects. An increase in heart rate increases compression of the intramyocardial blood space. This, in turn, causes transiently increased arterial pressure at constant flow or transiently decreased flow at constant pressure.

Comparison of the panels clearly shows that the rate of response of the index is faster at constant perfusion pressure than at constant flow perfusion. Also, it is obvious from the figure that at constant flow perfusion, the level of flow has almost no effect on the dynamic response. However, an effect of the level of pressure is found at constant pressure perfusion. At lower pressure, 80 mm Hg, the response is faster than at higher pressure, 120 mm Hg. In other words, the response at constant flow is consistent with a linear control system, while at constant pressure perfusion the system acts in a nonlinear fashion.

The experiments confirmed the finding of Belloni and Sparks [3] that rate of change of the coronary index BCI is a little faster if heart rate is increased than if this is decreased. The time needed for half the response to be completed is about 9% shorter when heart rate is increased. In Figure 9.2, the directional sensitivity is neglected and the results from an increase in heart rate are pooled with the responses to a decrease in heart rate.

9.3.2 Rate of change of autoregulation

The dynamic changes of normalized pressure–flow relations in response to the pressure and flow changes for 7 goats with a total of 113 interventions are summarized in Figure 9.3. At constant pressure perfusion, a decrease in pressure will initiate a vasodilation. As the dynamic response to heart rate change, BCI exhibits an initial reversed response of flow adjustment; the index first decreases, later followed by an increase. Again, this initial reversed response is the combined effect of the emptying of the intramyocardial compliance vessels due to the decreased arterial pressure and increased resistance as a result of the decreasing volume of the arterial bed. The initial reversed response in the other interventions can be explained by the same combination of compliance and resistance changes. It is clear from this figure that step changes in perfusion have a profound directional effect on the BCI response of goats. Especially at constant pressure perfusion, the response to a decrease in pressure is completely different from the response to an increase in pressure. If pressure is decreased, the index rises sharply after the initial dip and elicits an overshoot. The directional sensitivity is also present at constant flow perfusion, albeit less pronounced. The overshoot is not seen in the response to a reduction of flow with flow perfusion. The directional effect will be discussed in section 9.7.

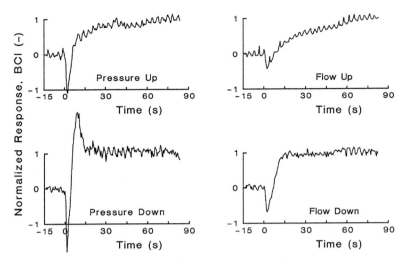

Figure 9.3: *Summary of the dynamic change of normalized pressure/flow ratios as a result of pressure and flow step changes. BCI is defined by Equation [9.2]. Left panels depict the results with constant pressure perfusion and right panels with constant flow perfusion. Upper panels show the averaged results of all experiments with a step-up in perfusion and the bottom panels with a step-down in perfusion. (Redrawn from Dankelman et al. [10].)*

9.3.3 Summary of t_{50} values

The response rates of flow adjustment and autoregulation were characterized by the time the pressure or flow responses needed to reach half of their final values; BCI = 1/2. These t_{50} values for the goat are summarized in Figure 9.4. The t_{50} values for the different interventions are purposely grouped according to perfusion condition (4 bars with constant pressure perfusion and 4 bars with constant flow perfusion) first, and then in a combination of perfusion change and heart rate change. Four pairs of bars can be recognized in this figure. Each pair should relate to either vasoconstriction or vasodilatation, e.g., an increase in perfusion and decrease in heart rate should both result in vasoconstriction. If a single control loop were responsible for the flow control, the t_{50} values could be expected to be the same for the paired responses. This seems to be true for the vasoconstriction induced by perfusion increase or heart rate decrease. However, vasodilation induced by a perfusion decrease is much faster than when it results from a heart rate increase under the same perfusion condition.

As is clear from the diagram, the rates of response of autoregulation when perfusion is increased are equivalent to the rate of response of flow adjustment. However, the index changes more rapidly if this is induced by a reduction in

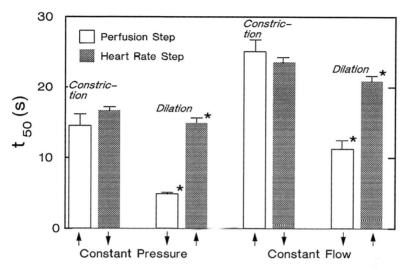

Figure 9.4: Bar diagram summarizing the t_{50} values of the index response in goat hearts to the different interventions. The left four bars are the results of experiments with constant pressure perfusion, the right four bars with constant flow perfusion. The arrow under the bar indicates whether the bar refers to an increase (arrow ↑) or decrease (arrow ↓) of perfusion or heart rate. Bars are grouped in pairs according to resulting vasoconstriction or vasodilatation and should be equal if controlled by the same control loop. t_{50} with a decrease in perfusion differed significantly from t_{50} with an increase in heart rate under the same conditions (denoted by *).

perfusion, and especially at constant pressure perfusion.

The interpretation of the condition dependency of the rate of change of the coronary index will be postponed until after the models on coronary flow control have been discussed. Recently, the same protocols were repeated in the anesthetized dog, applying the same techniques. It appeared that the general picture outlined above also holds for the dog but that the t_{50} values for the dog are about 2 to 3 times smaller than for the goat. No cause for this large discrepancy in dynamic behavior has yet been identified. In this respect, it must be underlined that the steady behavior of flow control for the dog is no different from that of the goat and that the differences in control behavior are specific for the dynamics of the control system.

The rates of metabolic adaptation and autoregulation are not compatible with the rapid responses in diastolic coronary index induced by a single ventricular extra activation [48] or a brief diastolic occlusion [47] respectively. Part of these rapid responses might have been due to the changes in coronary arterial pressure that may induce a change in index without change in arteriolar tone as was discussed in relation to Figure 1.6.

9.4 Rate of change in myocardial oxygen consumption

For the interpretation of the dynamics of flow adjustment to metabolism it is necessary to have some insight into the rate by which oxygen consumption changes. To this end, we studied the rate of change in myocardial oxygen consumption in the goat induced by cardiac arrest [57]. Periods of cardiac arrest could be induced by cessation of pacing since the bundle of His had been destroyed by the injection of Formalin. We chose to use cardiac arrest as an intervention in order to maximize the absolute values of oxygen consumption change to improve the signal to noise ratio. The preparation was essentially similar to that used in the experiments above, except that here an extra cannula was inserted in the great cardiac vein. The difference between coronary arterial and venous oxygen saturation was continuously measured, using an AVOX-instrument [49]. Since oxygen consumption and flow are changing, the Fick principle may not be applied to calculate oxygen consumption. Steady state is a major requirement for this application.

9.4.1 Model for the correction of changing oxygen buffers

The calculation of steady state oxygen uptake from flow and arterial-venous oxygen content difference is known as the Fick method. The Fick equation yielding the oxygen consumption can be written as

$$\mathrm{MVO_2} = \mathrm{CBF}[\mathrm{O}_{2a} - \mathrm{O}_{2v}] \qquad [9.3]$$

where:

$\mathrm{MVO_2}$ is the oxygen consumption in ml $\mathrm{O}_2 \cdot \mathrm{s}^{-1}$,
O_{2a} and O_{2v} are the arterial and venous oxygen contents, in ml O_2 per ml blood,
CBF   is the coronary flow in ml $\cdot \mathrm{s}^{-1}$.

However, the Fick equation may not be applied during dynamic conditions. In dynamic conditions, the amounts of oxygen stored in tissue and coronary blood may change and erroneously be interpreted as changes in oxygen consumption. A model taking the dynamic changes of the amount of stored oxygen into account was presented by Vergroesen and Spaan [57] and also by VanBeek and Elzinga [53]. The first method will be given here.

The model by which the transients in flow and arterial–venous oxygen content differences can be interpreted is depicted in Figure 9.5. The model distinguishes

9.4 Rate of change in myocardial oxygen consumption

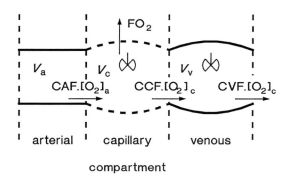

Figure 9.5: A model of the coronary circulation allowing the calculation of the dynamic change in oxygen consumption from time varying arterial flow and arterial-venous oxygen content difference. Apart from the tissue compartment the model also distinguishes two blood compartments, the capillary and venous compartments. The rotor blades indicate that the compartments are well-mixed. The FO_2 is the rate by which oxygen leaves the capillary space and apart from small changes in tissue oxygen content equals total mitochondrial oxygen consumption (MVO_2). It is assumed that oxygen pressure is so high that myoglobin remains saturated with oxygen. For abbreviations see text.

three compartments. The first is the tissue compartment in which oxygen is consumed. The second is the capillary compartment in which oxygen exchange occurs with the tissue compartment. The third and last compartment is the venous compartment. This compartment acts as dead space. Dynamic mass balance equations can be derived for the two vascular compartments. For the capillary compartment, the following oxygen balance equation can be derived:

$$FO_2 = CAFO_{2a} - CCFO_{2c} + \frac{d(V_c O_{2c})}{dt} \qquad [9.4]$$

where:

FO_2	is the oxygen leaving the capillary space and entering the tissue space,
CAF and CCF	are the flow entering and leaving the capillary space,
O_{2a} and O_{2c}	are the arterial and capillary oxygen content,
V_c	is the volume of the capillary blood space.

On the right hand side of the equation, the first term represents the oxygen flow into the capillary space and the second term the oxygen flow leaving the capillary space. The third term is the rate of change of the amount of oxygen contained within the capillary blood.

The oxygen balance equation of the third compartment is quite similar to that of the capillary space, only here it is assumed that no oxygen leaves the compartment by diffusion:

$$0 = \text{CCFO}_{2c} - \text{CVFO}_{2v} + \frac{d(V_v O_{2v})}{dt} \qquad [9.5]$$

where:

V_v is the volume of the venous bed,
O_{2v} is the venous oxygen content,
CVF coronary venous flow.

A mass balance equation also holds for the tissue compartment. However, this equation does not contain a term related to convective oxygen transport.

$$\text{MVO}_2 + \frac{d(V_t O_{2t})}{dt} = \text{FO}_2 \qquad [9.6]$$

where:

V_t is the volume of tissue,
O_{2t} is tissue oxygen content.

The above equations are complicated by the need to account for the volume change in the different compartments [50], which is due to different circumstances. The equations, however, can be simplified because the volume changes are small and the rate of change in the oxygen content of tissue is generally small compared to oxygen consumption. These simplifications are discussed in Appendix C. The resulting equation is

$$\text{MVO}_2 = \text{CAF}[O_{2a} - O_{2v}] - [V_v + V_c]\frac{dO_{2v}}{dt} - \frac{V_v V_c}{\text{CVF}} \frac{d^2(O_{2v})}{dt^2} \qquad [9.7]$$

9.4.2 Transients in oxygen consumption

The oxygen consumption as a function of time after arresting the heart can be calculated using Equation [9.7] from the time dependent coronary arterial flow and arterial-venous oxygen content difference. Results are summarized in Figure 9.6. As is clear from the top panel of this figure, coronary venous oxygen saturation in the transient condition is not a good representation of the capillary oxygen saturation. Obviously, the discrepancy is a function of the magnitude of coronary flow. At higher values of coronary flow this difference is smaller than at lower values of coronary flow. However, it was found that the rate of change in oxygen consumption was not really dependent on the level of coronary flow, which is a strong point in favor of the analysis. There is no physiological reason for the rate of change in oxygen consumption to be dependent on flow rate.

9.5 Rate of change in myocardial oxygen consumption

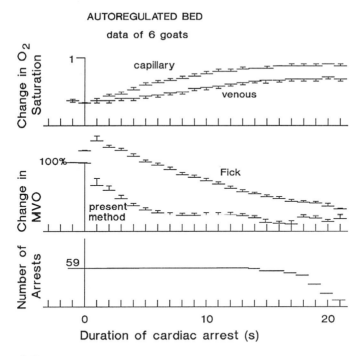

Figure 9.6: *The decrease of oxygen consumption during long diastoles in the goat. Bottom: Number of long diastoles used in calculating the average values in the top panels as function of time. Middle: The time dependency of oxygen consumption corrected for the rate of change of buffered oxygen in capillary and venous blood (mean ± S.E.). The line indicated by 'Fick' is the calculated oxygen consumption without correction for the change of buffered oxygen. Top: Average decrease in measured coronary venous oxygen saturation. Also shown is the calculated time dependency of capillary oxygen saturation (Redrawn from Vergroesen [57].)*

As is clear from Figure 9.6, myocardial oxygen consumption changes slowly, with a time needed to reach half of its maximum change in the order of 3.8 seconds. This value is close to the one reported by VanBeek and Elzinga [53] estimated on Tyrode perfused rat hearts.

In the experimental series discussed in this section, oxygen consumption decreased to about 20% of the control value before cardiac arrest. In absolute numbers, the oxygen consumption of the nonworking heart was 15 μl $O_2 \cdot [100\ g]^{-1} \cdot s^{-1}$. This is about the same as reported by Gibbs et al. [20] for the potassium arrested heart.

9.5 Oxygen model of coronary flow control

9.5.1 Model definition and equations

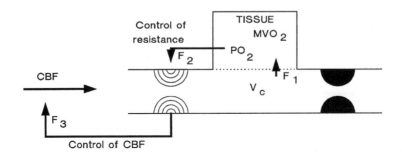

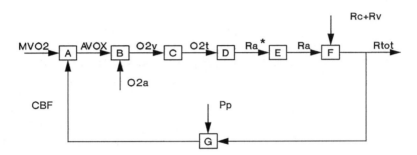

Figure 9.7: *Oxygen control model of the coronary circulation. The top panel depicts a schematic of the signals involved. F1 is the oxygen supply from blood to tissue. F2 represents the adaptation of the arteriolar resistance to a change in tissue P_{O_2}. F3 represents the change in CBF after a change in resistance. Bottom panel shows a block diagram of the control loop. For explanation see text.*

In the oxygen model presented here [8, 12, 55], tissue P_{O_2} is assumed to be the controlled factor. A further basic assumption is that tissue P_{O_2} determines coronary resistance. It has not been specified whether P_{O_2} controls resistance directly [18] or by means of a metabolic intermediate [19].

Coronary regulation is thought to take place as illustrated in the top panel of Figure 9.7. The resistance is thought to be related to the tissue P_{O_2}. It is assumed that the tissue can be described as a well-mixed compartment, so that coronary venous P_{O_2} reflects tissue P_{O_2}. Autoregulation can then be explained in the following way. Tissue P_{O_2} is affected by coronary flow. An increase in flow is equivalent to an increase in oxygen supply, which means that tissue P_{O_2} will increase. Hence, if coronary flow is increased by a disturbance above an equilib-

9.5 Oxygen model of coronary flow control

rium value, coronary resistance will increase so that flow is once again reduced to its equilibrium value. Flow adaptation to metabolism will be effectuated as follows. An increase in metabolism will cause tissue P_{O_2} to decrease and hence result in a lowering of coronary resistance in order to increase flow to match the increased oxygen demand.

The bottom panel in Figure 9.7 depicts the stream diagram of the signals. The equation related to block A is

$$\frac{\text{MVO}_2}{\text{CBF}} = \text{AVOX} \qquad [9.8]$$

with AVOX = the arterial–venous oxygen content difference.

In block B the arterial–venous difference is subtracted from the arterial oxygen content, yielding the venous oxygen content. In steady state, the venous oxygen pressure equals the tissue oxygen pressure; however, this equilibration will take some time. This is illustrated by block C in the diagram. The effect is simulated by a first order process. A step change in venous oxygen pressure will result in an exponential response of tissue oxygen pressure, ending in the equality of both quantities. Tissue oxygen pressure is the controlling signal for the coronary resistance. However, resistance will lag behind a change in this controlling signal because of the time required for the process of adjustment of smooth muscle tone (block D). This adjustment process is also simulated by a first order process (block E). The time constant of this process is 15 s. Total coronary resistance is the sum of the arteriolar resistance and the resistance of the capillary and venous resistances. This addition is illustrated by the summation block F. Block G illustrates how coronary flow and total resistance are related via the perfusion pressure,

$$\text{CBF} = \frac{P_p}{R_{\text{tot}}} \qquad [9.9]$$

The loop is now closed since flow forms the input for block A that has been discussed above.

9.5.2 Steady state solutions

In steady state the model equations result in the same equation as the empirical Equation [9.1] describing autoregulation curves at different oxygen consumption rates. These curves run parallel, depending on the factor a. Similarly, the curves relating coronary flow to oxygen consumption at various different perfusion pressures also run parallel. Equation [9.1] was fitted to experimental results obtained in dogs and goats by Vergroesen *et al.* [56]. Experimental values of the three coefficients are provided in Table 9.1.

9.5.3 Dynamic solutions of the oxygen model

In addition to the parameters needed for the steady state solution, the dynamic solution requires estimates of the two time constants. The time constant for the equilibration of tissue P_{O_2} can be estimated from the ratio between the oxygen buffering capacity of the heart tissue and the rate of oxygen influx. The oxygen buffering capacity of tissue can be calculated from the oxygen stored by the blood and the oxygen stored in the extravascular space. The amount of capillary blood in 100 g heart tissue is about 6 ml. With an oxygen carrying capacity of 10 ml $O_2 \cdot$ [100 ml blood]$^{-1}$, the oxygen storage capacity of blood in 100 g tissue is about 0.6 ml O_2. The solubility of oxygen in tissue is about 2.8×10^{-5} ml $O_2 \cdot$ ml tissue$^{-1} \cdot$ mm Hg^{-1}. Hence the storage capacity of the tissue by solubility is 0.01 ml $O_2 \cdot$ [100 g tissue]$^{-1}$. The storage capacity of myoglobin (see Chapter 11) in the tissue is not taken into account because we assume that the tissue P_{O2} will remain at such a level that these stores will always remain full. The flow of oxygen into the heart is assumed to be 0.16 ml $O_2 \cdot s^{-1} \cdot$ [100 g tissue]$^{-1}$. By dividing oxygen storage capacity by oxygen flow we arrive at a value of 4 s for this time constant. Obviously, this value is only an estimate and depends on the flow rate.

The second time constant must account for the rate by which arteriolar resistance adapts to a change in P_{O_2}. There is not much data on this point. We quite arbitrarily assumed a value of 20 sec [8]. Solutions of the model to a sudden

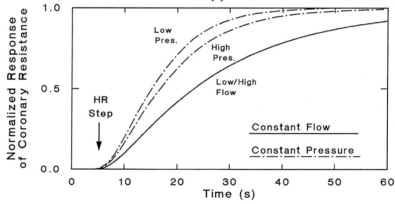

Figure 9.8: *Response of the coronary resistance to a change in oxygen consumption according to the oxygen model of coronary control. Dotted curves are normalized responses at two levels of pressure perfusion. The lower solid curve shows the response at two levels of flow perfusion. Constant pressure perfusion shows a faster response and is dependent on the level of pressure. Constant flow perfusion shows a slower response with the speed independent of the level of flow. (Redrawn from [8].)*

change in MVO_2 are presented in Figures 9.8 and 9.9. In order to facilitate the

9.5 Oxygen model of coronary flow control

comparison with the experimental results, the model predictions are presented in terms of the coronary index and are plotted as a function of time. Figure 9.8 depicts the model prediction for the dynamic response of flow adjustment to a change in metabolism. The dynamic responses of autoregulation are depicted in Figure 9.9. Two perfusion conditions were studied: constant flow and constant pressure perfusion.

The dynamic responses of both flow adjustment and autoregulation differ from the experimental results in that they lack the initial reversed response. This difference is due to a limitation of the model, because the mechanical interaction between myocardial contraction and coronary flow is not accounted for. Apart from the initial period, the model does predict the dependence of the rate of response in experimental conditions. In the first place, the response at constant pressure perfusion is faster than at constant flow perfusion. In the second place, the model also predicts a response rate independent of the level of perfusion with constant flow perfusion. As with the experiments, the rate of response at constant pressure perfusion is faster at lower perfusion pressure than at high perfusion pressure.

In the model, the cause of the different responses is easily found. At constant pressure perfusion, the response can be faster than at constant flow perfusion because of feedback. The feedback signal is responsible for the change of resistance and is faster when flow is allowed to vary freely. With constant flow perfusion, the flow is fixed and, as a result, the feedback limited. The model predicts a response rate independent of the level of flow at constant flow perfusion because the control model for flow perfusion is linear. Hence the responses behave according to the rules of a linear system, which would imply independence of the magnitude of flow. However, the model is not linear with constant pressure perfusion because of blocks A and G in the control diagram. The resistance is a nonlinear element when calculating flow from pressure. It is this nonlinearity which causes the pressure dependency of the response at constant pressure perfusion only.

The model prediction for the dynamic response of autoregulation is in line with the prediction generated by the model for flow adjustment. Because the feedback present at constant pressure perfusion is absent at constant flow perfusion, the response at constant pressure perfusion is faster than at constant flow perfusion. The model again predicts that at constant flow perfusion, the response rate will be independent of the level of flow, whereas at constant pressure perfusion, the response will be faster at lower pressure than at higher pressure. Moreover, the response times are of the same order as with flow adjustment under similar conditions.

The most remarkable difference between the model and experiments is the difference found in response to a lowering of pressure or flow at constant pressure perfusion and constant flow perfusion respectively. The reduction of perfusion pressure in the experiments resulted in a flow response which was completely

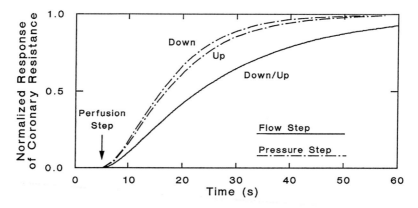

Figure 9.9: The model predictions for the dynamic response of autoregulation. Note that the model predicts a faster response for constant pressure perfusion than for constant flow perfusion. With constant pressure perfusion, the response is a little faster when pressure is decreased. (Redrawn from Dankelman [10].)

different and much faster than predicted by the model. The conclusion that must be drawn is that the model still lacks an element which is essential for explaining this experimental finding.

9.5.4 Oxygen dose–response curves

Arterioles are sensitive to oxygen in their environment and blood flow in small arterioles can cease completely at an artificially increased level of P_{O_2} [51]. The relation between tissue oxygen pressure and coronary resistance, further referred to as the oxygen dose–response curve, is one that is crucial to the oxygen model. However, little is known of this relationship. From our experiments on the steady state relation between coronary flow and myocardial oxygen consumption on the one hand and perfusion pressure on the other hand, coronary resistance was calculated as a function of the coronary venous P_{O_2}. As will be discussed in Chapter 11, coronary venous P_{O_2} needs not be a good representation of tissue P_{O_2}. However, its variation might be considered to reflect the variations in tissue P_{O_2}. The experimentally found relation between coronary venous P_{O_2} and coronary resistance is depicted in the left panel of Figure 9.10. The data in the right panel are calculated from arteriolar diameter measurements obtained in hamster cheek pouch [13] and hamster cremaster muscle [21]. Relative resistance variations were obtained by applying Poiseuille's law. Actual resistance was divided by the calculated resistance at maximal vasodilation. Comparison between the experimental results on single vessels and the coronary bed as a whole exhibits quite a difference in sensitivity for oxygen.

An important reason for the discrepancy is that the minimum resistance of

9.5 Oxygen model of coronary flow control

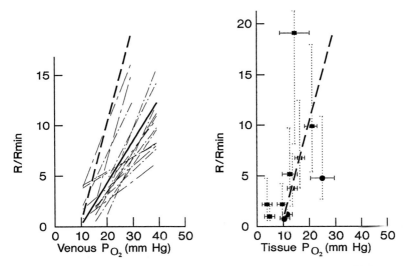

Figure 9.10: Oxygen dose–response curves. Left panel: Venous P_{O_2}–resistance relations as calculated from the data of Vergroesen et al. [56]. The heavy curve is the average of the experimental data. The broken line is the estimated curve for $R/R_{\min}$ for the coronary resistance vessels assuming that 30% of $R_{\min}$ is within the coronary capillaries and vein s. Right panel: Tissue P_{O_2}–resistance relation as calculated from the data of Gorczynski and Duling [21] (■) and of Duling [13] (●) on isolated single arterioles. Resistance was calculated from their diameter measurements using $R/R_{\min} = [D/D_{\max}]^4$. The broken line is the same as in the left panel.

the coronary bed does not only reflect the minimal resistance of the coronary arterioles but also the resistance distal to these vessels. As is illustrated in Figure 2.9 [7], a reasonable estimate of this resistance is 30% of the total. Recalculating the mean coronary oxygen dose–response curve, taking this 30% distal resistance into account, results in the broken line depicted in both panels of Figure 9.10. Hence, these broken lines represent the relative change of the coronary resistance vessels and is above the heavy line in the left panel since $R_{\min}$ for these vessels alone is smaller than for the coronary bed as a whole. Indeed, this correction does improve the agreement between the data of two so different experiments.

Our reasoning on the oxygen dose–response curves must be seen as an order of magnitude estimation. There is considerable scatter in both data sets. Moreover, in recent studies coronary resistance was studied as function of coronary venous P_{O_2}, P_{CO_2} and pH [5, 6]. These studies demonstrate that there is no unique relation between coronary resistance and coronary venous oxygen pressure. The oxygen dose–response curve is modulated by other factors.

9.6 Myocardial contraction and dynamics of coronary flow control

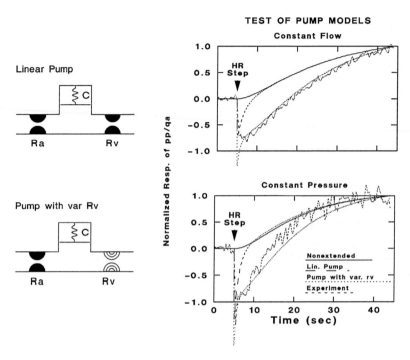

Figure 9.11: The linear and nonlinear pump models (left) evaluated for their prediction of the initial reversed response of the coronary index induced by a heart rate change (right). The noisy curves represent experimental data. The solid lines are the theoretical curves given in Figure 9.8. From the two model curves it is clear that compliance alone can not explain the initial phase completely. A resistance component depending on heart contraction is needed.

The control model based on tissue oxygen pressure did not account for the initial reversed response which was found experimentally and which must be attributed to the mechanical interaction between cardiac contraction and coronary flow. As is clear from the earlier chapters, the mechanism of interaction has not yet been established. For interpretation of the dynamics of coronary flow control, however, this interaction is crucial, not only as explanation of the reversal of index but also for the quantification of rate of vasomotor response. If the reversal can be explained completely by capacitive effects, then indeed the reference value at the start of the response, $\overline{P_i}/\overline{Q_i}$ in Equation [9.2], should be based on the pressure and flow ratio before the change in heart rate or perfusion. However,

9.6 Myocardial contraction and dynamics of coronary flow control

if the intervention induces a sudden and persisting effect on coronary resistance, then $\overline{P_i}/\overline{Q_i}$ of the first beat after initiation of the response should be taken as initial reference value. The estimates of t_{50} are strongly affected by such choice. In order to evaluate the magnitude of the dependency of t_{50} on the choice of the mechanical model, Dankelman et al. [9] quantitatively evaluated the effect of several mechanisms, namely the linear intramyocardial pump model, the nonlinear intramyocardial pump model (or tissue pressure model) and the waterfall model.

This evaluation was done by modifications of the oxygen control model as depicted in Figure 9.7. The capillary space was incorporated to evaluate the effect of intramyocardial compliance and the distal resistance was either kept constant (linear intramyocardial pump model), was volume dependent (nonlinear intramyocardial pump model) or designed to behave as a waterfall (pure waterfall model or waterfall-intramyocardial compliance combination). The two intramyocardial pump models are illustrated and evaluated in Figure 9.11. The evaluations have been done only for the response to a sudden change in heart rate.

With the addition of the intramyocardial compliance, the model is able to explain the inverse response because the increase in heart rate augments the time averaged compression of the intramyocardial vessels. The higher compression is expressed in a transiently reduced inflow at constant pressure perfusion and an increase in arterial pressure at constant flow perfusion. However, as was illustrated in Chapters 1 and 7, the characteristic time for events related to intramyocardial volume changes is about 1.5 s. As is clear from the measurements on transients in the coronary index BCI, the index becomes positive only after at least 4 seconds. If only compliance effects were involved, the index would have been positive much sooner, as illustrated by the model predictions in Figure 9.11.

The model with intramyocardial compliance can be extended by assuming that the outflow resistance of the model depends on volume, just as in the nonlinear intramyocardial pump model which was discussed in Chapter 6. Here we chose to have the outflow resistance to depend on volume. As was discussed in Chapter 6, the venules form the vascular compartment where the interaction between contraction and coronary flow is the strongest, which justifies the application of volume change only in this compartment. The addition of the volume dependent venous resistance allows the response of the coronary index to be described in a far better way as is illustrated in Figure 9.11. The simulation result can be understood quite simply. In addition to the compliance effect, venous resistance and therefore the total coronary resistance increases rapidly when a change in heart rate occurs. If this concerned only the resistance change, the effect could be interpreted as a sudden change in reference resistance of the coronary bed. The pressure/flow ratio just after the change of heart rate should be taken as reference instead of the ratio prior to the change in heart rate. A much more rapid response of coronary tone would then be determined than when using

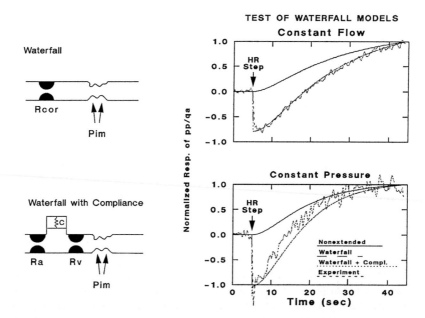

Figure 9.12: *The waterfall model with and without compliance (left) evaluated for their prediction of the initial reversed response of the coronary index induced by a heart rate change (right). The noisy curves are experimental results. The solid lines are the theoretical curves shown in Figure 9.8. The waterfall model fits the experimental data quite well but compliance has an effect only in the very beginning of the response at constant pressure perfusion. These two theoretical curves fall together except the very beginning.*

the pressure/flow ratio prior to the heart rate change. However, since the magnitude of the initial dip in pressure/flow ratio and index is due to the summation of the compliance and resistance alteration effect, the reference value, taking into account the initial change in resistance, can not be estimated without additional information on compliance.

With the addition of the waterfall element (Figure 9.12), the control model predicted the response of the coronary index as well as did the model with the nonlinear intramyocardial pump model. The explanation of the initial reversed response follows the same line of reasoning. At the moment a change in heart rate occurs, the pressure/flow ratio decreases suddenly because of the reduction in diastolic time fraction. Again, this would argue for the use of the pressure/flow ratio just after the heart rate change as reference value.

From the above we conclude that the initial reversed response of beat averaged index cannot be explained by intramyocardial compliance. It can equally well be explained by a resistance increase over the whole cardiac cycle or a decrease in diastolic time fraction. The spike in the index just after the change in heart rate is due to compliance and prevents an accurate determination of how much the altered mechanical events change the index at the moment the pacing rate is altered. It is also obvious from the simulations that the estimate of the rate of change of arteriolar tone strongly depends on the definition of the control condition. Without a correct understanding of the mechanical events one can only arrive at an under and upper bound for the t_{50} of change in arteriolar resistance; these bounds may differ as much as 50%. The sudden change of the index to a change in heart rate illustrates the importance of the clarification of the effect of cardiac contraction on coronary flow for the estimation of the rate of change in arteriolar resistance induced by a change in metabolism.

The initial reversed response of the coronary index BCI as a result of a change in perfusion pressure at constant pressure perfusion or a change in flow at constant flow perfusion can also be explained by the control models extended with an element for describing the mechanical interaction between myocardial contraction and coronary flow. Here again, two effects occur in combination, compliance and a changing resistance or compliance and waterfall element. The initial reversal is more pronounced with constant pressure perfusion than with constant flow perfusion, which points in the direction of a significant compliance effect. This has, however, not been evaluated further.

9.7 The directional effect in dynamic responses of autoregulation

The strong directional effect of the dynamic response of autoregulation deserves some emphasis. It points to characteristics that are hard to explain with our present knowledge. Since a decrease of pressure considerably speeds up the response rate compared to a change in metabolism, a facilitating mechanism of a nonmetabolic nature is indicated. The obvious mechanism to think of is a mechanical response of smooth muscle to a decrease in perfusion pressure. However, in this response, too, a flow sensitive mechanism is probably active. The constant flow perfusion experiments were performed in such a way that the sudden change in pressure related to the step change in flow was of the same magnitude as the changes occurring with the pressure steps during constant pressure perfusion. Therefore, if the facilitation of the response depended only on a mechanical stimulus of the arterioles, the index response at constant flow perfusion would be more similar to the one obtained at constant pressure perfusion. In view of the response to a decrease in perfusion, a feedback loop mediated by flow is likely. Flow mediated vasodilatory response is not likely to be the mechanism since the most rapid response is found with constant pressure perfusion where flow is most strongly reduced.

In general, the relaxation of smooth muscle induced by decreasing wall stress or wall stretch is referred as a myogenic response. This myogenic response was discussed in Chapter 8. However, the rate of response of the isolated arterioles is much slower than the rate of response of the coronary index induced by the decrease of perfusion pressure [23, 52]. Moreover, no directional sensitivity of the response was found. In a number of papers, the myogenic response was studied in skeletal muscle. Although some directional sensitivity of the response was reported, the rate of change was slower than presently found [22, 23, 24].

The directional effect with autoregulation is in accordance with the finding that the response of flow adjustment is faster when heart rate is increased than when heart rate is decreased. An increase in heart rate results in an increase of compression of the arterioles and hence a lowering of transmural pressure. Hence, the effect of increasing heart rate can be compared with the effect of a reduction in perfusion pressure. However, the experimentally found directional effect is much larger when perfusion pressure is decreased than when heart rate is increased. Part of this difference in magnitude may be understood by transmural differences of change in tissue pressure when heart rate is changed. This is in accordance with the classical concept that tissue pressure decreases from cavity pressure at the endocardium to atmospheric pressure in the epicardium. Hence, a possible facilitating effect at the subendocardium is attenuated by the more peripheral layers. Obviously, this interpretation does not hold when explaining the mechanical interaction by a varying elastance model.

9.8 Myogenic response in the coronary circulation

We argued above that the directional sensitivity of the coronary response to a change in perfusion could be classified as myogenic since it is most likely to be induced by a change in transmural pressure of the arterioles. Studies on the myogenic response in the coronary circulation have been reviewed recently by McHale et al. [37]. Studies cited by these authors as providing possible evidence for a myogenic response, however, neglect the possible effect of intramyocardial compliance. In the study of Eikens and Wilcken [15], reactive hyperemia as a result of short occlusions was studied. They showed that the repayment of flow after 2 cycles of occlusion was greater and lasted longer than after 1 cycle of occlusion. This could not be explained by a metabolic mechanism. Eikens and Wilcken concluded from these measurements that the myogenic properties of vascular smooth muscle may be important. However, venous outflow continues after coronary arterial occlusion, raising the possibility that the increase in reactive response could be due to a larger capacitance effect of the emptied intramyocardial vessels.

In the study of Sadick *et al.* [44] a balloon was inserted in the aorta of conscious dogs with a Formalin-induced heart block. Rapid inflation and deflation of the balloon resulted in a transient increase (durations of 300 and 500 ms) in diastolic aortic pressure and coronary flow. The diastolic coronary resistance index, mean diastolic pressure divided by mean diastolic flow, in the subsequent beats were analyzed. Only in the first beat an increase of index of 6 and 11% respectively was found. This was explained as vasoconstriction. However, mean diastolic aortic pressure in the first beat after intervention was decreased by 4.5% and 5.3% respectively. As discussed in Chapter 1, Figure 1.6, a decrease in coronary pressure at constant tone will in itself result in an increased diastolic resistance index. Hence, one may doubt the conclusion that this transient response of index of only one beat duration is sufficient evidence for a myogenic mechanism. Similar reasoning can be applied to the interpretation of other studies [47, 48]

As was illustrated above by means of models, the combination of effects such as compliance and volume dependent resistances on the one hand and change of vasomotor tone on the other hand makes it difficult to define a change of tone alone. Until now, no proper attention has been paid to the problems related to these interactions.

9.9 Adenosine model

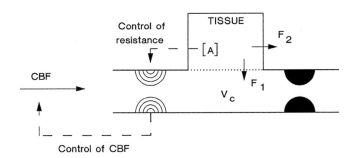

Figure 9.13: *Illustration of the adenosine hypothesis. F1 represents the adenosine washout, and [A] the adenosine concentration in tissue. CBF = coronary blood flow and V_c = capillary volume. F_1 = Flow of adenosine from tissue to blood and washout. F_2 = amount adenosine disappearing per unit time by chemical reactions in tissue.*

The same type of analysis that has been performed above for oxygen, a vasoconstrictor, can be performed for adenosine, a vasodilator. The vasodilator action of adenosine was first described by Gerlach and Dreisbach [19] and Berne [4]. Adenosine has long been considered as the possible mediator for coronary flow control [4, 43]. The adenosine mediated mechanism for control would largely follow the same lines as that of oxygen. The explanation of flow adjustment would be that an increase in metabolism releases more adenosine resulting in an increase of [A] causing such a vasodilation that the balance between oxygen supply and oxygen demand would once again match. Autoregulation would then come into play through the flow dependent washout of adenosine. An increase in flow would wash away interstitial adenosine, F_1, resulting in an increase in vasomotor tone and the reduction of flow. A decrease in flow would result in a vasodilation due to an accumulation of interstitial adenosine. This adenosine hypothesis is illustrated in Figure 9.13.

As with the oxygen hypothesis the adenosine hypothesis can be translated into mathematical equations. These equations follow the schematic of Figure 9.13.

$$\text{CBF} = [P_a - P_v] K_A \, [A] \qquad [9.10]$$

where:

P_a and P_v are the arterial and venous pressures,
K_A is a constant,
$[A]$ is the adenosine concentration.

In steady state adenosine loss equals adenosine production:

$$\text{CBF}\,[A] + K_2\,[A] = K_3 \text{MVO}_2 \qquad [9.11]$$

where:

K_2 and K_3 are constants.

The mathematical formulation of the adenosine model does not result in a prediction of linear autoregulation curves, and they show no parallel shift. Hence, although the adenosine model seems plausible enough in words, its mathematical expression does not result in a relationship between pressure, flow and metabolism which agrees with the experimental findings.

A somewhat different adenosine hypothesis was formulated by Granger et al. [25, 26]. They postulated that the adenosine production might be proportional to the supply and demand ratio. At values of this ratio lower than unity the adenosine production would increase, resulting in vasodilation. With a ratio larger than one, the adenosine pool would shrink and result in vasoconstriction. The model equations then yield:

$$\text{CBF}\,[A] + K_4\,[A] = K_5 \frac{MVO_2}{[\text{CBFO}_{2a}]} \qquad [9.12]$$

where K_4 and K_5 are constants.

However, this model fails to predict the parallel shift of autoregulation curves [55]. A parallel shift can, however, be obtained when the first term of

Equation [9.12], washout of adenosine, is replaced by a constant. A combination of this adenosine mass balance with a linearized [A]-resistance relation:

$$R = R_{\max} - K_6[A] \qquad [9.13]$$

yields a linear relation between CBF, MVO_2 and perfusion pressure such as in Equation [9.1]. Hence, this model does predict the characteristic parallel shift of the autoregulation curves when oxygen consumption is altered. However, there would be no washout of adenosine by flow. This would not appear to be a very realistic assumption [2, 14, 46].

9.9.1 Adenosine dose–response curves

In order to establish whether adenosine might have the potential for controlling coronary flow, Olsson et al. [42] measured the relation between peak reactive hyperemic coronary conductance and tissue adenosine concentration. Additionally, the coronary conductance was measured as a function of the adenosine concentration of coronary arterial blood, which was altered by coronary infusion of a concentrated adenosine solution. The dose–response curves are compared in Figure 9.14. At first sight, one might conclude that, indeed, tissue adenosine concentrations are in the range where coronary conductance can be altered [31]. There are, however, two important points to consider with respect to the significance of the tissue dose–response curve. First, since the cited study of Olsson et al. [42], it has been established that adenosine in tissue is distributed over compartments and hence the measured amount per wet weight of tissue does not reflect the interstitial adenosine concentration. Second, 5 and 15 seconds of coronary occlusions are ischemic stimuli. Hence, the adenosine production and consequently, the relation between tissue adenosine concentration and conductance, might hold under ischemic conditions, but what is needed, however, is a relation between tissue adenosine concentration obtained by altering oxygen consumption and/or perfusion pressure (see below).

When coronary flow conductance is made dimensionless such that the relative change in conductance is calculated as a function of blood adenosine concentration, the relationship depicted in Figure 9.14 is transformed into the one depicted in Figure 9.15. In our laboratory VanBavel [52] measured the relation between the cross-sectional area of isolated coronary arterioles as a function of bath adenosine concentration. When recalculating these results in terms of relative dependence of arteriolar resistance on adenosine concentration, a relation is found which closely resembles that obtained for the coronary system as a whole. As is clear from Figure 9.15, there is a fair agreement between the two dose–response curves, implying that the response of arterioles is sensitive enough to explain the dose–response relation of adenosine for the coronary circulation as a whole.

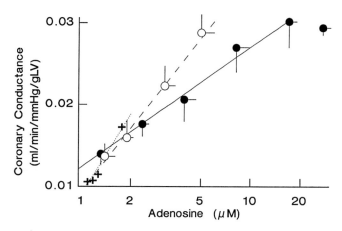

Figure 9.14: Adenosine dose–response curves. These depict the relationship between coronary conductance and tissue adenosine concentration during reactive hyperemia following 5 s (+) or 15 s (o) of coronary occlusion. Shown also is the relationship between coronary conductance and adenosine concentration during intracoronary infusion of this nucleoside (●). Vertical and horizontal bars represent ± SEM. (Redrawn from Olsson et al. [42].)

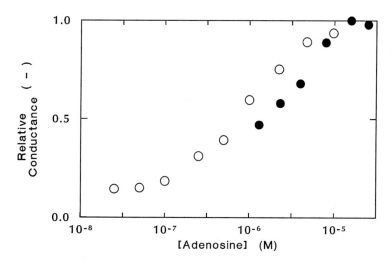

Figure 9.15: An adenosine dose–response curve obtained from adenosine infusion in coronary arteries from data provided in Figure 9.14 (●), compared to those obtained from isolated coronary small arteries (o). For both curves, the response is expressed as the relative change in conductance, having a value 0 in the control state and 1 at maximal dilation. (Data on isolated vessels from VanBavel [52].)

9.9.2 Experimental evidence for and against the adenosine hypothesis

Many studies have been directed at illustrating the relationship of adenosine production to the level of metabolism [43, 46]. Indeed, pericardial adenosine concentration does increase with oxygen consumption. A few experiments have been directed at showing a relation between perfusion pressure and adenosine production within the heart [46]. Other studies into this relationship show an absence of such an effect (e.g., [11]). The interpretation of experiments on tissue adenosine became very complicated after it was established that most of the tissue adenosine is not free in the interstitium but restricted to intercellular compartments [41].

The adenosine hypothesis can be tested by carrying out experiments with the infusion of the enzyme adenosine deaminase (ADA). Intracoronary infusion of this enzyme must affect interstitial adenosine concentration. However, different groups have established that the addition of ADA has no effect on coronary flow control [28, 32]. If coronary arterial pressure is kept constant, coronary flow is not affected by the administration of ADA, nor is the relation between coronary flow and oxygen consumption [1]. On the one hand, tissue adenosine concentration is in the range where it may affect arteriolar tone. Moreover, it may be possible that because of matters related to the affinity of the enzyme and compartmentalization of adenosine the ADA experiments were not interpreted correctly. On the other hand, one would expect some effect of ADA administration on flow when adenosine is involved in the normally active control process. Therefore, these ADA experiments leave little support for the theory of a role of adenosine in coronary flow control within the physiological range.

It has been shown that the intracoronary infusion of adenosine deaminase decreases the reactive hyperemic response after coronary occlusion [45]. Hence, there could be a role for adenosine as a sort of safety valve, an additional vasodilator in ischemia. Obviously, adenosine might play a role in other processes such as, for example, vasogenesis [25]. Moreover, adenosine has been shown to inhibit neutrophil infiltration in models of ischemia.

9.10 Discussion

9.10.1 Adaptation of coronary flow in animals and humans

Coronary flow is adapted to the metabolic needs of the heart. This adaptation could be quantified by the sensitivity of flow to oxygen consumption. However, coronary flow is also determined by coronary arterial pressure. This dependency could also be quantified by means of a sensitivity. The relation between flow on the one hand and oxygen consumption and coronary arterial pressure on the other hand yielded the formula

$$\text{CBF} = a\text{MVO}_2 + bP_p + c \qquad [9.14]$$

The values of the constants a, b and c, in so far they could be determined from studies of our own and of others, are summarized in Table 9.1. We looked at various studies in order to establish species differences and the effect of anesthesia. Moreover, since studies on local coronary flow control are often performed in a cannulated coronary artery, the possible effect of cannulation was assessed in the anesthetized goat by repeating the studies without cannulation. The constants b and c could not be determined from some of these studies as pressure was not controlled.

As is clear from the table, apart from the data on trained dogs published by VonRestorff et al. [58], the sensitivities of coronary flow for oxygen consumption a are all close, ranging between 1.37 to 1.68. Hence, the steady state behavior of coronary flow control seems to be the same whether it concerns anesthetized animals, anesthetized humans or conscious humans. It seems as if the data of VonRestorff et al. differ from the other studies both in terms of the sensitivity of flow to oxygen consumption as well as to coronary arterial pressure. The study of VonRestorff was on awake chronically instrumented dogs divided into three groups: trained mongrels, untrained pointer mates and highly trained pointer mates. The data of the study in our table are an average of all three groups since they seem to have behaved very similarly in their coronary flow adaptation program. It is not clear to us why these data are so different from the other studies which also contain mongrel dogs and trained humans.

Table 9.1: *Experimental estimates for the parameters a, b, c of Equation [9.14]. CBF and MVO_2 were expressed in ml $\cdot$ min^{-1} $\cdot$ g^{-1} and P_p in mm Hg. Data from Kitamura [29], VonRestorff [58], Vergroesen [56], and VanWezel (personal communication). VanWezel used nifedipine or nitroprusside to keep P_{aorta} constant, so b could not be estimated in this study.*

Author	Species	a	$b \times 10^{-2}$	c	r^2
Kitamura	Human awake, exercise	1.37	0.25	-	.93
VonRestorff	Dog awake, exercise	1.02	0.11	-0.003	.993
VanWezel	Human anesth., nifedipine	1.48	-	-	.92
VanWezel	Human anesth., nitroprusside	1.53	-	-	.93
Vergroesen	Dog anesth. artificial perf.	1.40	0.34	-0.167	.92
Vergroesen	Goat anesth. artificial perf.	1.68	0.52	-0.25	.91
Vergroesen	Goat anesth. natural perf.	1.52	0.30	-0.16	.95

9.10.2 Evaluation of pharmacological coronary vasodilators

Coronary flow may be increased by drugs. It is important to establish that when a drug is administered to increase oxygen supply to the myocardium this increase is not secondary to an increase in oxygen consumption or an increase in arterial pressure. If the drug increases oxygen consumption and the increase in flow measured can be explained on the basis of this oxygen consumption increase, the drug should not be referred as to a vasodilator. Moreover, in circumstances where supply is critical, the administration of such a drug is detrimental. Consequently, in evaluating the vasodilator capacity of a drug, oxygen consumption and arterial pressure should be controlled factors.

In the context of a study of the efficacy of preventing poststernotomy hypertension [54] in the Academic Medical Center in Amsterdam, the relation between oxygen consumption and oxygen supply was measured in patients undergoing open heart surgery.[1] Coronary flow was measured in the coronary sinus with a continuous thermodilution method [17]. Oxygen saturation as well as hemoglobin content were determined from blood samples. The protocol was as follows. Ten minutes after initiation of anesthesia the measurements were performed and will be referred to as control values. After baseline measurement, infusion of either nitroprusside or nifedipine was initiated. The second measurement was taken before incision and the third after sternotomy. The infusion rate of the drugs was adjusted such that systemic arterial pressure remained between 80% and 120% of control. Correlation between oxygen consumption and coronary flow of pooled data would be improved by the variation in heart weights, which were not estimated. In order to avoid this, the differences between measurement 2 and control and 3 and control were plotted in Figure 9.16a and b for nitroprusside and nifedipine respectively. The decrease in flow and oxygen consumption with the first measurement can be attributed to reduction in systemic pressure, the increase of these quantities in the second measurement due to stress induced by sternotomy.

Regression was done on the pooled data of each figure and resulted in a slope for the nitroprusside data of 1.53 and for nifedipine of 1.48. These numbers agree fairly well with the sensitivities for flow on oxygen consumption presented in the table above. It had already been concluded that the sensitivities of awake humans closely resembled those of anesthetized animals. Hence, we may conclude from the data that neither nifedipine nor nitroprusside changed the relation between oxygen consumption and coronary flow in the range studied. Consequently these drugs had no primary vasodilator capabilities under the circumstances described; had they had such an action, coronary flow would have been increased to a larger

---

[1] Measurements were done by Dr. HB VanWezel, Department of Anesthesiology, who kindly provided permission to include the data in this chapter.

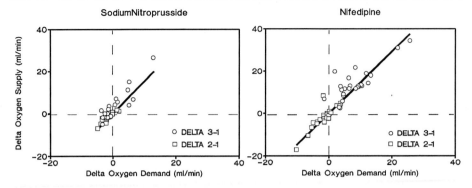

Figure 9.16: Relation between oxygen supply and oxygen demand in anesthetized humans. Left: Changes under influence of nitroprusside. Right: Changes under influence of nifedipine. Increase in demand is due to stress induced by sternotomy. Open circles: difference between sternotomy (3) and control (1), open squares: difference between infusion of drug under study (2) and control.

amount than predicted by the rise in oxygen consumption. This example shows that vasoactivity of a coronary drug cannot be studied without a proper control of arterial pressure and oxygen consumption.

9.10.3 Flow adaptation and oxygen extraction

It is often stated that coronary blood flow has to increase to meet oxygen demand since myocardial oxygen extraction is already maximal. This is, however, not generally true and oxygen extraction frequently increases with oxygen consumption. In the past, the interventions performed to study the relation between supply and demand most certainly influenced the myocardial oxygen consumption as well as the systemic pressure. Since oxygen consumption and systemic pressure decreased concomitantly the relation between supply and demand will pass through the origin.

As was illustrated in this chapter, supply varies linearly with demand. However, because of the arterial pressure effect the relationship intercepts the supply axis at a value different from zero. The effect of such an intercept on oxygen extraction is illustrated in Figure 9.17. Two curves representing experimental results are depicted in the figure. These curves represent the data of VonRestorff *et al.* [58] and Vergroesen *et al.* [56] and are determined by their lower and upper limits of oxygen demand. Also, four proportional relationships are shown, giving the theoretical relation between demand and supply if extraction were constant. Because of the offset of the experimental demand and supply relations, mainly caused by the direct arterial pressure effect, the experimental relations will cross the curves of constant extraction such that extraction increases with increasing

9.10 Discussion

demand. Note that the two experimental curves differ considerably and that the extraction in the experiments of VonRestorff is extremely high.

From Figure 9.17 one may conclude that an increase in oxygen demand is met for a major part by an increase in supply. However, oxygen extraction is certainly not maximal under resting working conditions of the myocardium. Hence, supply does not increase merely because extraction is maximal. Coronary venous saturation is probably closely related to the error signal responsible for flow control. The increased extraction at increased oxygen consumption induces vasodilation but may not be referred to as an ischemic stimulus. Extraction can still increase a certain amount above control without signs of ischemia.

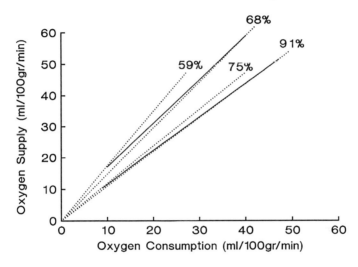

Figure 9.17: *Relation between oxygen demand-supply relationships and oxygen extraction. Two realistic demand-supply relations at an arterial pressure of approximately 100 mm Hg are depicted by solid lines, describing the results of VonRestorff et al. [58] (lower line) and Vergroesen et al. (upper line) (see Table 9.1). These relationships are linear but do not pass through the origin and hence are not proportional relationships. The dotted lines are theoretical supply and demand relations at constant extraction. Because of the offset in supply caused by the pressure term, the experimental demand and supply curves will cross the reference curves of higher extraction.*

9.10.4 Integration of different possible mechanisms for controlling coronary flow

Several factors affecting coronary resistance have been discussed above, including the myogenic response, oxygen and adenosine. Recently, flow dependent relaxation was studied at the level of isolated coronary resistance vessels [33] and was shown to be significant. The endothelial cells have the potential to produce endothelin, a very powerful vasoconstrictor. P_{CO_2} and pH have been suggested as mediators in the regulation of coronary flow. Recently, Broten et al. [5, 6] showed that the relation between coronary venous P_{O_2} and coronary resistance as proposed by Drake-Holland et al. [12] is modulated by arterial and venous P_{CO_2}. The question now arises whether all these factors are involved and the extent of interplay between them.

One has to start by concluding that when a certain substance has been shown to have an effect on coronary vascular resistance, this does not necessarily imply that this substance plays a role in the normal control of coronary blood flow. Each substance may have a special function which has nothing to do with the control of blood flow. It is quite possible that, for example, adenosine only plays a role in ischemia of the heart and functions as a safety valve. Although the experiments with adenosine deaminase point in that direction, the fact remains that normal tissue levels of adenosine are in the range where small arterioles are sensitive. Hence, if adenosine is not important in flow control, there should be a mechanism overruling the adenosine effect.

There may be several mechanisms involved in the regulation of a certain quantity, the effects of which must be carefully tuned. Central heating is a simple example which may serve to clarify this necessity. If a temperature control valve is mounted on the heat exchanger in the room which also contains the main thermostat for the heating system, the temperature control in the house will almost certainly malfunction. If the temperature setting on the exchanger is set at 18^0 centigrade and the thermostat at 20^0 centigrade, the heating system will heat up the rest of the house, since the valve will shut to keep the temperature below the thermostat temperature setting.

With respect to the control of coronary flow, it is clear that the system is designed to maintain P_{O_2} at such a level that the mitochondria can be supplied by oxygen. Hence, one way or the other, the error signal for control of resistance has to come from the metabolic machinery. It is not difficult to understand that the smallest arterioles are under the direct control of the metabolism in the surrounding myocytes. However, the small arteries with diameters of between 100 and 200 μm may not be in intimate contact with the parenchyma and, thus, not under direct metabolic control. Myogenic tone and flow dependent relaxation may play a role in tuning the effects at such upstream control sites. A dilation of the smallest arterioles results in an increased flow which then in turn will increase vasodilation in more proximal vessels [33] increasing flow to a higher level which would not be obtainable by dilation of the smaller arterioles alone. A similar reasoning holds for the myogenic response. Dilation of the distal vessels reduces pressure at this level, inducing myogenic relaxation in the more proximal small arteries. If the upstream dilation is too large, the metabolic signal to the smallest arterioles will induce a vasoconstriction and the propagation of the control signal upstream will be reversed. Hence, the flow dependent dilation and myogenic response may act as amplifiers of the control signal of the smallest arterioles.

The study of interaction of the different mechanisms should include the definition of strength, working range and mutual modulation of these factors. Studies directed to these interactions are in progress.

In resting cremaster muscle, myogenic constriction may still be induced in conditions one normally would expect vasodilation: low flow rates and low perivascular P_{O_2} [39]. Whether this still will be the case at high metabolic rates as in the heart still remains to be proven. It recently has been found that the myogenic response in isolated coronary arterioles is independent of endothelium [34]. Sympathetic vasoconstriction via α- receptors can reduce a coronary flow increase, normally found by increased metabolism, by about 30% [40]. Recently, evidence has been provided that α-tone, tone induced by the α-receptor, strongly interacts with myogenic tone [16]. Moreover, α-tone is very sensitive to local parameters as, e.g., pH [38]. The local dependency of α-tone is different for small and large resistance vessels. For this moment one has to conclude that a single perspective in which all these different mechanisms and interaction are related is still lacking.

9.10.5 The use of models on flow control

The oxygen model is a simple example of how the analysis of a model for flow control could be done. It puts statements about a mechanism into formulas and allows a quantitative test of a hypothesis. For example, tests of the adenosine hypothesis did not result in a model which could describe both flow adjustment and autoregulation without some unrealistic assumptions of the washout of adenosine. In fact, in a very early study performed on the basis of a simple model, Laird et al. [35] questioned whether adenosine was able to describe both flow adjustments and autoregulation at the same time. Experimental evidence against the adenosine hypothesis came much later [11, 28, 32].

A very important conclusion of the oxygen model is that, indeed, both autoregulation and metabolic flow adjustment can be controlled by a single mechanism. This obviously is not proof for the oxygen model. However, the two phenomena on coronary flow control are often independently approached in experiments. For example, the myogenic response was seen to be responsible for autoregulation without considering the consequence of such a response for metabolic flow adjustment. A different, useful outcome of the oxygen model is that it unifies many observations on the static and dynamic behavior of the coronary flow control. The coronary response to a decrease in perfusion was a distinct exception, making it unlikely that this response is dominated by a metabolic factor. The next stage in the development of models should be to include more specific properties of, for example, myogenic response. Some propositions can be found in the literature: e.g., [30].

In the aggregate, coronary physiologists have still not identified the exact mechanisms of local flow control. The use of models may facilitate development of hypotheses, as well as critical testing of these ideas. Moreover, model studies may be helpful as framework in elucidating the role and interactions of different mechanism.

9.11 Summary

Coronary flow is adjusted to the metabolic needs of the hearts by a local control mechanism. At constant coronary arterial pressure coronary flow varies linearly with oxygen consumption. However, when oxygen consumption is kept constant flow does depend on coronary arterial pressure. Hence, the match between flow and oxygen consumption is not perfect. The adaptation of flow to oxygen consumption is referred to as flow adaptation although in the literature terms like metabolic regulation or exercise hyperemia can be encountered. The phenomenon of flow being relatively independent of coronary arterial pressure is referred to as autoregulation. It can be demonstrated, on the basis of a simple control model that assumes tissue oxygen pressure to be the controlled variable, that theoretically both phenomena of flow control can be accomplished by a single mechanism.

It is shown that the rate of change of oxygen consumption as established after cardiac arrest can be characterized by a t_{50} of 4 s. The rate of change of coronary resistance in the anesthetized goat is slower with a t_{50} of about 14 s. The rate of change of tone is not constant but depends on the manner of perfusion. When perfusion pressure is kept constant change of resistance is faster than when flow is kept constant. Moreover, at constant pressure perfusion the rate of change of resistance induced by a heart rate change does depend on the level of perfusion pressure while at constant flow this rate is independent of the magnitude of flow. These findings are consistent with the oxygen control model. The rate of change of coronary resistance can also be described by the oxygen model when the change is induced by an increase in perfusion pressure or flow, but not when a reduction of perfusion pressure of flow is the cause. This points in the direction of a specific mechanism directed to a fast response when the perfusion of the heart is endangered.

Adenosine formation and degradation were also described by a mathematical model. However, this model could only be made to describe control of flow when it was assumed that adenosine cannot be washed out by coronary flow. This assumption seems not very realistic in the light of experimental evidence. Experiments applying the infusion of adenosine deaminase give evidence against an important role of adenosine in the control of flow. Flow adaptation to an increased oxygen demand as well as the response of flow to changes in coronary arterial pressure are hardly or not at all affected by the infusion of this enzyme.

However, arterioles are sensitive to levels of adenosine concentration estimated from interstitial fluids, suggesting that adenosine plays a role under physiological conditions.

The control of coronary flow as established in anesthetized animals is comparable with conscious dogs during exercise although the latter exhibit a larger oxygen extraction. The quantitative studies on the effect of sodium nitroprusside and nifedipine on coronary resistance show that the dilatory effects on the coronary circulation may be secondary to changes in myocardial oxygen consumption. Hence, in the strict sense these substances are not vasodilators in the doses studied in this chapter.

References

[1] BACHE RJ, DAI XZ, SIMON AB, SCHWARTZ JS, HOMANS DC (1987) Effect of adenosine deaminase on coronary vasodilation during exercise. *Circulation* **76** *Suppl.* IV: 146.

[2] BARDENHEUER H, SCHRADER J (1986) Supply-to-demand ratio for oxygen determines formation of adenosine by the heart. *Am. J. Physiol.* **250** (*Heart Circ. Physiol.* **19**): H173–H180.

[3] BELLONI FL, SPARKS HV (1977) Dynamics of myocardial oxygen consumption and coronary vascular resistance. *Am. J. Physiol.* **233** (*Heart Circ. Physiol.* **2**): H34–H43.

[4] BERNE RM (1963) Cardiac nucleotides in hypoxia: possible role in regulation of coronary blood flow. *Am. J. Physiol.* **204**: 317–322.

[5] BROTEN TP, ROMSON JL, FULLERTON DA, VANWINKLE DM, FEIGL EO (1989) Oxygen carbon dioxide control of coronary blood flow. *FASEB J.* **3**: A973.

[6] BROTEN TP, FEIGL EO (1990) Role of oxygen and carbon dioxide in coronary autoregulation. *FASEB J.* **4**: A403.

[7] CHILIAN WM, LAYNE SM, KLAUSNER EC, EASTHAM CL, MARCUS ML (1989) Redistribution of coronary microvascular resistance produced by dipyridamole. *Am. J. Physiol.* **256** (*Heart Circ. Physiol.* **25**): H383–H390.

[8] DANKELMAN J, SPAAN JAE, STASSEN HG, VERGROESEN I (1989) Dynamics of coronary adjustment to a change in heart rate in the anaesthetized goat. *J. Physiol. Lond.* **408**: 295–312.

[9] DANKELMAN J, STASSEN HG, SPAAN JAE (1990) System analysis of the dynamic response of the coronary circulation to a sudden change in heart rate. *Med. Biol. Eng. Comp.* **28**: 139–148.

[10] DANKELMAN J, SPAAN JAE, VANDERPLOEG CPB, VERGROESEN I (1989) Dynamic response of the coronary circulation to a rapid change in its perfusion in the anaesthetized goat. *J. Physiol. Lond.* **419**: 703–715.

[11] DOLE WP, YAMADA N, BISHOP VS, OLSSON RA (1985) Role of adenosine in coronary blood flow regulation after reductions in perfusion pressure. *Circ. Res.* **56**: 517–524.

[12] DRAKE-HOLLAND AJ, LAIRD JD, NOBLE MIM, SPAAN JAE, VERGROESEN I (1984) Oxygen and coronary vascular resistance during autoregulation and metabolic vasodilation in the dog. *J. Physiol. Lond.* **348**: 285–299.

[13] DULING BR (1972) Microvascular responses to alterations in oxygen tension. *Circ. Res.* **31**: 481–489.

[14] EDLUND A, FREDHOLM BB, PATRIGNANI P, PATRONO C, WENNMALM A, WENNMALM M (1983) Release of two vasodilators, adenosine and prostacyclin, from isolated rabbit hearts during controlled hypoxia. *J. Physiol. Lond.* **340**: 487–502.

[15] EIKENS E, WILCKEN DEL (1974) Reactive hyperemia in the dog heart: Effects of temporarily restricting arterial inflow and of coronary occlusions lasting one and two cardiac cycles. *Circ. Res.* **35**: 702–712.

[16] FABER JE, MEININGER GA (1990) Selective interaction of α-adrenoceptors with myogenic regulation of microvascular smooth muscle. *Am. J. Physiol.* **259** (*Heart Circ. Physiol.* **28**: H1126–H1133

[17] GANZ W, TAMURA K, MARCUS HS, DONOSO R, YOSHIDA S, SWAN HJC (1971) Measurement of coronary sinus blood flow by continuous thermodilution in man. *Circulation* **44**: 181–195.

[18] GELLAI M, NORTON JM, DETAR R (1973) Evidence for direct control of coronary vascular tone by oxygen. *Circ. Res.* **32**: 279–289.

[19] GERLACH E, DREISBACH RH (1963) Der nucleotid-Abbau im Herzmuskel bei Sauerstoffmangel und seine mögliche Bedeutung fur die Coronardurchblutung. *Naturwiss* **50**: 228–229.

[20] GIBBS CL, PAPADOYANNIS DE, DRAKE AJ, NOBLE MIM (1980) Oxygen consumption of the non-working and potassium chloride-arrested dog heart. *Circ. Res.* **47**: 408–417.

[21] GORCZYNSKI RJ, DULING BR (1978) Role of oxygen in arteriolar functional vasodilation in hamster striated muscle. *Am. J. Phsyiol.* **235** (*Heart Circ. Physiol.* **4**) : H505–H515.

[22] GRANDE PO, LUNDVALL J, MELLANDER S (1977) Evidence for a rate-sensitive regulatory mechanism in myogenic microvascular control. *Acta Physiol. Scand.* **99**: 432–447.

[23] GRANDE PO, MELLANDER S (1978) Characteristics of static and dynamic regulatory mechanisms in myogenic microvascular control. *Acta Physiol. Scand.* **102**: 231–245.

[24] GRANDE PO, BORGSTROM P, MELLANDER S (1979) On the nature of basal vascular tone in cat skeletal muscle and its dependence on transmural pressure stimuli. *Acta Physiol. Scand.* **107**: 365–376.

[25] GRANGER HJ, HESTER RK, HAENSLY WA (1982) Biochemistry and

metabolism of coronary vessels. In: *The Coronary Artery*. Ed. KALSNER S. Oxford University press, New York: 168–186.

[26] GRANGER HJ, SHEPHERD AP JR (1973) Intrinsic microvascular control of tissue oxygen delivery. *Microvasc. Res.* **5**: 49–72.

[27] GREGG DE (1963) Effect of coronary perfusion pressure or coronary flow on oxygen usage of the myocardium. *Circ. Res.* **13**: 497–500.

[28] HANLEY FL, GRATTAN MT, STEVENS MB, HOFFMAN JIE (1986) Role of adenosine in coronary autoregulation. *Am. J. Physiol.* **250** (*Heart Circ. Physiol.* **19**): H558–H566.

[29] KITAMURA K, JORGENSEN CR, GOBEL FL, TAYLOR HL, WANG Y (1972) Hemodynamic correlates of myocardial oxygen consumption during upright exercise. *J. Appl. Physiol.* **32**: 516–522.

[30] KOCH AR (1964) Some mathematical forms of autoregulatory models. *Circ. Res.* **15** *Suppl.* I: 269–278.

[31] KROLL K, SCHIPPERHEYN JJ, HENDRIKS FFA, LAIRD JD (1980) Role of adenosine in postocclusion coronary vasodilation. *Am. J. Physiol.* **238** (*Heart Circ. Physiol.* **7**): H214–H219.

[32] KROLL K, FEIGL EO (1985) Adenosine is unimportant in controlling coronary blood flow in unstressed dog hearts. *Am. J. Physiol.* **249** (*Heart Circ. Physiol.* **18**): H1176–H1187.

[33] KUO LD, DAVIS MJ, CHILIAN WM (1990) Endothelium-dependent, flow-induced dilation of isolated coronary arterioles. *Am. J. Physiol.* **259** (*Heart Circ. Physiol.* **28**): H1063–H1070.

[34] KUO L, CHILIAN WM, DAVIS MJ (1990) Coronary arteriolar myogenic response is independent of endothelium. *Circulation* **66**: 860–866.

[35] LAIRD JD, BREULS PNWM, VANDERMEER P, SPAAN JAE (1981) Can a single vasodilator be responsible for both coronary autoregulation and metabolic vasodilation. *Basic Res. Cardiol.* **76**: 354–358.

[36] LANSMAN JB (1988) Endothelial mechanosensors. Going with the flow. *Nature* **331**: 481–482.

[37] MCHALE PA, DUBÉ GP, GREENFIELD JC JR (1987) Evidence for myogenic vasomotor activity in the coronary circulation. *Prog. Cardiovasc. Dis.* **30**: 139–146.

[38] MCGILLIVRAY-ANDERSON KM, FABER JE (1990) Effect of acidosis on contraction of microvascular smooth muscle by α_1 and α_2-adrenoceptors. Implications for neural and metabolic regulation. *Circ. Res.* **66**: 1643–1657.

[39] MEININGER GA, MACK CA, FEHR KL, BOHLEN HG (1987) Myogenic Vasoregulation overrides local metabolic control in resting rat skeletal muscle. *Circ. Res.* **60**: 861–870.

[40] MOHRMAN DE, FEIGL EO (1978) Competition between sympathetic vasoconstriction and metabolic vasodilation in the canine coronary circulation. *Circ. Res.* **42**: 79–86.

[41] OLSSON RA, SAITO D, STEINHART CR (1982) Compartmentalization of the adenosine pool of dog and rat hearts. *Circ. Res.* **50**: 617–626.

[42] OLSSON RA, SNOW JA, GENTRY MK (1978) Adenosine metabolism in canine myocardial reactive hyperemia. *Circ. Res.* **42**: 358–362.

[43] RUBIO R, BERNE RM (1975) Regulation of coronary blood flow. *Prog. Cardiovasc. Dis.* **18**: 105–122.

[44] SADICK N, MCHALE PA, DUBÉ GP, GREENFIELD JC JR (1987) Demonstration of coronary artery myogenic vasoconstriction in the awake dog. *Basic Res. Cardiol.* **82**: 585–595.

[45] SAITO D, STEINHART CR, NIXON DG, OLSSON RA (1981) Intracoronary adenosine deaminase reduces canine myocardial reactive hyperemia. *Circ. Res.* **42**: 1262-1267.

[46] SCHRADER J, HADDY FJ, GERLACH E (1977) Release of adenosine, inosine and hypoxanthine from the isolated guinea pig heart during hypoxia, flow-autoregulation and reactive hyperemia. *Pflügers Arch* **369**: 1–6.

[47] SCHWARTZ GG, MCHALE PA, GREENFIELD JC JR (1982) Hyperemic response of the coronary circulation to brief diastolic occlusion in the conscious dog. *Circ. Res.* **50**: 28–37.

[48] SCHWARTZ GG, MCHALE PA (1982) Coronary vasodilation after a single ventricular extra-activation in the conscious dog. *Circ. Res.* **50**: 38–46.

[49] SHEPHERD AP, BURGAR CG (1977) A solid state arterio-venous oxygen difference analyzer for following whole blood. *Am. J. Physiol.* **232** *(Heart Circ. Physiol.* **1**): H437–H440.

[50] SPAAN JAE (1985) Coronary diastolic pressure-flow relation and zero flow pressure explained on the basis of intramyocardial compliance. *Circ. Res.* **56**: 293–309.

[51] SULLIVAN SM, JOHNSON PC (1981) Effect of oxygen on blood flow autoregulation in cat sartorius muscle. *Am. J. Physiol.* **241** *(Heart Circ. Physiol.* **10**: H807–H815.

[52] VANBAVEL E (1989) *Metabolic and myogenic control of blood flow studied on isolated small arteries.* PhD Thesis. University of Amsterdam, The Netherlands.

[53] VANBEEK JHGM, ELZINGA G (1986) Response time of mitochondrial O_2 consumption to heart rate changes in isolated rabbit heart. Abstract *Proc. Int. Union Physiol. Sci.* **16**: 485.

[54] VANWEZEL HB, BOVILL JG, KOOLEN JJ, BARENDSE GAM, FIOLET JWT, DIJKHUIS JP (1987) Myocardial metabolism and coronary sinus blood flow during coronary artery surgery: Effects of nitroprusside and nifedipine. *Am. Heart J.* **113**: 266–273.

[55] VERGROESEN I, DANKELMAN J, SPAAN JAE (1990) Static and dynamic control of the coronary circulation. In: *Coronary circulation, basic mechanism and clinical relevance.* Eds. KAJIYA F, KLASSEN GA, SPAAN JAE,

HOFFMAN JIE. Springer-Verlag Tokyo: 221–232.
[56] VERGROESEN I, NOBLE MIM, WIERINGA PA, SPAAN JAE (1987) Quantification of O_2 consumption and arterial pressure as independent determinants of coronary flow. *Am. J. Physiol.* **252** (*Heart Circ. Physiol.* **21**): H545–H553.
[57] VERGROESEN I, SPAAN JAE (1988) Rate of decrease of myocardial O_2 consumption due to cardiac arrest in anesthetized goats. *Pflügers Arch.* **413**: 160–166.
[58] VONRESTORFF W, HOLZ J, BASSENGE E (1977) Exercise induced augmentation of myocardial oxygen extraction in spite of normal coronary dilatory capacity in dogs. *Pflügers Arch.* **372**: 181–185.

Chapter 10

Water balance within the myocardium

ISABELLE VERGROESEN, YVES HAN, JENNY DANKELMAN and JOS AE SPAAN

10.1 Introduction

ONE OF THE ROLES OF THE MICROCIRCULATION is to maintain the water balance between plasma and interstitium in the myocardium. Judged by the number of papers related to the interstitium and to the mechanics of coronary flow, the interstitium is a neglected field of research.

Obviously, the interstitium has a role in the transfer of substrates and metabolites between the capillaries and the myocytes. However, in relation to the study of coronary flow, the mechanics of the interstitium are of great importance. In the discussion on models of coronary flow mechanics, tissue pressure was a crucial quantity. Since tissue pressure is assumed to behave like liquid pressure it is implicitly assumed that there is an interstitial space containing free movable water in which pressure is transmitted according to one of the basic laws of hydrostatics [2]. It remains to be seen whether this is true. Moreover, in discussing compliance, which is especially important in studies on coronary flow dynamics, it is as yet unclear whether volume changes in the microcirculation are appropriately distinguished from volume changes within the interstitial space.

Apart from the relevance for basic insight in coronary flow mechanics, more knowledge of water exchange and edema formation may be important for the mechanical function of the heart. Myocardial edema may cause cardiac dysfunction [24]. Moreover, an increase in diastolic wall stiffness due to edema might impair cardiac function [21]. Since anoxia tremendously increases lymph flow [19], the enlargement of the interstitial fluid space may be an important factor in the deteriorating process of ischemia.

Water transfer between capillary and interstitium has been studied in different organs and various elegant single capillary studies in mesentery have been published (e.g., Michel et al. [17]). The capillary transmural pressure is an important parameter in the balance of water over the capillary walls. This pressure difference between interstitium and capillary blood is time variant in the myocardial wall and might be quite different at the subendocardium compared to the subepicardium. Experimental data on subendocardial capillary pressure are totally unavailable and much confusion surrounds the topic of subendocardial tissue pressure.

There is not much difference between the walls of capillaries and venules. Hence, exchange processes will also occur at the venular level. However, for convenience it is assumed that exchange of substances only occurs at the capillary level.

Obviously, the properties of the capillary wall are important in determining the exchange of substances between capillary and interstitium. Water passes easily through this barrier and the rate of flow through this wall is determined by the difference of hydrostatic pressure between capillary lumen and interstitium on the one hand and the osmotic pressure difference on the other hand. Small molecules which dissolve in water are able to flow with the water through the capillary wall. Consequently their concentrations are the same in plasma as in interstitial fluid. However, large molecules like proteins do not pass easily through the walls of the capillaries. Consequently, the protein concentration measured in lymph is lower than plasma concentration and decreases with the magnitude of the lymph flow.

The interstitium is subjected to compressive forces which may be generated by left ventricular pressure and propagated by the tissue fluids or generated in a distributed way by myocytes interwoven in the system which are able to vary their elastance or geometry. The mechanisms involved are quite similar to those discussed in relation to the effect of cardiac contraction on the microvessels within the myocardium. The prediction of the effect of cardiac contraction on the transfer of water over the capillary wall is not trivial. If both fluid filled compartments are closed, contraction can have no effect on the transmural pressure difference since both capillary blood pressure and interstitial pressure will increase by the same amount. Since blood can leave the capillary relatively easily, thereby lowering capillary blood pressure, one might expect extrusion of water from the interstitium into the capillaries. However, in diastole the opposite would occur and the net effect is hard to predict. It becomes even more difficult if one includes the possible cyclic resistances changes in the venules due to cardiac contraction.

As far as experimental evidence goes for the moment, cardiac contraction helps to prevent myocardial edema. The weight of the isolated and perfused rabbit heart is stable when the heart is beating but increases after during arrest [27]. This is consistent with an increase of lymph flow with increasing the work load of the heart [28].

Important to the analysis of the interstitial water content, as well as to the mechanics of coronary flow, is the compliance of the interstitial space, defined as the amount of volume by which the interstitium is increased through an increase in interstitial pressure. As with the compliance of the blood vessels, one might expect to find a pressure dependency. Although the compliance of the vascular compartment was determined by the mechanics of the vessel walls, the compliance of the interstitium is determined by the structure of its boundaries, walls of vessels and myocytes, as well as by the connective structures within the interstitial space. Research directed at quantifying the relative importance of these effects is barely under way.

10.2 Myocardial interstitium and lymph

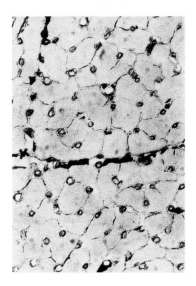

Figure 10.1: Histological picture of a cross section of the dog left ventricle illustrating the geometry of the interstitium. The section was 8 μm thick and silver methenamine stain was applied. Note the little space in between myocytes. (Photograph kindly provided by Dr. SR Kayar, Dept. of Physiology, UMDNJ-Robert Wood Johnson Medical School.)

The interstitium is the space left over by blood, lymph vessels and myocytes. As a result, its geometry is variable as is illustrated by Figure 10.1. In the normal heart the interstitial volume is around 20 volume % [22]. This is larger with edema but lower with hypertrophy [4].

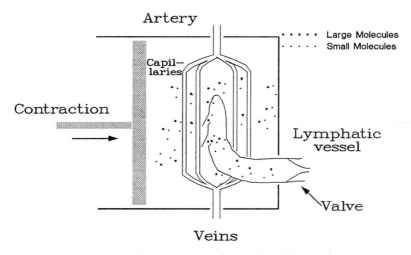

Figure 10.2: Schematic illustration of the origin of lymph capillaries with the valves at the inlets and in larger lymphatics. Valves in transmural lymph vessels are sparse and much less frequent than in epicardial lymph vessels. Molecules may pass capillary walls as they do with blood capillaries (Figure 10.3) but also through valve like structures. As is suggested by the piston all structures within the myocardium are subjected to compression. Note that the density of large and small dots do not relate quantitatively to concentrations.

The myocardial interstitium contains 3 to 7 g collagen per 100 ml interstitial space [2, 4]. The function of the collagen is to resist changes in tissue configuration and volume. It also forms a matrix for glycosaminoglycans, GAG's, which can bind water. The water binding capacity is so large that the GAG's occupy about 1000 times more space when bound to water compared to their unhydrated structure. These hydrated GAG's give the interstitium a gel-like ground substance which is enmeshed in a network of collagen fibers. As a result, the free water space is much smaller than the total interstitial space.

The interstitium is considered as a closed compartment, although it drains into the lymphatic system via lymph capillaries. The lymph system is closed at one end, with lymph capillaries originating in the interstitial space (Figure 10.2). At the inlet a valve structure is supposed to guarantee a one-way flow direction. The lymph capillaries form at each layer of the heart muscle a plexus, which drains into larger vessels. The cardiac lymph is collected in the larger lymph vessels running on the epicardium along the epicardial arteries and veins. Lymph vessels contain valves to prevent backflow and normally form anastomoses at all levels. In the steady state, it may be assumed that the composition of lymph will reflect that of the interstitial space.

In general, compression of the lymphatics by myocytes is assumed to be an important driving force for lymph flow. Moreover, contraction of smooth muscle in the walls of larger lymphatic vessels has been observed. Because of valves in the lymphatic vessels, both these compressive forces contribute to maintaining lymph flow. Obviously, lymph flow can be maintained only by sufficient net flux of water and solutes out of the capillary blood. Since all myocardial structures are subjected to compression by the beating of the heart as illustrated in Figure 10.2 it is not yet clear what the net effect is of compression on water transfer out of the blood capillaries into the lymphatic system.

Lymph capillaries have a much wider diameter than blood capillaries: 45 μm versus 5 μm. Intercapillary distance of lymph capillaries is much greater than for blood capillaries: 300 μm versus 20 μm [9, 18]. Hence, the capillary density of the lymph collecting system is much lower than that of the blood capillary system. The branching structure of the lymph tree has not yet been established quantitatively in terms of, e.g., Strahler orders, branching ratios or segment length ratios. Nothing is known about the resistance of the lymph system. Lymph flow rate in the normal dog heart is about of 3 ml $\cdot$ hr^{-1} $\cdot$ [100 g]$^{-1}$ [19]. This flow rate is very low compared to the interstitial volume of 20 vol%, and this implies that it would take 7 hours for the interstitium to be drained completely by the lymphatic system once. This time constant is very long compared to the one minute needed for all the blood in the cardiovascular system to circulate once. The contrast is even stronger if the lymph drainage time is compared with the residence time of blood cells in the coronary vascular system. However, transcapillary water transport is much larger than lymph flow and can be estimated at 3 ml $\cdot$ min^{-1} $\cdot$ [100 g]$^{-1}$ [16], assuming that the capillary filtration coefficient equals (rabbit heart) 0.35 ml $\cdot$ min^{-1} $\cdot$ [100 g]$^{-1}$ $\cdot$ mm Hg^{-1}. A large amount of water, originally drained into the interstitial space from a capillary, is reabsorbed by the blood.

Lymph consists mainly of water, salts and proteins [19]. The concentration of protein in the lymph is normally about 3 to 4 g $\cdot$ [100 ml]$^{-1}$ which is about 66 to 86% of plasma protein concentration [1, 12, 19]. However, lymph protein concentration decreases with increasing lymph flow as will be discussed below (e.g., Figure 10.4).

10.3 Transport of water and proteins across the capillary membrane

10.3.1 Routes

As Figure 10.3 illustrates, the handbook of physiology [6] lists several ways for substances to cross a capillary wall.

Water and lipophilic substances may diffuse across the endothelial cell, crossing two membranes and the cytoplasm. Lipophilic substances may dissolve in the cell membrane and diffuse within the membrane layer to the other side of the endothelial cell. Junctions between endothelial cells contain pores of different sizes. All these pores can be used for the transport of water, lipids and small molecules, whereas proteins can cross the endothelial layer by means of the larger pores only. The endothelial cells may contain fenestrae which may be open or closed by a single membrane layer. These fenestrae offer passage to water, lipids, small molecules and proteins. Vesicles are specifically for the transport of proteins and other large molecules.

The special interest of this chapter is with the transcapillary transport of water. In theory, water can use all the routes but the relative contributions are not equal. Intuitively, the pores and the transcellular pathways can be considered to be the most important for water transport in the heart. However, the relative contributions of these two has not been quantified.

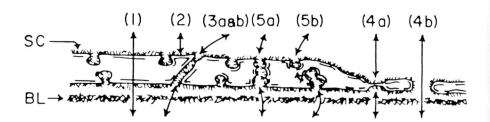

Figure 10.3: *Transport pathways in capillary endothelium. SC: cell surface coat, BL: basal lamina. 1: endothelial cell pathway, 2: lateral membrane diffusion pathway, 3: intercellular junction pathway (a: small pores impermeable to proteins, b: large pores permeable to proteins), 4: endothelial cell fenestrae pathway (a: specialized openings, b: membranes are fused, bypassing aqueous cytoplasmic phase), 5: endothelial cell vesicles pathway (a: moving vesicles, b: transient communication between vesicles). (From [6], by permission of the authors and the American Physiological Society.)*

For this book, especially, the dynamics of water transport are of importance and it would be worthwhile to know which pathway offers the least resistance. In general, transport flux by convective flow through the pores is faster than by diffusion. However, the surface area of the pores is much smaller than the cellular membrane surface and hence it is not obvious which pathway is dominant. In relation to flow dynamics, the relative speed of water flow over the endothelial layer in comparison to the convective vascular flow is of importance. In the past, it was assumed that membrane transport was so fast that blood flow was the rate limiting process in obtaining equilibrium of the interstitial balance [13, 33]. However, there is some evidence that at high flow rates (i.e., during vasodilation), the transport of water is limited by the membrane itself [3, 7].

10.3.2 Driving forces

In the analysis of water transport through the capillary membrane in general two forces are considered, namely the differences in hydrostatic pressures and the osmotic pressures difference across the membrane. The osmotic pressure is generated by all the solutes within the fluids considered. However, the small molecules pass the capillary membrane almost as easily as water and hence, due to differences in the concentration of the larger molecules, an osmotic gradient will be left in steady state. The driving force generated by this concentration difference of, especially, proteins is referred to as oncotic pressure. Since the capillary membrane is not absolutely impermeable to the larger molecules, only part of the oncotic pressure gradient caused by concentration gradients can be used to generate transmembrane flow. This factor is taken into account by the so-called reflection factor, σ, which is unity if the membrane is absolutely impermeable and zero if the membrane offers no resistance to transfer of the solute. The transport of water (solvent) through the capillary membrane is described by the Starling hypothesis, which mathematically can be expressed by [16, 26]:

$$J_v = L_p S_A [P_{tr} - \sigma \pi_{tr}] \qquad [10.1]$$

where:

J_v is volume flow across the capillary wall, $[J_v] = \text{ml} \cdot \text{s}^{-1} \cdot [100 \text{ g}]^{-1}$,
P_{tr} is hydrostatic pressure difference across the capillary wall or transmural pressure, $[P_{tr}] = \text{mm Hg}$,
π_{tr} is colloid osmotic pressure difference across the capillary wall or transmural osmotic pressure, $[\pi_{tr}] = \text{mm Hg}$,
L_p is hydraulic conductivity or filtration coefficient, $[L_p] = \text{ml} \cdot \text{s}^{-1} \cdot \text{cm}^{-2} \cdot \text{mm Hg}^{-1}$
S_A is capillary surface area, $[S_A] = \text{cm}^2 \cdot [100 \text{ g}]^{-1}$,
σ is reflection coefficient (dimensionless value between 0 and 1)

As is clear from Equation [10.1], it is not possible to understand the water balance of the interstitium without knowledge of the determinants of the protein concentration in the interstitium. These interstitial proteins originate predominantly from the blood plasma.

There are two major factors involved in the protein transfer across the capillary wall: diffusion and convection. The former process is determined by the concentration difference of the proteins between blood plasma and interstitial fluid and the latter by the flow of water through the pores in the capillary walls. In mathematical form these processes are described by the Kedem-Katchalsky [14] formulation.

$$J_s = P_A S_A C_{tr} + [1 - \sigma] J_v C_s \qquad [10.2]$$

with

J_s is net transport of solute, $[J_s] = $ mol $\cdot$ s^{-1} $\cdot$ [100 g]$^{-1}$,
P_A is permeability of membrane to substance, $[P] = $ cm $\cdot$ s^{-1},
C_{tr} is mean concentration difference across the capillary wall, $[C_{tr}] = $ mol $\cdot$ ml^{-1},
C_s is mean solute concentration in the capillary plasma, $[C_s] = $ mol $\cdot$ ml^{-1}.

The first term in the right hand side of this equation accounts for the diffusive transport of solute and the second term for the convective transfer. Note that the product $P_A S_A$ is equal to the PS product discussed in Chapter 3.

The blood plasma and interstitium contain proteins of different molecular weights. In principle, one may superimpose the effects of the individual molecules, taking into account their respective reflection coefficients. Below, the effect of the reflection coefficient on the ratio between interstitial and plasma protein concentration will be analyzed in relation to the magnitude of lymph flow.

10.3.3 Lymph flow and protein concentration

It may be assumed that the driving force of lymphatic flow is the difference between interstitial fluid pressure and the systemic venous blood pressure since in the end lymphatics drain into the venous system. The oncotic pressure difference across the capillary membrane has been estimated as 7 mm Hg under normal conditions. Hence mean capillary blood pressure has to be at least above this value before lymph flow can occur.

In the heart, capillary blood pressure can be most easily increased by increasing coronary venous blood pressure. The effect of venous pressure on coronary lymph flow and total lymph protein concentration when the myocardial lymphatic system is cannulated is illustrated in Figure 10.4 which was redrawn from Laine and Granger [15]. The collecting cardiac lymph was cannulated proximal to the cardiac lymph nodes and lymph flow was collected by counting the drops from the cannula. Interstitial pressure was measured by the insertion of a microtip pressure cannula. Although there are drawbacks to this method of measuring

10.3 Transport of water and proteins across the capillary membrane

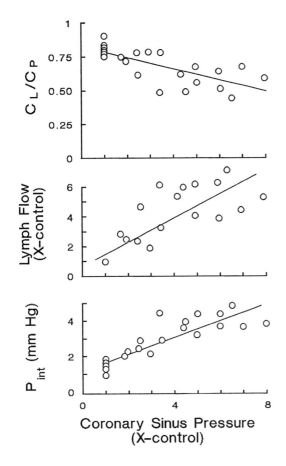

Figure 10.4: Effect of coronary sinus pressure on the ratio between lymph protein concentration C_L and plasma protein concentration C_P (top panel), lymph flow (middle panel) and diastolic interstitial pressure P_{int} (bottom panel). Lymph flow is expressed relative to its value under control venous pressure. (Redrawn from Laine and Ganger, [15].)

true interstitial fluid pressure, these will not be further discussed here. Coronary venous pressure was elevated by inflating a balloon in the coronary sinus. Figure 10.4 shows that increasing the coronary venous pressure results in an increase in interstitial pressure and lymph flow. Since both quantities are linearly related to each other, lymph flow is linearly related to interstitial pressure.

It is important to note that the total concentration of protein in lymph decreases with the magnitude of lymph flow. This decrease is due to the fact that water passes the blood capillary wall much faster than do the proteins. This results in a dilution of the interstitial solution and hence a decrease in the interstitial protein concentration. The interstitial protein concentration, however, cannot be reduced to zero. This is illustrated in Figure 10.5 for β-lipoprotein, which has a large molecular weight compared to albumin and consequently a high reflection coefficient. If hydrostatic pressure is increased the convective flux of proteins through the capillary wall will be much larger than the diffusive flux, allowing the latter to be disregarded.

In steady state, the amount of protein to cross the capillary wall per unit time must equal the amount of protein leaving by lymph per unit time. Moreover, lymph flow must equal the transcapillary solute flow. These two conditions yield:

$$J_s = C_l J_v \qquad [10.3]$$

Substitution of Equation [10.3] into Equation [10.2] results in

$$\frac{C_l}{C_p} = 1 - \frac{\sigma J_v}{J_v + P_A S_A} \qquad [10.4]$$

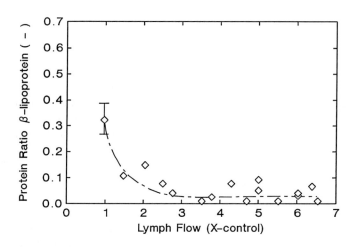

Figure 10.5: *The effect of lymph flow on the ratio between β-lipoprotein concentration in lymph and plasma. The ratio at higher flow rates indicates the reflection coefficient. (Redrawn from Laine and Granger, [15].)*

The effect of lymph flow on β-lipoprotein is illustrated in Figure 10.5. In contrast to the dependency of total protein concentration ratio shown in Figure 10.4, the ratio of this larger molecule levels off and this final ratio provides the reflection coefficient of the protein as could be expected from Equation [10.4].

10.4 Dynamic changes in interstitial volume and pressure

There are several reasons to be interested in the dynamics of interstitial volume and pressure. The obvious reason is that the beating of the heart is a dynamic process. Consequently the dynamics of all processes related to the function of the heart are of interest. A more practical reason is that in the study of coronary flow mechanics it is important to have knowledge about the compliance of the vascular bed. These compliance effects are hard to distinguish from those of the interstitium since the capillaries are so permeable for water. In this section, a number of studies focussing on the dynamics of the interstitial water balance are discussed. We have recently started experiments on the dynamics of coronary lymph pressure to investigate the behavior of interstitial pressure measured in a natural cavity within the heart. Although these experiments are still at the preliminary stage, the report on some observations may stimulate the discussion and research on the volume and pressure balance of this important fluid compartment in the heart.

10.4.1 Heart weight and vascular volume experiments

Several experimental techniques have been employed to study the rate of transcapillary solute flux. Examples are heart weight changes induced by osmotic transients and dye dilution techniques [29, 30, 31]. The interpretation of the experimental findings is complicated by the interaction between a compliant microcirculation and compliant interstitium. In most studies it is assumed that intramyocardial compliance can be neglected, in order to simplify the analysis. However, the assumption of a negligible vascular compliance would not appear to be justified. The problems regarding the interpretation of dynamic signals related to the transcapillary membrane transfer will be illustrated by some experimental data of Vargas and Blackshear [31].

The experiments of Vargas and Blackshear were performed with a Ringer perfused rabbit heart according to Langendorff. The heart was mounted in the perfusion system with the apex up in order to facilitate drainage of the ventricles. The heart was continuously weighed during perfusion and weight changes resulting from a sudden change in plasma osmotic pressure were registered. These osmotic transients were induced by adding sucrose to the perfusate. In some experiments radioactive labeled red cells were added and the total vascular volume changes were estimated by monitoring the radiation from the heart by a gamma camera. Perfusion flow was controlled during the interventions. However, due to bubble traps in the perfusion system, the interventions were not done at real constant flow as was done with the experiments described in Chapter 9. The perfusion system had a rather high compliance, as is obvious from the flat perfusion pressure signals presented in the paper discussed. A typical result of the study is reproduced in Figure 10.6.

The left panels relate to the injection of a highly concentrated sucrose solution with an additional osmotic pressure of 420 mm Hg. Due to the reflection coefficient of sucrose at the capillary membrane of 0.16, the effective increase in osmotic pressure is 67 mm Hg. As is clear from the top tracing, the change in

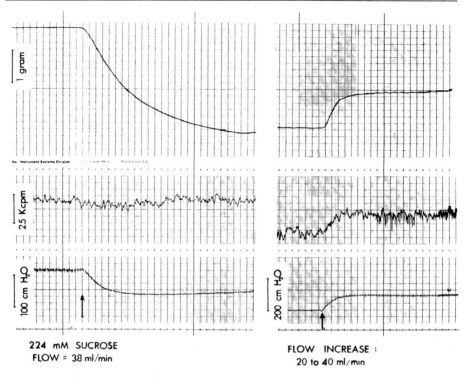

Figure 10.6: *Responses of total heart weight (top panel) and total intramyocardial blood volume as measured by radioactivity counting (middle panel) to rapid changes in plasma osmotic pressure (left panels) and change in perfusate flow (right panels). Experiments were done at constant flow. Resulting perfusion pressure is shown in the bottom panels. Average heart weight in these experiments during control conditions was 8 g. Note that blood volume is hardly affected by the osmotic transient but is strongly affected by a change in flow. Response of heart weight to a change in flow has fast and slow changes. The rapid change is explained by changes in vascular volume and the slow change by water flow into the interstitium. (From Vargas and Blackshear, [31], by permission of authors and American Physiological Society.)*

heart weight is tremendous, considering that the average heart weight in control condition did not exceed 8 grams. From the radioactivity count one has to conclude that the number of labeled red cells within the heart was hardly affected by the intervention. Assuming the hematocrit remained constant, it must be concluded that the entire weight change is attributable to the change in interstitial water content and probably in cellular water content. Since coronary flow was kept constant, the reduction in perfusion pressure represents a decrease in

10.4 Dynamic changes in interstitial volume and pressure

coronary resistance. In contrast to the suggestion of the authors, it is not likely that this reduction in coronary resistance is due to control of vascular smooth muscle. As was shown in Chapter 9, the rate of change of coronary tone is not fast enough to explain such a rapid change in perfusion pressure. Moreover, the gradual increase in perfusion pressure later in the tracing of the response indicates an increase in tone to restore coronary resistance (see Chapter 9). The mechanical effect of a reduced interstitial pressure on resistance is as could be expected. A decrease in interstitial volume must be accompanied by a reduction in interstitial pressure and a widening of the microvessels. However, one would have expected to see such an effect on total vascular volume.

The experimental results from the osmotic transients are all the more puzzling when compared to the changes induced by a change in perfusate flow depicted in the right panels of Figure 10.6. The doubling of flow resulted in a strong increase of perfusion pressure. Note that the initial response in perfusion pressure is rather slow, especially compared to those obtained with a more perfect constant flow perfusion system in Figure 9.3. Concomitant with the increase in perfusion pressure, vascular volume increased, which was most probably due to the compliance of the intramyocardial microcirculation. Since both flow and pressure changed during this intervention, it is unwarranted to conclude that coronary resistance decreased as a result of this increased vascular volume. The weight of the heart increased and the interpretation of the weight signal by the authors seems correct and relates the rapid change of weight in the first seconds to the change in blood volume while ascribing the following slower weight change to water transfer from the capillaries to the interstitium.

The responses of radioactivity (Figure 10.6) to a change in osmotic pressure (left panels) and a change in flow (right panels) seem to be contradictory. With the former response, one would expect a decrease in vascular volume in response to a change in osmotic pressure because of the decreasing perfusion pressure. However, the decrease in interstitial volume and therefore in interstitial pressure would tend to increase vascular volume. Since the radioactivity is rather constant the two effects could have completely cancelled out one another, which may, on the one hand seem rather accidental. However, on the other hand, the right panels clearly show that the vascular volume is pressure dependent. Consequently this capacitive effect must play a role in the osmotic transient experiment. Moreover, it should be kept in mind that, as the authors warned in their paper, the experimental method could not determine the redistribution of blood volume over vascular compartments and water over vascular and interstitial compartment. This question, however, is very relevant to the estimates of the rate of transfer of water over capillary membranes, since the models used for the interpretation of these results are all based on the assumption that the capillaries do not change volume during the interventions.

10.4.2 Lymphatic pressure

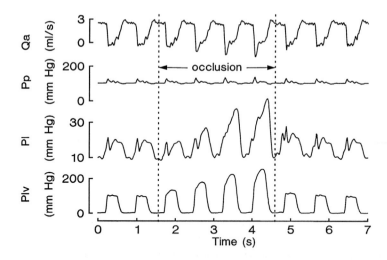

Figure 10.7: *Measurements of lymphatic pressure in an epicardial lymph vessel measured in an anesthetized open chest goat with cannulated left main coronary artery. P_{lv} = left ventricular pressure, P_l = lymph pressure, Q_a = coronary arterial flow and P_p = perfusion pressure. The absolute value is not representative for the pressure in the intramural lymph vessels because of anastomoses in the lymphatic system and because lymph flow obstruction will result in an unknown increase of pressure. However, one may assume that the relative variations are representative for intramural pressure variations [11]. Note the immediate response of lymphatic pulse pressure induced by an aortic occlusion.*

Although important conclusions may be drawn from dynamic measurements of myocardial lymph flow, lymphatic flow rates are so low that this is hardly possible. An alternative is to cannulate an epicardial lymphatic vessel and measure the pressure when lymphatic flow is obstructed, using a pressure transducer with a very low compliance. In this way, very rapid changes in lymphatic pressure can be registered. Obviously the lymph obstruction might increase interstitial fluid pressure in the area drained by the cannulated lymph. However, due to the many anastomoses in the epicardial lymphatic system, the obstruction will only be partial.

A typical result of such a lymphatic pressure experiment is illustrated in Figure 10.7. The preliminary results reported below were obtained from a cannulated epicardial lymph vessel in the anesthetized goat. A first investigation of the lymphatic pressure was directed at establishing whether any main determinants of interstitial pressure were indeed observable in the lymphatic pressure. The determinants looked at are left ventricular pressure (P_{lv}) and plasma oncotic

10.4 Dynamic changes in interstitial volume and pressure

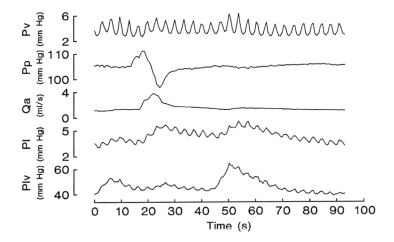

Figure 10.8: Effect of coronary bolus injection on coronary lymph pressure in a preliminary experiment. $P_{lv}=$ left ventricular pressure, $P_l=$ lymph pressure. $P_v=$ coronary venous pressure, $Q_a=$ coronary arterial blood flow and $P_p=$ coronary perfusion pressure. The rise in flow indicates the arrival of the bolus at the coronary resistance vessels. Coronary lymph pressure responds in seconds after the increase of flow. Note the increase in lymph pressure when mean left ventricular pressure increases, illustrating that the effect of the rise in left ventricular pressure is not a very short acting one.

pressure. P_{lv} has an immediate effect on lymphatic pressure as is illustrated in Figure 10.7. Lymph pressure is pulsatile and in phase with P_{lv}. A brief occlusion of the descending aorta shows a strong effect on the pulsatility of the lymphatic pressure. In this particular experiment the diastolic lymphatic pressure is about 10 mm Hg which is about the magnitude of the coronary venous pressure.

Since interstitial pressure forms an important determinant of lymphatic flow and since this interstitial pressure depends on transcapillary water transport, one would expect an increase in lymphatic pressure to be accompanied by a reduction in plasma oncotic pressure. The effect of a bolus injection of saline in the coronary perfusion line on lymphatic pressure is illustrated in Figure 10.8. All signals were averaged per beat. The periodic fluctuations in coronary venous pressure, lymphatic pressure and left ventricular pressure are caused by respiration. The injection of saline had hardly any effect on the perfusion pressure because of the pressure perfusion system. The arrival of the bolus at the resistance vessels is apparent from the sharp increase in the beat averaged coronary arterial flow. Lymphatic pressure reacted within seconds with a rising slope and recovered more slowly than the coronary arterial flow signal.

The delay between the rise in flow and the rise in lymphatic pressure indicates that volume variations measured by the integration of the difference between arterial and venous flow with a time constant of less than two seconds are most probably due to blood volume variations [32] and that interactions with the interstitial space are not rapid enough to affect estimates of intramyocardial vascular compliance. Although heart rate was kept constant, beat averaged left ventricular pressure increased after recovery of the coronary flow signal and caused another increase in lymphatic pressure.

The potential for measuring rapid transients in interstitial variables with the aid of the technique of lymphatic cannulation is obvious from these first results. Further quantitative interpretations of these experiments are in progress.

10.5 Numbers on permeability, surface area and reflection coefficients

The permeability of capillaries for water is high, since water moves through the entire capillary surface area, which allows rates that are 10–100 times faster than the rates of solutes that diffuse only through interendothelial clefts [5, 20, 23]. The permeability of water has been found to be between 60 and 150×10^{-5} cm $\cdot$ s^{-1}. Michel [16] reports a capillary filtration coefficient in the rabbit heart of 0.35 ml $\cdot$ min^{-1} $\cdot$ mm Hg^{-1} $\cdot$ [100 g]$^{-1}$. This means that at a net pressure difference of 9 mm Hg the water transport across the capillary membrane amounts to 3 ml $\cdot$ min^{-1} $\cdot$ [100 g]$^{-1}$.

The capillary surface area, expressed in units cm^2 $\cdot$ g^{-1} wet.wt., is not the same in the different organs. The lungs have a very large capillary surface area (3000–3500) compared to heart muscle (500–575). Although the experimental techniques used to estimate these numbers are quite crude, this difference is probably significant [5].

Reflection coefficients (1 = impermeable, 0 = no barrier) for the heart capillary endothelium range from 0.8 for albumin to 0.07 for NaCl [5].

10.6 Compliance of the interstitial space

The compliance of the interstitial space can be defined as the change in interstitial fluid volume (V_{IF}) divided by the change in interstitial pressure (dP_i). The determination of both these quantities is controversial [2]. Determination of dV_{IF} has been done by using the change in total organ weight as a measure for the change in V_{IF}, possibly including changes in vascular volume. The measurement of P_i was done with needle, wick or capsule. Each of these techniques has its own pitfalls and difficulties [2, 8, 10]. In the heart, compliance has been measured in the Tyrode perfused Langendorff preparation, using the change in weight as a measure of V_{IF} and a 27-gauge needle introduced in the heart muscle directly to measure dP_i [30]. The change in V_{IF} was induced by a change in the osmotic or hydrostatic pressure gradient across the capillary wall under the same general experimental conditions.

Because of all these technical difficulties, one has to conclude that at present no reliable data on interstitial compliance are available. The data that are presented in the literature are referred to as hydrostatic compliance and osmotic compliance. The former is established by a step in perfusion pressure and the latter by an osmotic transient. Both these interventions are illustrated in Figure 10.6. Typical values are 0.064 ± 0.013 ml $\cdot$ [cm H_2O]$^{-1}$ $\cdot$ [10 g]$^{-1}$ for the hydrostatic compliance and 0.27 ml [cm H_2O]$^{-1}$ $\cdot$ [10 g]$^{-1}$ for the compliance due to hyperosmolarity. The difference was attributed to the loss of water from the cardiac cells during the osmotic pressure changes which may be absent during the hydrostatic pressure changes. In units more convenient to coronary flow mechanics, the hydrostatic compliance amounts 0.85 ml $\cdot$ [100 g]$^{-1}$ $\cdot$ mm Hg^{-1}. This is in the same range as intramyocardial compliance of the blood space. However, in the interpretation of the data the authors have not properly taken into account the compliance of the blood compartment. Hence the high value of interstitial hydrostatic compliance found may be explained to a great extent by vascular compliance. On the other hand, with the estimation of compliance of the vascular space, interstitial compliance was neglected. On the basis of time scale, however, one would attribute rapid changes (time constant smaller than 2 s) in heart weight to vascular compliance and slower changes to interstitial compliance. Since intramyocardial compliance was calculated from fast responses one might assume that this compliance has been estimated correctly but that the hydrostatic compliance of the myocardial interstitium is overestimated by the numbers provided above. More specific experiments should be designed to distinguish between microvascular and interstitial compliance in the heart.

10.7 Transcapillary water transport and cardiac contraction

A prediction of water balance within the interstitium requires a prediction of capillary pressure. Such a prediction may follow from models accounting for the interaction between the mechanics of the circulation and the interstitium, based on the water exchange between these two compartments. In principle, the models presented for the analysis of the coronary circulation can be extended to do so.

As was discussed in Chapter 7, none of the models is capable of fully describing the coronary flow mechanics. Hence, the importance of the model analysis is not that this can yield an exact prediction of transmural pressure, but that insight into the possible mechanisms that should be considered is gained. Contraction increases interstitial fluid pressure, which leads the interstitium to empty into the capillaries. On the other hand, contraction will increase resistance to venous outflow from the myocardium and hence increase capillary blood pressure, resulting in a tendency of the interstitium to fill. The linear intramyocardial pump model, the waterfall model and nonlinear intramyocardial pump model provide a means to assess the importance of this interaction. In the first model, time averaged capillary pressure is independent of contraction. In the waterfall model contraction increases capillary blood pressure in systole but systole and diastole do not affect each other. In the nonlinear pump model contraction will increase capillary blood pressure as well but additionally accounts for diastolic–systolic interaction.

A proper extension of the models to account for water exchange should also take into account the exchange of substances across the capillary membrane. However, these modifications would be laborious and do not come within the scope of this chapter. Only the behavior of transmural capillary pressure, as an important determinant of the water flow over the capillary membrane, will be analyzed for the subendocardium, as has been done before by Spaan and Dankelman [25].

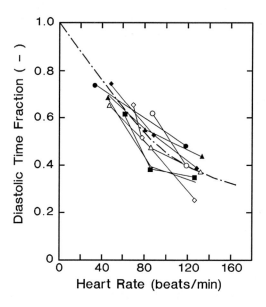

Figure 10.9: Relation between diastolic time fraction and heart rate as assumed for the simulation of effect of intramyocardial tissue pressure on capillary transmural pressure (broken curve). The data points are from series of dogs used for a different purpose. Duration of diastole was decided from a threshold value of 10% of the diastolic-systolic pressure difference.

For all three models of the subendocardial layer, transcapillary pressure has been calculated as a function of time. To make matters simple, it was assumed that tissue pressure had the shape of a square wave, a diastolic pressure of 0 mm Hg and a systolic pressure of 100 mm Hg. The relation between the diastolic time fraction and heart rate, illustrated in Figure 10.9, then defines the phasic tissue pressure completely as a function of heart rate. The time averaged transcapillary pressure was subsequently calculated as a function of coronary arterial pressure and time averaged tissue pressure. The latter was altered by assuming different heart rates.

10.7.1 Waterfall model and linear intramyocardial pump model: effect of coronary arterial pressure

Although the predictions for capillary transmural pressure are quite different, the behavior of the two models can be easily analyzed in conjunction with each other. The subendocardial vasculature is subdivided into two compartments, one proximal and one distal. The pressure at the node (the junction of the two compartments) is assumed to equal mean capillary blood pressure. In the waterfall model the distal compartment contains the waterfall element in series with a proximal resistance. The latter represents half of the resistance of the capillary bed plus the venous resistance. In the linear pump model, the distributed compliances and resistance of the proximal and distal parts of the vascular beds have been lumped together in the two compartments. However, since our interest is in the time averaged flow and the model is linear, the compliances are immaterial. The values for the proximal and distal resistances in the two models were taken as equal, with the former equal to 15% and the latter to 85% of total coronary resistance.

For the arrested state the two models are identical, since the waterfall element is not active, due to the fact that tissue and venous pressure are equal, and the compliances in the linear model play a role only during transients. The blood pressure at the connecting node, P_b, is then easily calculated since it depends on the ratio between distal resistance, R_{dis}, and total resistance, $R_{dis} + R_{prox}$, on the one hand, and the arterial and venous pressure on the other, which is written as:

$$P_b = \frac{R_{dis}}{R_{prox} + R_{dis}}[P_{art} - P_{ven}] + P_{ven} \qquad [10.5]$$

For the transmural pressure in the arrested heart:

$$P_{tr} = -P_{tis} + P_b \qquad [10.6]$$

Because of the same distal resistance in the two models, both have the same arterial pressure–transmural pressure curve, which is depicted in Figure 10.10. The slope of this curve represents the ratio between the distal resistance and total resistance.

For the continuously contracted heart, capillary blood pressure remains the same in the linear intramyocardial pump model since it is once again steady state. The arterial pressure versus transmural pressure curve is shifted parallel to the curve for the arrested heart by a distance which is equal to the tissue pressure.

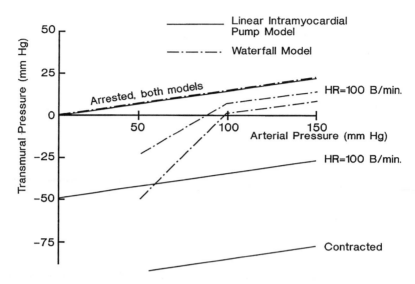

Figure 10.10: *Arterial pressure–transmural pressure curves as predicted by the waterfall and linear intramyocardial pump models (solid lines). Results are shown for the states of permanent arrest, permanent contraction and the heart beating at 100 beats min^{-1}. For the permanent arrested state the parameters were chosen such that the curves for the two models coincide (top solid and dash-dotted lines).*

For the waterfall model, we have to distinguish between two conditions: one where tissue pressure exceeds arterial pressure and the other where arterial pressure is higher than tissue pressure. For arterial pressures equal or lower than tissue pressure, there can be no flow according to the waterfall hypothesis (see Chapter 6). Consequently, capillary blood pressure will equal arterial pressure. With arterial pressure equal to tissue pressure, transmural pressure will be zero. When arterial pressure increases above tissue pressure, a driving pressure, which is the difference between arterial pressure and tissue pressure, will cause the flow of blood. Assuming that the waterfall function acts at the most distal part of the circulation, the capillary blood pressure can be calculated with Equation [10.5] after substitution of P_{ven} by P_{tissue}. This explains why the transmural arterial pressure curve for arterial pressures higher than tissue pressure has the same slope as in the arrested heart.

For the beating heart, the predictions of the two models are obvious as well. In a steady beating condition, the linear model predicts time averaged relations independent of compliance values since compliance effects are averaged out. As a result, the slope of the arterial pressure–transmural curve is always the same but runs parallel to the arrested situation with a difference in transmural pressure equal to the time averaged tissue pressure. With the waterfall model, we can consider the diastolic and systolic period independently. The time averaged transmural pressure difference follows from the difference between the time averaged capillary blood pressure and time averaged tissue pressure. The arterial pressure–transmural pressure curve is split up into two straight lines which intersect at an arterial pressure equal to systolic tissue pressure. For $P_{art} \geq P_{tissue}$ the slope is equal to the arrested and permanent contraction state. For $P_{art} < P_{tissue}$ the slope is determined by the duration of systole and diastole respectively.

10.7.2 Nonlinear intramyocardial pump model: the effect of arterial pressure

The nonlinear intramyocardial pump model allows the development of hypotheses about the role of the systolic–diastolic interaction of the venular compression on the transcapillary pressure. In this section, we present simulation results only of the model with intramyocardial pressure as the compressive force. The results presented were obtained with the standard pressure–volume relation of the venular compartment. The prediction using the alternative pressure–volume relation depicted in Figure 7.3 showed very similar results. For the tissue pressure, the parabolic-shaped pressure was used with a systolic maximum of 90 mm Hg.

The results with arterial pressure as the independent variable are depicted in Figure 10.11. For the arrested heart, the arterial pressure–transmural pressure relation, although quite linear, does not pass through the origin. In permanent systole, this relation exhibits a similar course to the waterfall model prediction for arterial pressures lower than systolic pressure. For a permanent contraction, the nonlinear intramyocardial pump pressure also predicts closure of the venules in the subendocardium. There is a difference, however, for arterial pressures higher than systolic tissue pressure. The model also predicts near closure in this condition.

The predictions for the beating heart are essentially different from the predictions by the two other models as is illustrated in Figure 10.11. Because of the systolic–diastolic interaction, the dependency of transmural pressure on arterial pressure in the beating condition is very similar to that of the arrested heart for arterial pressure above 50 mm Hg. For arterial pressures below this threshold, the transmural pressure drops sharply. The similarity between the relations of the arrested and beating heart are caused by the relative short duration of systole. For arterial pressures above 50 mm Hg, systole is not long enough to empty the venules. This explanation is in accordance with the time varying volume of the venular compartment illustrated in Figure 6.12.

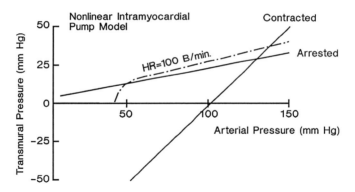

Figure 10.11: *Relations between time averaged capillary transmural pressure and arterial pressure simulated by the nonlinear intramyocardial pump model (Chapter 6). For the arrested heart the relation is almost linear. For the permanent systole (contracted), the venules are predicted to be completely closed. Note that for the beating heart the relation is quite similar to that of the arrested heart for arterial pressures above 50 mm Hg whereas below this threshold the transmural pressure drops readily. Since oncotic pressure difference between plasma and interstitium is about 7 mm Hg, net water transfer will be out of the capillary space for transmural pressure above this value.*

10.7.3 Simulated transmural pressure as function of heart rate at constant arterial pressure

Obviously, transmural pressure is not only a function of arterial pressure, but also of the time averaged tissue pressure. The model dependency of the latter relationship was evaluated for the different models. The tissue pressure was altered by changing the simulated heart rate. For the waterfall model and linear intramyocardial pump model, a square wave for the tissue pressure was assumed with a systolic value of 100 mm Hg. For the nonlinear pump model, parabolic tissue pressure was again assumed with a peak value of 100 mm Hg. The simulation results are presented in Figure 10.12.

The waterfall and linear intramyocardial pump models predict a linear decrease in transmural pressure with arterial pressure. For the linear intramyocardial pump model this decrease is trivial since capillary blood pressure is independent of tissue pressure and is only a function of arterial pressure, which is constant. The linearity is also to be expected from the waterfall model. Arterial pressure is lower than systolic tissue pressure and hence in systole the capillary blood pressure will be equal to arterial pressure, which was kept constant. Diastolic capillary blood pressure is also constant. Hence, both time averaged capillary blood pressure and time averaged tissue pressure will increase linearly

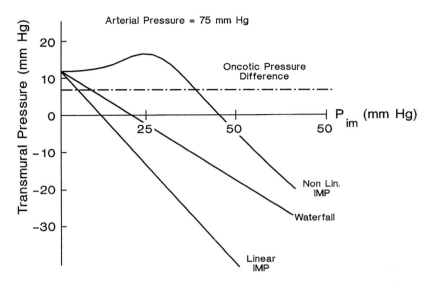

Figure 10.12: Simulation results of the dependency of transmural pressure on time averaged tissue pressure, P_{im}, according to the different models for the subendocardium. Tissue pressure was altered by changing the simulated heart rate. 'Linear IMP' refers to the linear intramyocardial pump model. 'Non Lin. IMP' refers to the nonlinear intramyocardial pump model. All models predict transfer of water out of the interstitium into the capillaries when the heart is arrested since transmural pressure is higher than oncotic pressure difference (dash-dotted line). Note the trajectory of tissue pressure over which transmural pressure is relatively constant for the nonlinear pump model.

with the systolic time fraction, but the latter pressure will increase more rapidly than the former pressure.

The tissue-transmural pressure curves predicted by the nonlinear intramyocardial pump model behave quite differently. With tissue pressure increasing from zero, the transmural pressure first increases or stays rather constant, depending on the pressure–volume relation for the venular compartment. The tissue pressure at which the transmural pressure becomes negative is much higher than with the other two models. The 50 mm Hg at which this happens coincides with a simulated heart rate of 100 beats · min^{-1}. The oncotic pressure difference between plasma and interstitium is about 7 mm Hg, as was discussed above. The horizontal dash-dotted line in Figure 10.12 refers to this oncotic pressure difference. For transmural pressures above this value, water is transferred out of the capillary space into the interstitium. For lower values, net water transfer takes place in the direction of the capillary space and the net force subsequently tends to empty the interstitium. The several interacting forces involved in establishing a water balance will further be discussed below.

10.8 Discussion

Under a wide variation of conditions, the interstitium is a stable compartment with respect to its water content, as was established from continuous weighing of the heart, and with respect to its constitution, as measurement from the lymph composition. However, volume and protein concentration of the interstitium may vary widely. Important determinants of the interstitial balance of water and oncotic pressure are similar to those in other organs. These have been discussed thoroughly by others [2, 6, 16]. Important factors are the interstitial compliance and dilution of interstitial proteins in the control of interstitial water content. Both reduce the driving forces for water flow from the blood capillaries into the interstitium. Undoubtedly there are extra factors to be considered when discussing the balances within the myocardium. For the time being, one can only guess about the differences in balances between subendocardium and subepicardium in a beating heart.

10.8.1 Transmural differences in water balance

The first question to be addressed is whether transmural exchange between subendocardium and subepicardium of lymph and/or interstitial fluid can occur. The presence of valves in the lymphatic system should prevent backflow within the lymph vessels. Even so, plasma water may still be extruded from the capillary blood in the subendocardium, which is then absorbed by the capillary blood in the subepicardium. Hence, a low lymphatic flow might be the cause of such an subepicardial-subendocardial interaction and not reflect a low net water transfer across the capillary membrane. In order to assess such a possible mechanism one has to know the potential of the total capillary membrane for transferring water in reference to the magnitude of myocardial lymph flow on the one hand and total coronary flow on the other hand. As was discussed above, water transfer across the total capillary wall area is about 5% of averaged coronary flow. In turn, under these same conditions, lymph flow is about a fraction of this water flow capacity across the capillary walls. Apart from the presence of valves in the lymphatic system this small lymphatic flow seems to point to an almost perfect match with exchange of interstitial fluid by the lymphatic system, if present, between subendocardium and subepicardium.

It is generally assumed that time averaged tissue fluid pressure is higher in the subendocardium than in subepicardium. As was discussed above, at a typical heart rate of $100 \cdot min^{-1}$, this difference in tissue pressure might be about 40 mm Hg. This is a considerable difference, taking into account the fact that the equivalent driving pressure for water flux in other organs is estimated to be about 10 mm Hg. Since plasma oncotic pressure is about 20 mm Hg and interstitial oncotic pressure is about 75% of this value, it is unlikely that differences in transmural tissue pressure can be compensated for by differences in interstitial oncotic pressures. Not much is known about transmural differences in interstitial compliance. Theoretically, there is a possibility that transmural differences in this parameter compensate for differences in tissue pressure.

10.8.2 Stabilizing mechanisms in transmural capillary pressure

The pressure dependent venous resistances and compliances of the different vascular compartments suggest a stabilizing mechanism for capillary transmural pressure. In this respect, the fact that the venular compartment does not show an open and shut behavior, as is assumed with the waterfall model, is important. The nonlinear intramyocardial pump models couple systole with diastole in the sense that diastole is too short to open the venular compartment completely. This increased venular resistance in the model impedes the flow through the myocardial system but also leads to a higher diastolic capillary blood pressure than occurs with a complete opening of the venular compartment. As is clear from Figure 10.12, this mechanism of variable venular resistance causes what is more or less a plateau in the relation between transmural pressure and tissue pressure. This reduces the range in endocardial–epicardial transmural pressure variations to be accounted for by other factors.

Obviously, the range of transmural pressure variation left to be compensated for depends on the assumed pressure–volume relations, and especially those of the venous compartments. There is much uncertainty in this respect. In fact, the assumed relationships are not much more than educated guesses. However, simulations with alternative pressure–volume relations showed similar results, suggesting that the basic mechanism is not overly sensitive to the exact course of the relation between pressure and volume in the venular compartment.

As noted in the introduction to this chapter, the beating of the heart results in a maintenance of heart weight [27]. Because of the small amount of lymph flow one has to conclude that in the beating heart the hydrostatic capillary pressure difference is smaller than the oncotic pressure difference. The nonlinear intramyocardial pump model predicts a larger difference and tends to predict edema formation. It will be clear, however, that the prediction of the exact level of the plateau in the intramyocardial pressure–transmural pressure relation depends on the assumed parameters.

10.8.3 Tissue pressure versus time varying elastance and water balance

We have not yet analyzed the prediction by the time varying elastance version of the intramyocardial pump model. However, from the simulation results presented in Chapter 6, we concluded that venular resistance was not greatly affected by heart contraction. Hence, with respect to capillary blood pressure, this model will behave somewhere between the nonlinear and linear intramyocardial pump models. Assuming that tissue fluid pressure depends on left ventricular pressure, as has been established by measurements of tissue pressure, this would imply that contraction will increase interstitial pressure more than capillary blood pressure and result in a net force for emptying the interstitial space. From this line of reasoning the probability for edema formation is lower when the coronary microcirculation is affected by contraction via time varying elastance than via tissue pressure secondary to left ventricular pressure. However, as discussed above, tissue pressure measurements as performed up to now are difficult to interpret. It is likely that capillary blood and interstitial fluid are both affected by the same compressive mechanism. Hence, a model for water transport based on the time varying elastance concept should incorporate an interstitial compartment analogous to the capillary compartment in which pressure variations are caused by time varying elastance. Without model calculations, predictions of this effect are difficult to make.

10.9 Summary

The lymphatic system is the natural drainage system of the interstitium. The interstitium is irregularly shaped and located in between the myocytes and around the vessels. The interstitial space is filled with gel and free movable water. The water content of the interstitium is determined by differences in oncotic and hydrostatic pressures between blood plasma and free interstitial water. There are several pathways for water and solutes. Water can diffuse through the endothelial cells and flow through the endothelial clefts. The larger molecules can be transported through the clefts as well as cellular vesicles.

An increase in coronary sinus pressure increases lymphatic flow, resulting in a decrease in the ratio between protein concentration in the lymph and blood plasma, illustrating the lower rate of transfer of these proteins as compared to water. This impediment of protein flux is described by the reflection coefficient. Data on interstitial pressure are confusing because the methods to measure this tend to disturb the interstitial structure. Recent measurements of stopped flow epicardial lymphatic pressure may offer an alternative but are still waiting a fuller interpretation. It has been calculated that transcapillary water transfer is about $3 \text{ ml} \cdot \text{min}^{-1} \cdot [100 \text{ g tissue}]^{-1}$, which is about 3% of the level of coronary flow.

Lymphatic flow is in the order of $3 \text{ ml} \cdot \text{hour}^{-1} \cdot [100 \text{ g}]^{-1}$ and is a fraction of the total transcapillary water transport possible. Hence, in agreement with the classic concept of Starling, it is to be expected that water will leave the capillaries at some locations and enter the capillaries at others.

The models on coronary flow mechanics were evaluated for their predictions on transcapillary pressure difference. When systolic–diastolic interaction was allowed as formulated by the nonlinear intramyocardial pump model, the transcapillary pressure in the beating heart behaved quite similar to that in the arrested heart. This in contrast to the waterfall model and linear intramyocardial pump model.

References

[1] ARESKOG NH, ARTURSON G, GROTTE G, WALLENIUS G (1964) Studies on heart lymph. II. Capillary permeability of the dog's heart, using dextran as a test substance. *Acta Physiol. Scand.* **62**: 218–223.

[2] AUKLAND K, NICOLAYSEN G (1981) Interstitial fluid volume: local regulatory mechanisms. *Physiol. Rev.* **61**: 556–643.

[3] BOLWIG TG, LASSEN NA (1975) The diffusion permeability of water of the rat blood-brain barrier. *Acta Physiol. Scand.* **93**: 415–422.

[4] CHVAPIL M (1967) Physiology of Connective Tissue. London, Butterworth: 417.

[5] CRONE C, LEVITT DG (1984) Capillary permeability to small solutes. In: *Handbook of Physiology. The cardiovascular system.* Eds. RENKIN EM, MICHEL CCH. Am. Physiol. Soc., Bethesda, **2 (IV)** chapter 10: 411–466.

[6] CURRY FE (1984) Mechanics and thermodynamics of transcapillary exchange. In: *Handbook of Physiology. The cardiovascular system.* Eds. RENKIN EM, MICHEL CCH. Am. Physiol. Soc., Bethesda, **2 (IV)** chapter 8: 309–374.

[7] EICHLING JO, RAICHLE ME, GRUBB JR RL, TER-POGOSSIAN MM (1974) Evidence of the limitations of water as a freely diffusible tracer in brain of the rhesus monkey. *Circ. Res.* **35**: 358–364.

[8] ELIASSEN E, FOLKOW B, HILTON SM, ÖBERG B, RIPPE B (1974) Pressure volume characteristics of the interstitial fluid space in the skeletal muscle of the cat. *Acta Physiol. Scand.* **90**: 583–593.

[9] FELDSTEIN ML, HENQUELL L, HONIG CR (1978) Frequency analysis of coronary intercapillary distances: site of capillary control. *Am. J. Physiol.* **235** (*Heart Circ. Physiol.* 4): H321–H325.

[10] GUYTON AC (1965) Interstitial Fluid pressure: II. Pressure volume curves of interstitial space. *Circ. Res.* **16**: 452–460.

[11] HAN Y, VERGROESEN I, SPAAN JAE (1990) Myocardial interstitial pressure is mainly caused by left ventricular pressure. Abstract. *Circulation* **82** *Suppl.* III: 380.
[12] HARRIS TR, GERVIN CA, BURKS D, CUSTER P (1984) Effects of coronary flow reduction on capillary-myocardial exchange in dogs. *Am. J. Physiol.* **234** (*Heart Circ. Physiol.* **3**): H679–H689.
[13] HEVESY G, JACOBSEN CF (1940) Rate of passage of water through capillary and cell walls. *Acta Physiol. Scand.* **1**: 11–18.
[14] KEDEM O, KATCHALSKY A (1958) Thermodynamic analysis of the permeability of biological membranes to non-electrolytes. *Biochem. Biophys. Acta* **27**: 229–246.
[15] LAINE GA, GRANGER HJ (1985) Microvascular, interstitial and lymphatic interactions in normal heart. *Am. J. Physiol.* **249** (*Heart Circ. Physiol.* **18**): H834–H842.
[16] MICHEL CCH (1984) Fluid movements through capillary walls. In: *Handbook of Physiology. The cardiovascular system.* Eds. RENKIN EM, MICHEL CCH. Am. Physiol. Soc., Bethesda, **2 (IV)** chapter 9: 375–409.
[17] MICHEL CC, MASON JC, CURRY FE, TOOKE JE, HUNTER P (1974) A development of the Landis technique for measuring the filtration coefficient of individual capillaries in the frog mesentery. *Q. J. Exp. Physiol.* **62**: 1–10.
[18] MILLER AJ (1982) *Lymphatics of the Heart.* Raven Press, New York.
[19] MILLER AJ, ELLIS A, KATZ LN (1964) Cardiac lymph: flow rates and composition in dogs. *Am. J. Physiol.* **206**: 63–66.
[20] PERL W, SILVERMAN F, DELEA AC, CHINARD FP (1976) Permeability of dog lung endothelium to sodium, diols, amides, and water. *Am. J. Physiol.* **230**: 1708–1721.
[21] POGATSA G, DUBECZ E, GABOR G (1976) The role of myocardial edema in the left ventricular diastolic stiffness. *Basic Res. Cardiol.* **71**: 263–269.
[22] POLIMENI PI (1974) Extracellular space and ionic distribution in rat ventricle. *Am. J. Physiol.* **227**: 676–683.
[23] ROSE CP, GORESKY CA, BACH GG (1977) The capillary and sarcolemmal barriers in the heart: an exploration of labeled water permeability. *Circ. Res.* **41**: 515–533.
[24] SALISBURY PF, CROSS CE, RIEBEN PA (1962) Intramyocardial pressure and strength of left ventricular contraction. *Circ. Res.* **10**: 608–623.
[25] SPAAN JAE, DANKELMAN J (1989) Prediction of dynamic transcapillary pressure difference in the coronary circulation. In: *Analysis and simulation of the cardiac system-Ischemia.* Eds. SIDEMAN S, BEYAR R. CRC Press Boca Raton, Florida: 265–275.
[26] STARLING EH (1896) On the absorption of fluids from the connective tissue spaces. *J. Physiol. Lond.* **19**: 312–326.
[27] STUBBS J, WIDDAS WF (1959) The interrelationship of weight change and

coronary flow in the isolated perfused rabbit heart. *J. Physiol. London* **148**: 403-416.
[28] TAIRA A, MATSUYAMA M, MORISHITA Y, TERASHI I, KAWASHIMA Y, MARUKO M, ARIKAWA K, MURATA K, AKITA H (1976) Cardiac lymph and contractility of heart. *Jap. Circ. J.* **40**: 665–670.
[29] VARGAS FF, BLACKSHEAR GL, MAJERLE RJ (1980) Permeability and model testing of heart capillaries by osmotic and optical methods. *Am. J. Physiol.* **239** (*Heart Circ. Physiol.* **8**): H464-H468.
[30] VARGAS FF, BLACKSHEAR GL (1981) Secondary driving forces affecting transcapillary osmotic flows in perfused heart. *Am. J. Physiol.* **240** (*Heart Circ. Physiol.* **9**): H457–H464.
[31] VARGAS FF, BLACKSHEAR GL (1981) Transcapillary osmotic flows in the in vitro perfused heart. *Am. J. Physiol.* **240** (*Heart Circ. Physiol.* **9**): H448–H456.
[32] VERGROESEN I, NOBLE MIM, SPAAN JAE (1987) Intramyocardial blood volume change in first moments of cardiac arrest in anesthetized goats. *Am. J. Physiol.* **253** (*Heart Circ. Physiol.* **22**): H307–H316.
[33] YUDILEVICH DL, ALVAREZ OA (1967) Water, sodium and thiourea transcapillary diffusion in the dog heart. *Am. J. Physiol.* **213**: 308–314.

Chapter 11

Oxygen exchange between blood and tissue in the myocardium

Jos AE Spaan and Peter A Wieringa

11.1 Introduction

OXYGEN TRANSPORT TO THE MYOCYTES has been recognized as a factor of utmost importance to cardiac metabolism and control of blood flow for many decades. On a macroscopic scale, the problem seems simple since supply and demand are normally matched, as discussed in Chapter 9. However, as discussed in Chapters 1 and 3, both flow and oxygen pressures may vary widely in the myocardium at the microscopic level and in tissue units of milligrams and grams.

Two basic physical principles which determine the supply of oxygen to the mitochondrial machinery in the cardiac cells may be distinguished: convection and diffusion. Convection of oxygen refers to transport by the flow of the fluid in which it is dissolved, such as blood, interstitial fluid and intercellular fluid. Diffusion is the result of Brownian motion of the molecules. The net transport by diffusion is induced by concentration gradients, which for oxygen are caused by the oxygen consumption within the cells. Convection and diffusion of oxygen always occur. However, in certain parts of the circulation and in tissues, one of the two means for transport may be dominant. A simplification of the problem can be reached by, on the one hand, neglecting the diffusion component in the transfer of oxygen by blood and, on the other hand, by neglecting the convection of oxygen in the interstitial and intercellular space. After these simplifications a system is left in which still many significant subprocesses can be recognized. A list of these processes, by no means exhaustive, includes: red cell spacing in capillaries, capillary network geometry, capillary spacing, and a possible diffusion barrier to oxygen at the capillary or cellular interface. Moreover, in red muscle, myoglobin acts as an extra oxygen buffer, but may also facilitate oxygen transport in the tissue [27]. In fact, the same holds true for hemoglobin within the red cells [24, 26, 36, 47, 48]. The degree of complexity of the analysis of oxygen delivery to myocardial tissue starts to grow when these factors are added. Studies have been undertaken on many of these processes but we are far from understanding the interactions of all these mechanisms. A large obstacle to this understanding is due to the difficulty of studying the coronary microcirculation. Again, the subendocardium is the most important region to be studied because of its vulnerability, but using current approaches, in situ studies are impossible. As a result, the investigations of oxygen transfer into tissues have always been strongly theoretically oriented. This chapter will be restricted to the theoretical analysis of three major questions:

1. how much tissue can be supplied by oxygen from a single capillary,

2. how strong is the interaction in oxygen exchange between neighboring capillaries, and

3. what is the impact of the capillary network of the heart and especially its interconnectedness on oxygen distribution?

The oxygen diffusion from a single capillary was elegantly analyzed by Krogh in 1919 [28, 29], in a study which described the potential of a capillary to supply oxygen to its surroundings. The second problem has received some attention in the last decades by the work of Popel [39, 40, 41] and Grunewald and Sowa [17]. Here, the results of a numerical solution to the two-dimensional diffusion equation will be discussed. These results were obtained by our own group, and described by Wieringa in his PhD thesis [53]. The interaction of O_2 diffusion is restricted to capillaries one to two intercapillary distances away. However, because all neighboring capillaries interact, the oxygen exchange of one capillary theoretically affects the exchange of all other capillaries in the network. The solutions to this two-dimensional problem are then applied to predict the distribution of oxygen in tissues that have a capillary network as described in Chapter 3. The theoretical method is briefly explained in this chapter and the reader is referred to Wieringa's thesis for the detailed analysis. The conclusions of the study are highly relevant to the issue of heterogeneity in oxygen transport.

A theoretical diffusion problem relevant to many in vitro experiments, but also to the exchange of oxygen between the left ventricular cavity and the subendocardium, is the diffusion of oxygen from a space containing oxygen into a layer of tissue. This theory was partly developed by Hill in 1929 [19] and will be evaluated in this chapter as well. The spherical symmetrical diffusion problem will not be treated in this chapter. The specific implications of different geometrical boundary conditions has been studied by Boag [3].

The analysis of oxygen transfer from a single capillary, intercapillary shunting, and transfer from the ventricular cavity will be subjected to a few major assumptions. It is assumed that oxygen, bound and dissolved, is homogeneously distributed within the blood and that oxygen consumption is homogeneously distributed within the tissue. The assumptions related to the oxygen distribution in blood will not be discussed in detail below. On the basis of geometrical considerations, these assumptions are not unreasonable. The capillary radius is small compared to half the intercapillary distance, and the dimensions of the red cells as well as the distance between adjacent red cells in the capillaries are small compared to the capillary length. Moreover, because of capillary blood flow, the spatial inhomogeneity will be averaged out in time. It is more difficult to rationalize the plausibility of the assumption of homogeneous oxygen consumption in tissue. Oxygen consumption is restricted to the mitochondria that occupy a significant space of the tissue, about 20%. Therefore, the error introduced by this assumption on homogeneous oxygen consumption will receive some special attention below. Moreover, the intracellular oxygen gradients, facilitated diffusion by myoglobin, and the possible resistance of the capillary wall to oxygen consumption will be discussed.

11.2 Experimental data on oxygen distribution in the myocardium

Extracellular devices, cellular constituents, and diffusible tracers have been used to probe the oxygen tension. Gayeski [10] gives a short summary of the different techniques. The most frequently used O_2 probe is the oxygen electrode. Oxygen electrodes make use of the property that a suitable polarizing voltage, applied to a precious metal in the presence of O_2, generates a current, while reduction of O_2 occurs at the electrode's surface. One of the sources of error in the application of these electrodes is due to the formation of some hydrogen peroxide (H_2O_2) which causes disturbance of the measurement. The initial problems with the bare electrode tip have been overcome by covering the tip by a membrane, resulting in a better environment for the reaction. However, a diffusion barrier is introduced in this way [46, 51, 52]. Among the technical difficulties are the oxygen consumption of the electrode that influences the local O_2 tension, and the residual current in the absence of oxygen. For an electrode with a tip of 1 μm, the consumption is negligible. Grunewald [16] estimated that the diffusion field of such electrodes should be around 10 μm. Hence, the P_{O_2} signal obtained will reflect a volume average around the electrode which for the heart has geometrical dimensions which are at least about half the intercapillary distance. The response time of oxygen electrodes is from several seconds to one minute.

Whalen [51] measured oxygen tension in the beating cat heart using a gold-silver electrode. Possible P_{O_2} variations throughout a heart beat were not reflected by his measurements which might have been due to the slow response time of the electrode. Spatial variations were between 0 and 31 mm Hg (obtained from 8 cats) with a skewed distribution and a mean of 6-9 mm Hg in both left and right ventricles. The P_{O_2} was significantly higher in the subepicardial layers (10 mm Hg) than in deeper layers (5 mm Hg). It is impossible to conclude whether the P_{O_2} values measured [32, 51] reflect those of small blood vessels, intra- or intercellular spaces. This uncertainty is due to the badly defined position of the oxygen sensitive element within the tissue. Purely based on chance one might expect that the contribution of these different compartments are proportional to their percentage of volume in the tissue. Since about 70% of the tissue volume are myocytes, one might expect that this compartment dominates the P_{O_2} measurements.

Optical methods make use of the differences in light absorption of myoglobin and/or hemoglobin at different oxygen saturation levels. In 1937, Millikan [34] designed experiments to study the kinetics of the physiology of myoglobin in situ. A major problem with the optical methods is the interference of light absorption of hemoglobin and myoglobin. These problems have to be solved by either applying many wavelengths or even continuous spectra, or a very high spatial resolution.

Grunewald and Lubbers [15] and Holz et al. [20] used a cryomicrophotometric method to determine hemoglobin saturation of capillaries in the rabbit heart. Small samples (2-3 mm) were removed in situ and rapidly frozen. Thin, 10 – −12 μm, microslices 2-3 mm from the epicardium were made at −60 ^{0}C and hemoglobin saturation was measured at −100 ^{0}C in a vacuum isolated microscope cooling chamber. The histograms of HbO_2 saturations had maxima between 20 and 47% and minima between 0 and 10%. The arterial HbO_2 saturation in femoral artery was 98% at the moment of freezing the heart. The distribution histogram was less skewed than to be expected from the P_{O_2} histograms found by Whalen [51].

Coronary venous oxygen pressure has been measured in vitro [9] on isolated dog hearts using oxygen electrodes. Results from Weiss and Sinha [50] on oxygen saturation in small coronary veins, measured by means of a microspectrophotometric method are presented in Figure 11.1. Mean venous saturations were 51.7±3.5% (SE) for subepicardial and 33.8±3.0% (SE) for subendocardial veins. The subendocardial and subepicardial distributions were also quite differently affected by an increase in left ventricular systolic pressure. The P_{O_2} histograms showed a rather uniform distribution.

11.2 Experimental data on oxygen distribution in the myocardium

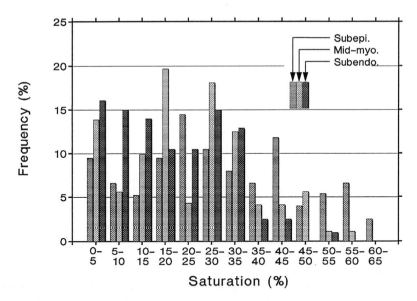

Figure 11.1: *The distribution of oxygen saturation of small veins over the myocardial wall as estimated by cryomicrospectrophotoscopy. Note the significant number of veins with oxygen saturation close to zero. (Redrawn from Weiss and Sinha [50]).*

In general one might expect that the oxygen pressures calculated from capillary red cell oxygen saturations overestimated the space averaged capillary oxygen pressure. The diffusion of oxygen out of the red cells requires an oxygen gradient and hence plasma P_{O_2} will be lower than red cell P_{O_2} [12].

Recently, Nakamura et al. [37] applied a P_{O_2} sensor at the paraconal interventricular branch of the left coronary artery. Taking arterial oxygen pressure as 100% they measured an oxygen pressure of 70% in the subendocardial myocardium, 15% in the mid-ventricular wall and 9% in the subepicardial layers. Hypoxia following an occlusion first occurred at the mid-myocardium. The author suggests that oxygen is supplied directly from the left ventricular cavity to subendocardial areas.

Obviously, each technique has its strong and its weak points. The advantage of measuring oxygen saturation of either hemoglobin or myoglobin is that direct information on the oxygen content of blood or myoglobin is obtained. Relating oxygen tissue pressure to oxygen content requires the additional knowledge of local factors as pH, $P_{C_{O_2}}$ and for blood, $_{2,3}$DPG concentration. On the other hand, tissue oxygen pressure is the driving force for oxygen diffusion. A complete picture of the local state of, and potential for, oxygen transport requires more than just the measurement of one variable. Apart from these conceptual problems, there are also technical problems inherent to each method. Insertion of oxygen electrodes has the disadvantage of introducing a foreign object into the tissue. It is clear that cell damage, and occlusion of capillaries and arterioles may be the immediate result of the penetration of an electrode and that vasoconstriction and vasodilation due to inflammation will influence the local P_{O_2} within several minutes. The cryogenic methods for the determination of hemoglobin and myoglobin saturations have the disadvantage that first the tissue has to be frozen. The freezing front has to enter the tissue from the epicardium and at best from epi- and endocardium together. A freezing front proceeds at a rate declining with the inverse of the square root of the tissue thickness already frozen. It takes seconds to freeze a layer of 1 cm thick. As soon as the epicardium is frozen, blood stops flowing into and out of the myocardial wall and blood in the deeper layers will have some time left to redistribute while oxygen consumption continues. However, although some uncertainty exists with respect to the quantification, a key message of all these studies is that oxygen pressure and oxygen saturations are quite heterogeneously distributed. All studies, regardless of whether local oxygen tension or local saturations were measured, exhibit a wide range of values. Moreover, each method shows a significant amount of tissue with low oxygen pressure or saturation. The histogram of Figure 11.1 indicates that 10–15% of myocardial tissue has a venular oxygen saturation of 0–5%. Understanding oxygen distribution at the microscopic level indeed requires understanding of the oxygen delivering capacity of a single capillary as a function of its oxygen pressure as well as the potential of diffusional interaction between capillaries.

11.3 Oxygen transfer from a single capillary without intercapillary exchange

The potential of a capillary to provide surrounding tissue with oxygen can be studied by solving the diffusion equation for the situation depicted in Figure 11.2 where a capillary surrounded by tissue is being considered. The tissue forms a cylinder with radius R_K which may be infinite. It is assumed that the oxygen pressure everywhere in the capillary is the same and equal to P_c. Oxygen consumption per unit tissue weight is denoted by M and constant as long as oxygen partial pressure is greater than zero. For the radius where $P = 0$ the oxygen consumption is zero as well. The problem is cylindrically symmetrical, reducing it to one dimension: the radial dimension.

The derivation of the diffusion equation and its solution are provided in Appendix D. In this section only the solutions will be presented and the importance of the parameters will be discussed.

The oxygen partial pressure distribution can best be presented in its dimensionless form by

11.3 Oxygen transfer from a single capillary without intercapillary exchange

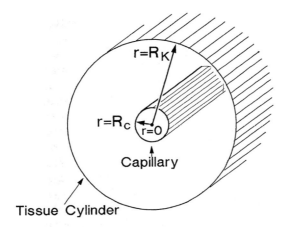

Figure 11.2: Illustration of the diffusion of oxygen from a capillary to surrounding tissue. A capillary with radius R_c is surrounded by a tissue cylinder which can either extend to infinity or have a radius R_K. The latter is referred to as the Krogh cylinder. The solution discussed in this section requires the definition of either P_{O_2} or flux, for example, at the capillary wall and/or outer tissue radius. Two such boundary conditions are required.

$$P^*(r^*) = M^* r^{*2} + K_1 \ln(r^*) + K_2 \qquad [11.1]$$

where:

$P^*(r^*)$	is the dimensionless oxygen pressure defined by Equation [11.3],
$\ln(r^*)$	is the natural logarithm of the dimensionless radius r^*, defined by Equation [11.2],
K_1, K_2	are integration constants to be determined from the boundary conditions.

The dimensionless variables are defined as follows:

$$r^* = \frac{r}{R_c} \qquad [11.2]$$

which is the relative radius within the tissue with reference to the capillary radius, R_c.

$$P^*(r^*) = \frac{P}{P_c} \qquad [11.3]$$

is the oxygen pressure as fraction of the pressure at $r = R_c$ being P_c.

The dimensionless parameter M^* expresses the balance between oxygen demand, M, on the one hand and the factors determining the potential of the capillary to deliver oxygen on the other hand:

$$M^* = \frac{MR_c^2}{4\alpha D P_c} \qquad [11.4]$$

where:

> α is the solubility of oxygen in the tissue,
> D is diffusion coefficient of oxygen in tissue.

The advantage of the dimensionless notation is that the relative importance of physical parameters becomes clear and the presentation of results is facilitated.

11.3.1 Krogh solution

The classic problem applies to a tissue cylinder with radius R_K supplied with oxygen by the capillary in the center. This tissue cylinder, which is referred to as a Krogh cylinder [30], is assumed to be insulated for oxygen exchange from its surroundings. The two boundary conditions, needed to solve Equation [11.1], are

- oxygen pressure is prescribed at the wall of the capillary, and

- oxygen flux is zero at the outer wall of the tissue cylinder, and therefore also the oxygen pressure gradient is zero.

Translated into mathematical notations these boundary conditions are:

$$\begin{cases} r^* = 1 & P^* = 1 \\ r^* = R_K^* & \dfrac{dP^*}{dr^*} = 0 \end{cases} \qquad [11.5]$$

where R_K^* is ratio between the radius of the Krogh cylinder and that of the capillary.

Substitution of these boundary conditions in Equation [11.1] (see Appendix D) results in expressions for the integration constants

$$K_1 = -2M^* R_K^{*2} \qquad [11.6]$$

$$K_2 = 1 - M^* \qquad [11.7]$$

The resulting equation can now be written as

$$P^*(r^*) = M^*\left[r^{*2} - 2R_K^{*2}\ln(r^*) - 1\right] + 1 \qquad [11.8]$$

The oxygen pressure distribution clearly depends on the values of the parameters, M^* and R_K^*. In order to present relationships between the dimensionless variables relevant to physiological problems one needs estimates for the ranges of values of the dimensionless parameters. As has been discussed in Chapter 3, a

11.3 Oxygen transfer from a single capillary without intercapillary exchange

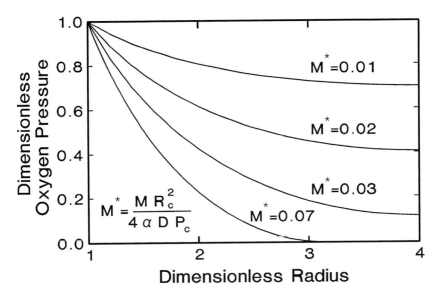

Figure 11.3: Solutions of the Krogh equation, $P^*(r^*)$ according to Equation [11.8], for several values of the dimensionless oxygen consumption assuming a Krogh cylinder radius of 4 times the capillary radius. Note that the shape of the curves for $M^* = 0.01$, 0.02 and 0.03 are similar since $1 - P^*$ is proportional to M^*. However, for $M^* = 0.07$ the shape is different since the Krogh radius is too large. The balance of factors expressed by M^* is too large for all the tissue to be supplied. This curve was calculated using boundary conditions expressed by Equation [11.9].

wide range of values of the capillary radius and intercapillary distance has been published. We will assume 2.5 μm and 20 μm respectively for these distances. The order of magnitude of the Krogh cylinder radius should be half the intercapillary distance, measured from capillary center to capillary center, which makes 10 μm a good estimate for the Krogh cylinder radius for the heart. This results in $R_K^* = 4$. An upper value of M^* requires the definition of an upper value of tissue oxygen consumption and minimal value of oxygen partial pressure. Taking 0.66 ml $O_2 \cdot s^{-1} \cdot [100 \text{ g}]^{-1}$ as an estimate for M and 10 mm Hg for P_c and substituting the values of $\alpha = 2.8 \times 10^{-3}$ ml O_2 mm Hg$^{-1} \cdot [100 \text{ g}]^{-1}$ and $D = 1.5 \times 10^{-5}$ cm^2 s^{-1}, we arrive at an upper limit for $M^* = 0.022$.

The distribution of the dimensionless oxygen pressure for four different values of M^* is illustrated in Figure 11.3. Note that the solutions can only be valid if the calculated oxygen pressure remains positive throughout the whole tissue cylinder. If negative values do occur, the derived integration constants are no longer valid and Equation [11.8] no longer holds. This is illustrated by the curve for $M^* = 0.07$ which was calculated applying an additional implicit boundary condition which is discussed below.

11.3.2 Maximal radius of the Krogh cylinder

In the classic Krogh problem the radius of the tissue cylinder is a preset geometrical constraint. It is of great practical interest to know how large this radius may be without generating an anoxic region in the outer shell. In other words, what is the maximal radius of a Krogh cylinder at a given oxygen consumption and capillary oxygen pressure?

The problem of the maximal radius of the Krogh cylinder can be treated in the following way. The maximal radius is defined as R_f^* without a priori knowledge of its magnitude. The oxygen pressure and oxygen flux at this boundary are known and should be zero here. In mathematical form, the boundary conditions become

$$\begin{cases} r^* = 1 & P^* = 1 \\ r^* = R_f^* & \begin{cases} \dfrac{dP^*}{dr^*} = 0 \\ p^* = 0 \end{cases} \end{cases} \qquad [11.9]$$

Substitution of these relations into the general solution, Equation [11.8], yields

$$K_1 = -2M^* R_f^{*2} \qquad [11.10]$$

$$K_2 = 1 - M^* \qquad [11.11]$$

$$M^*\left[R_f^{*2}[1 - 2\ln(R_f^*)] - 1\right] + 1 = 0 \qquad [11.12]$$

Equation [11.12] presents an implicit relation between the maximal Krogh radius as a function of the dimensionless oxygen consumption only. The oxygen partial pressure as a function of dimensionless radius remains as described by Equation [11.8], obviously only within the Krogh cylinder. Outside this cylinder oxygen pressure is simply equal to zero.

The relative maximal Krogh radius as a function of dimensionless oxygen consumption is depicted in Figure 11.4. As is to be expected, the Krogh radius goes to infinity when the oxygen consumption approaches zero.

Equation [11.12] provides an implicit relation between maximal Krogh radius and oxygen consumption. For practical purposes, it might be useful to have an explicit formula to calculate the Krogh radius. An empirical approximation of Equation [11.12] is formed by

$$R_f^* = 1.242 M^{*-0.35} \qquad [11.13]$$

11.3 Oxygen transfer from a single capillary without intercapillary exchange

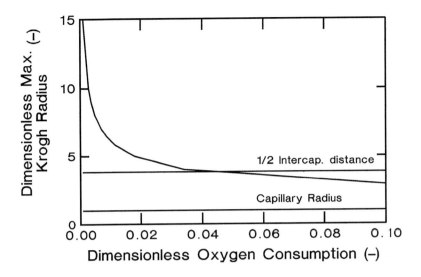

Figure 11.4: *Relationship between maximal dimensionless Krogh radius, R_f^* and dimensionless oxygen consumption as calculated from Equation [11.12]. Note the sharp increase for very small values of dimensionless oxygen consumption.*

The relative error in predicting the relative Krogh radius by this equation is a function of the dimensionless oxygen consumption and is graphically depicted in Appendix D. The relative error is within ± 3% and depends on the dimensionless oxygen consumption.

The solution of Equation [11.12] in realistic units is illustrated in Figure 11.5. The left panel gives the Krogh radius relative to capillary radius (2.5 μm) as a function of oxygen consumption for several values of capillary oxygen pressure, P_c. Realistic values for oxygen consumption of the arrested heart (arrest), heart under normal conditions (control) and in exercise (exercise) are indicated. The horizontal line indicates half of the intercapillary distance. As long as the maximal Krogh radius is longer than this distance it may be assumed that all tissue can be supplied by oxygen up to a sufficient amount. Note that this still is so during exercise at a capillary oxygen pressure of 10 mm Hg (curve not shown). An oxygen pressure of 10 mm Hg coincides, according to a standard oxygen dissociation curve, with a coronary venous oxygen saturation of about 20%. Hence, we may conclude that the capillary distance is small enough to supply all the tissue with sufficient oxygen. Note also that for oxygen consumption of the heart at control rate and an oxygen pressure of 50 mm Hg the maximal Krogh radius is 14.2 times the capillary radius, 3.6 times the radius of the tissue cylinder supplied by oxygen if the area of influence is restricted to one tissue cylinder per capillary

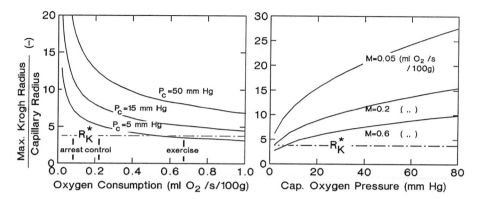

Figure 11.5: Dependency of the maximal dimensionless Krogh cylinder radius, R_f^*, on oxygen consumption for different values of capillary oxygen pressure (left panel) and as a function of capillary oxygen pressure, P_c, for different values of oxygen consumption (right panel). Horizontal lines indicate half the intercapillary distance. If the maximal Krogh radius becomes smaller than half the intercapillary distance, the capillary density is too low and an anoxic core may occur. The units of oxygen consumption, M, are ml $O_2 \cdot s^{-1} \cdot [100\ g]^{-1}$.

and 1.8 times the intercapillary distance. Hence, at this oxygen pressure a single capillary is able to supply oxygen to a tissue space normally supported by six more capillaries.

The dependency of the maximal Krogh radius on capillary oxygen pressure is illustrated in the right panel of Figure 11.5. Note that this dependency is modest. The reduction of the maximal Krogh radius at high oxygen consumption ($M = 0.6$ ml $O_2 \cdot s^{-1} \cdot [100\ g]^{-1}$) is only 30% with a reduction of oxygen pressure from 50 to 15 mm Hg. Obviously, the reduction in amount of tissue supplied is much more than 30%, namely 63%, since tissue volume within the Krogh cylinder is proportional to πR_f^2.

11.3.3 General solution to the Krogh problem

In the previous two sections the tissue cylinder had a prescribed radius, R_K, and calculations of maximal Krogh radius, R_f were made. These two conditions can be summarized in a general solution. In dimensionless notation this yields

$$P^* = M^*[r^* - 2R_t^{*2} \ln(r^*) - 1] + 1 \qquad [11.14]$$

with:

$$R_t^* = R_K^* \quad \text{if} \quad R_K^* < R_f^*$$
$$R_t^* = R_f^* \quad \text{if} \quad R_K^* > R_f^*$$

where:

> R_t is the radius of the tissue cylinder to which Equation [11.14] applies,
> R_K is the Krogh radius being fixed at half the intercapillary distance,
> R_f is maximal Krogh radius being the radius of tissue cylinder that maximally can be supplied by oxygen from a single capillary, given the physiological parameters, e.g., capillary pressure and oxygen consumption.

11.3.4 Decrease of oxygen partial pressure in a perfused capillary applying the Krogh model

So far, the decrease of oxygen pressure along a capillary was neglected. At high capillary blood flow and low oxygen consumption this may be a reasonable assumption, but it is certainly not true in general. Capillary oxygen pressure decreases with distance from the inlet. The rate by which it decreases depends on the flow of blood. The smaller the capillary blood flow the more rapid the capillary P_{O_2} decays with distance. The decay of capillary P_{O_2} can be predicted from mass balance considerations. Again, some simplifications have to be introduced in order to keep the mathematics manageable. It is assumed that oxygen diffusion in the axial direction can be ignored, both within the capillary and in the tissue. This assumption is not unrealistic considering the ratio between capillary length and Krogh cylinder radius and the much faster axial transport by convection as compared to diffusion.

The mathematical formulation of the problem is provided in Appendix D. The derivation is based on the division of the capillary with surrounding tissue into cylindrical slices. For each slice, the Krogh equation is solved. It is not difficult to see that when the maximal Krogh radius is larger than the assumed tissue radius, the oxygen pressure in the capillary will decrease linearly with distance z. The solution is

$$P(z) = P_i - \frac{M\pi[R_t^2 - R_c^2]}{Qh\beta} z \qquad [11.15]$$

where:

> P_i is the oxygen pressure at the capillary inlet, $[P_i]$ = mm Hg,
> Q is capillary flow, $[Q]$ = ml · s^{-1},
> h is the oxygen binding capacity, $[h]$ = ml O$_2$ · ml^{-1} blood,
> β is the slope of the oxygen saturation curve of hemoglobin, $[\beta]$ = mm Hg^{-1}.

The oxygen pressure in the tissue as a function of radius r and at given z can be calculated by the Krogh equation, Equation [11.14]. As is to be expected, the gradient in capillary oxygen pressure in the axial direction depends on the ratio between the oxygen consumption per unit length, $M\pi[R_t^2 - R_c^2]$, and the oxygen flow through the capillary $Qh\beta$. We will not elaborate on this solution any further but apply it in the analysis of heterogenous flow below.

11.4 Capillary interaction with blood–tissue oxygen exchange

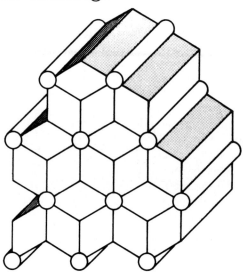

Figure 11.6: *Two-dimensional slab of tissue perforated by capillaries. The capillaries are stacked in a regular hexagonal structure. The tissue slab is divided into subunits, each bounded by two capillaries and referred to as elementary units. The two-dimensional diffusion equation will be solved for this plane with an arbitrary distribution of oxygen pressure in the capillaries. Gradients within the capillaries are assumed to be zero. Oxygen consumption is assumed to be constant.*

The Krogh cylinder analysis showed that oxygen may diffuse from a capillary to far over half the intercapillary distance into the cylinder of influence of neighboring capillaries. Hence, neighboring capillaries will affect each other's oxygen delivery to the tissue. Moreover, although capillaries may be stacked in an orderly and symmetrical manner, their oxygen pressures may be asymmetrical because of different perfusion conditions of the capillaries and different oxygen pressures of their inlets.

This section addresses the problem of quantifying the interaction in a system of parallel capillaries stacked in a hexagonal manner as is illustrated in Figure 11.6. We first will consider the condition where there are no axial gradients of oxygen pressure in either capillaries or tissue. Moreover, it is assumed that the oxygen pressure in a capillary unit is constant. The capillaries are represented by i, which has a value between 1 and N, N being the number of capillaries in the slab. The oxygen pressure of capillary i is referred to as P_i.

Because there is no cylinder symmetry, we now have to solve the diffusion problem in two dimensions. The two-dimensional diffusion equation is:

$$\left[\frac{\partial^2 P}{\partial x^2} + \frac{\partial^2 P}{\partial y^2}\right] = \frac{M}{\alpha D} \quad [11.16]$$

where x and y are orthogonal coordinates, also being orthogonal with z.

The derivation of this equation will not be discussed here. It follows simply from a mass balance of a slab of tissue with a small height and width. The boundary conditions are formed by the values of the oxygen pressure at the capillary walls defined as P_i and zero oxygen flux at the boundaries of the tissue slab. However, if a slab of tissue with a large length and height is considered, periodicity may be assumed if all capillaries have the same oxygen pressure resulting in boundary conditions at lines of symmetry around a capillary.

Analytic solutions to Equation [11.16] for the geometry as given by Figure 11.6 are hard to derive. The so-called finite element numerical technique provides tools for calculating the oxygen pressure distribution. Basically, one could solve the diffusion equation for the complete area. However, use may be made of the periodicity in the capillary lattice to reduce the computational effort. Without going into too much detail we will report some results derived by Wieringa [53] in his PhD thesis using a finite element method (AFEP) [44].

11.4.1 Oxygen pressure distribution

The oxygen pressure in the tissue is simply described by

$$P(x,y) = f(x,y)\frac{MR_c^2}{\alpha D} + \sum_i^N g_i(x - x_i, y - y_i)P_i \quad [11.17]$$

where P_i the is oxygen partial pressure in capillary i. The functions $f(x,y)$ and $g_i(x - x_i, y - y_i)$, in mathematical terminology, refer to the homogeneous solution and inhomogeneous solution of the diffusion equation respectively. Hence, the oxygen pressure distribution follows from the linear superposition of functions $f(x,y)$ and $g_i(x - x_i, y - y_i)$. These functions will now be discussed briefly.

Basically, the functions $f(x,y)$ and $g_i(x - x_i, y - y_i)$ are the same for all capillaries. The function $g_i(x - x_i, y - y_i)$ is equal to one at the wall of capillary i and zero at the walls of all other capillaries. The function $f(x,y)$ is zero at all capillary walls, including capillary i. Within the tissue, $P(x,y)$, the oxygen partial pressure, is positive, except for the condition of extreme oxygen consumption where the analysis does not hold. The function $f(x,y)$ is essentially negative within the tissue and zero at the capillary walls. The function is weighted, at

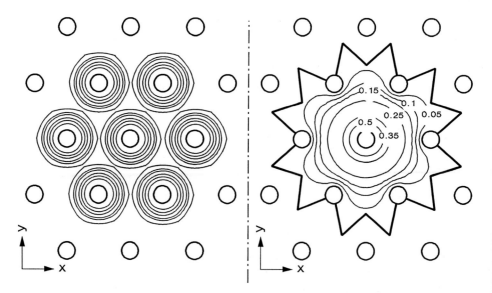

Figure 11.7: Partial solutions of the diffusion equation. Left: $f(x,y)$ which equals zero at the capillary walls and is solely determined by the ratio $MR_c^2/(\alpha D)$. The function is negative at all values for x, y. Note the symmetry in the solution which is due to the symmetry in the field. The contours correspond with 1/20, 1/10, 1/5, 1/4, 1/3 and 1/2 of the minimum value of $f(x,y)$ respectively. This minimum value is obtained at the center of gravity between three capillaries. Right: $g_i(x - x_i, y - y_i)$ which equals zero at all capillary walls except capillary i where it equals unity. The numbers indicate the value of $g_i(x - x_i, y - y_i)$: $g_i(x - x_i, y - y_i) = 1$ at the wall of the capillary in the center.

a giving geometry of capillaries and tissue, by the ratio between oxygen consumption and the product of solubility and diffusion coefficient. Each function $g_i(x - x_i, y - y_i)$ is positive in the tissue and is weighted by the oxygen partial pressure of capillary i.

The function $g_i(x - x_i, y - y_i)$ is not repetitive with each capillary because it has value one at the wall of capillary i but zero at all other capillaries. This function alone describes the oxygen diffusion from a single capillary when oxygen consumption is zero and all other capillaries are maintained at zero oxygen pressure. Hence, this function will approach zero at a large distance from capillary i, since oxygen is taken up by the capillaries at zero oxygen pressure. A realistic boundary condition to the two-dimensional diffusion equation that would result in the true function $g_i(x - x_i, y - y_i)$, is zero oxygen pressure at infinite distance of capillary i. However, we assumed zero oxygen pressure at a boundary indicated with the heavy line in the right panel of Figure 11.7. There were two reasons

11.4 Capillary interaction with blood–tissue oxygen exchange

why we assumed the function to be zero at such a limited distance from capillary i. The first is practical, since in this way the area over which the function had to be calculated was limited. More importantly, however, the limitation of the area for solving the diffusion equation limits the interaction of diffusion to its closest neighbors. This considerably facilitates the capillary network analysis below. Comparing the results of the limited area with a larger area showed only minor deviations induced by the restriction of the tissue area for solving the diffusion equation. Hence one may assume that the error introduced by restricting the area of calculation is limited.

The functions $f(x,y)$ and $g_i(x - x_i, y - y_i)$ are almost circularly symmetric around capillary i up to close to half the intercapillary distance. The function $g_i(x - x_i, y - y_i)$ deviates from circular at a larger distance from the capillary because of the sink function of the neighboring capillaries.

As is expressed by Equation [11.17], the oxygen distribution in a slab of tissue follows from a superposition of functions. On physical principles, the oxygen pressure must either be positive or equal to zero. Hence, at each arbitrary location the second term of the right side of this equation must exceed the first term. The function $g_i(x - x_i, y - y_i)$ expresses the possibility of interaction between neighboring capillaries which even may result in a net transfer of oxygen from one capillary to another. Hence, instead of delivering oxygen to tissue, a capillary can absorb oxygen from its surrounding tissue.

The extreme that allows comparison with the Krogh problem discussed above is when all capillaries have the same oxygen pressure. Because of symmetry the oxygen partial pressure and oxygen flux over the hexagonal boundaries should equal zero. As is clear from Figure 11.7, the elementary functions are circularly symmetric over an important fraction of the space in an hexagon around a capillary. The Krogh solution approximates the solution quite well under these conditions. However, with an uneven distribution of capillary oxygen pressure asymmetry is generated and interaction between capillaries should be taken into account.

Because of the assumed boundary around a capillary, indicated by the heavy lines in Figure 11.7, it is obvious that each capillary has an interaction between its 6 neighboring capillaries. However, in an indirect way a single capillary will theoretically affect the oxygen exchange of all other capillaries.

11.4.2 Average oxygen pressures in tissue units and oxygen flow through these

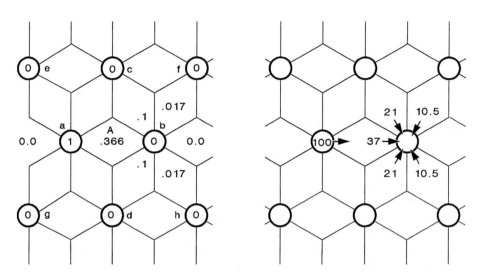

Figure 11.8: Average oxygen pressure in and flux through tissue units. Left: Values of contribution of the function $g_i(x - x_i, y - y_i)$ to the average oxygen pressure in tissue units. One unit has been denoted 'A'. Right: The flux of oxygen through the tissue units from capillary i to a neighboring capillary expressed in percent.

The hexagonal structure of capillary distribution allows tissue units to be defined by Figure 11.6 and Figure 11.8. The state of the oxygen supply to these units can be expressed by their average oxygen pressure. Because of the linearity of the equations, we can calculate the average tissue unit P_{O_2} as the sum of average values of the functions $g_i(x - x_i, y - y_i)$ and $f(x, y)$, weighted with the factors defined in Equation [11.17].

The oxygen consumption in a tissue unit results in an average oxygen pressure reduction of $-5.88 M R_c^2 [\alpha D]^{-1} \cdot$ mm Hg. The factor -5.88 follows from the function $f(x, y)$. From the left panel in Figure 11.8 it can be concluded that the oxygen pressure in each tissue unit is directly affected by 8 capillaries, denoted $a - h$ in the left panel, according to the respective functions $g_i(x - x_i, y - y_i)$. Adding all the effects one may write for the average oxygen pressure in a tissue unit, A,

$$P_A = -5.88 \frac{M R_c^2}{\alpha D} + 0.366[P_a + P_b] + 0.1[P_c + P_d] + 0.017[P_e + P_f + P_g + P_h] \qquad [11.18]$$

where $P_a - P_h$ are the oxygen pressures in capillaries $a - h$.

A simple check on the correctness of this equation follows by taking the oxygen pressures in the 8 capillaries equal to unity and the oxygen consumption zero. The average oxygen pressure in the tissue unit should then become equal to the oxygen pressure in the capillaries, which indeed is so. The calculated difference between capillary P_{O_2} and the average P_{O_2} in adjacent tissue units induced by oxygen consumption (the first term in the right side of Equation [11.18]) equals 1.31 mm Hg for control and about 4 mm Hg for exercise.

11.4.3 Tissue oxygen distribution in a network model inducing heterogeneous capillary flow

In Chapter 3 a model of the capillary bed was presented, taking into account the many capillary anastomoses found in the heart. We now define tissue slabs with a thickness equal to the elementary capillary segment length corresponding to this model. The anastomoses are thought to be within the boundary planes between adjacent slabs. The oxygen distribution within each slab can be calculated as a function of capillary P_{O_2}s. The mass balance for oxygen couples inlet and outlet P_{O_2} of the capillary segments under given conditions of perfusion and oxygen uptake. Because of the interaction between P_{O_2}s in adjacent capillaries, the outlet P_{O_2} of one capillary is not only a function of its own inlet P_{O_2} but also a function of the inlet P_{O_2}s of several other capillaries in the vicinity. Such interactions can be well described in matrix and vector equations [53].

When it is assumed that capillary flows are well mixed at capillary branchings, the mass balance for one layer can be combined with the mass balance for the previous and next layer. In order to limit the computational effort it also has been assumed that capillary hematocrits are constant. Thus a set of equations can be obtained for the entire network. The unknown capillary P_{O_2}s can be calculated using this set of equations with the known variables: capillary blood flows, oxygen consumption rate, and arteriolar P_{O_2}. It should be noted that this model does not account for a spatial and temporal variations in capillary hematocrit. The oxygen distribution under several conditions was calculated in a network consisting of 7 by 7 capillaries in width and 7 segments in length. The interested reader is referred to the thesis of Wieringa [53] for the mathematical details of this analysis. Here we will discuss some salient results of this analysis.

In our simulations we assumed that the arteriolar oxygen pressure was 50 mm Hg, the value at which, according to the linearized oxygen saturation curve, the blood is shown to have an oxygen saturation of 85%. This assumes that some oxygen has left the blood in the arterioles before it enters the capillary bed. An arteriolar P_{O_2} of 50 mm Hg is not unrealistic since such values have been found for the hamster cheek pouch [8]. A cross section through the network is depicted in Figure 11.9. Capillaries are indicated by small hexagons instead of circles to make drawing them easier. The rhombi, representing the tissue units, and the

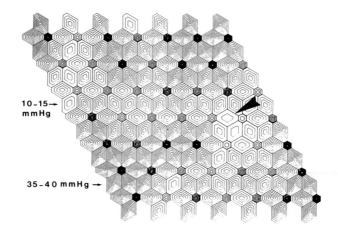

Figure 11.9: *Capillary and oxygen partial pressure in a cross section of the tissue. The capillaries are represented by hexagons. The tissue units are indicated by rhombi. The number of repetitions of hexagons and rhombi in each of the units indicates the level of the capillary and tissue unit P_{O_2} respectively. Each repetition corresponds to 5 mm Hg. Some pressures are indicated in the figure. The arrow indicates a tissue segment in which the oxygen pressure deviates strongly from a neighbor capillary. (Redrawn from Wieringa [53].)*

capillary hexagons are repeated for every 5 mm Hg of the level of the P_{O_2}.

Note the heterogeneous distribution of oxygen pressure over the tissue rhombi. Capillaries with low P_{O_2} may be alongside a capillary of high P_{O_2}. A further analysis of the role of shunting under a variety of conditions follows from the oxygen histograms calculated by the model.

11.4.4 Oxygen histograms

A means of obtaining an impression of the distribution of tissue oxygen pressure and the factors that influence this is the representation of the results in histograms. Tissue unit P_{O_2}s were grouped in ranges of 2.5 mm Hg and the frequency histograms were then composed. The effect of the absence of intercapillary shunting was studied by means of a slight modification to the model, such that oxygen exchange was limited to a hexagon around the capillaries. This, in fact, is the same condition as for the Krogh cylinder and it will be referred to as the Krogh network model. The effect of oxygen shunting on the oxygen distribution in tissue can now be evaluated by using the same capillary network for both conditions, with and without the potential for diffusional shunting. This comparison is provided in Figure 11.10.

Under standard parameter values for both models the variation of the oxygen

11.4 Capillary interaction with blood–tissue oxygen exchange

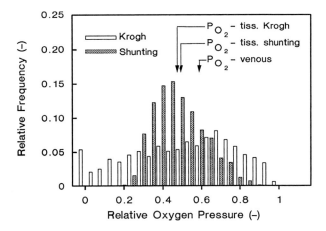

Figure 11.10: *Histograms of predicted oxygen pressure distribution. The range of P_{O_2} per bar = 2.5 mm Hg. A relative $P_{O_2} = 1$ corresponds to arteriolar P_{O_2}. Open bars are results from the distributed Krogh model. Each capillary segment has its own tissue cylinder to which to deliver oxygen since intercapillary shunting is prevented. Filled bars are results from the network model allowing for intercapillary shunting. Note that the network model applying the Krogh cylinder was not accommodated to decrease tissue cylinder diameter when the Krogh diameter exceeded max. tissue cylinder diameter that could be provided with oxygen. This resulted in the prediction of negative P_{O_2} for some segments. (Data from Wieringa [53].)*

pressure histograms can be reduced by as much as a factor of 2 if shunting is taken into account. The broadening of the histogram when shunting is excluded is to be expected since, if shunting is not feasible, the tissue around a capillary with low oxygen pressure will be deprived of oxygen, whereas it would otherwise receive oxygen from more distant capillaries. A second important conclusion is that the mean tissue oxygen pressure is lower than the venous oxygen pressure. This is due to the fact that some capillary pathways form a flow shunt with respect to others. The diffusional shunting has little impact on this finding, since the conclusion is the same when shunting is prevented. It is important to note that in the classic concept of parallel perfused capillaries draining into a collecting vein, the average oxygen tissue pressure is higher than venous oxygen pressure.

Obviously, the shape of the histograms depends on the value of the different parameters. For instance, if the blood flow is increased while the oxygen consumption rate is kept constant, the variation of the oxygen histograms will decrease and the mean value will increase. In an infinite flow rate the variation will be zero and the mean tissue P_{O_2} will equal the arteriolar P_{O_2}. Under such hypothetical conditions, the oxygen supplied by the blood outweighs the oxygen uptake by the tissue. On the other hand, decreasing flow at constant oxygen consumption will result in a decrease of the mean tissue P_{O_2} and an increase in variation. This reasoning holds for the conditions with and without shunting, albeit in different degrees.

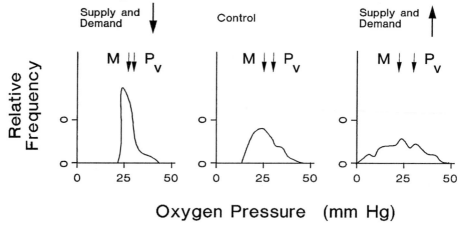

Figure 11.11: Effect of a concomitant increase in flow with oxygen consumption on the tissue oxygen pressure histograms of the model allowing for intercapillary shunting. The middle panel is the control histogram. The left panel is the result if both flow and oxygen consumption are reduced by a factor of two. The right panel shows the result where flow and oxygen consumption are increased by a factor of four. Note that the predicted venous oxygen pressure, P_v, is unaltered because of the macroscopic mass balance. The figure illustrates the dependence of possible capillary interaction on the level of oxygen consumption. The inverse of the width of the histograms indicates the magnitude of intercapillary oxygen shunting.

The effect of a concomitant change of flow and oxygen consumption is less obvious. Figure 11.11 shows the results obtained from a network (with oxygen shunting) in which oxygen consumption and overall flow through the network are varied proportionally. According to the Fick principle venous oxygen saturation should remain constant which, if we neglect altering influences on the oxygen saturation curve, implies a constant venous oxygen pressure. It was considered as a positive test of the model that indeed the predicted venous oxygen pressure remained constant and equal to the value resulting from the Fick principle. The model calculations predict a relatively small change in mean tissue oxygen pressure. However, the variation changes significantly. The concomitant increase of flow and oxygen consumption results in a broadening of the histogram and hence in an increased number of tissue units with very low oxygen pressures. The concomitant decrease of flow and oxygen consumption results in a smaller variation.

The cause of this relation between variation and oxygen consumption and flow must be looked for in the intercapillary oxygen shunting. As was discussed in relation to the Krogh cylinder, the radius within which a capillary affects oxygen transfer diminishes as oxygen consumption increases, and hence the potential for intercapillary shunting declines. The histogram yields the characteristics of the distributed Krogh model under this condition.

11.4.5 Oxygen pressure history of a red cell travelling through the capillary network

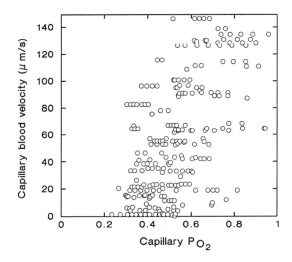

Figure 11.12: *Correlation between flow into and oxygen delivery by capillary segments in a network under control conditions. Note the poor correlation which is a result of the poor correlation between flow and distance travelled by the blood from an arteriole on the one hand and diffusional shunting on the other hand.*

In a model of homogeneous perfused parallel capillaries, flow is constant in all capillaries while oxygen pressure is gradually declining with distance from the capillary inlet. As a result, there will be no correlation between flow and capillary oxygen pressure. However, in a capillary network with interconnectedness as analyzed in this section, one would intuitively assume a correlation between capillary oxygen pressure and flow. A high flow suggests a path of low resistance and hence short travel time of red cells from the feeding arterioles. A test of these intuitions is provided for by a correlation between flow and oxygen pressure over capillary segments in our network model as is given in Figure 11.12.

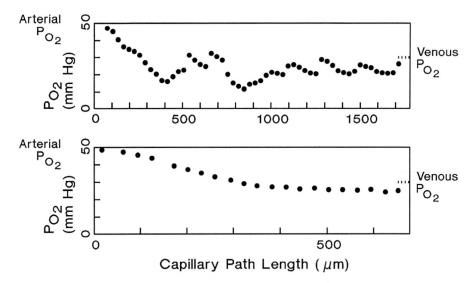

Figure 11.13: Oxygen pressure variations of red cells travelling through the capillary network along two different pathways. Each data point is the mean oxygen pressure in a capillary segment. The successive segments form a pathway for red cells to flow from an arteriole to a venule. In the bottom panel the decrease in oxygen pressure is gradual, in accordance with the classical school of thought. This holds for short paths. The top panel shows a pathway in which oxygen pressure decreases below the level of venous pressure, and then increases. The jumps in oxygen pressure are due to blood mixing at branch points. A gradual increase in oxygen pressure is due to oxygen shunted from adjacent capillaries.

Although there is some correlation, it is poor because of mixing of capillary blood at interconnections and diffusional shunting.

There are many possible capillary paths along which a red cell can travel from the arteriolar inlet to the venular outlet [43]. In the model two pathways were selected to construct Figure 11.13. The bottom panel depicts a pathway in which oxygen pressure decreases gradually from arteriole to venule. This is the classical theory; a gradual decline in oxygen pressure when the red cell travels further into the microcirculation. This decline is predicted by the Krogh model (Equation [11.15]). The top panel in Figure 11.13 shows a pathway about twice as long as the one in the bottom panel. Here, the course of oxygen pressure is more erratic. Our imaginary red blood cell increases its oxygen pressure a number of times when going from one segment to the other. This is due to blood with a different P_{O_2} mixing at capillary bifurcations. In some parts of the pathway, oxygen pressure shows a gradual increase instead of a decrease. This is due to a net oxygen intake from adjacent capillaries and can be predicted only by models allowing intercapillary shunting. Such conditions can occur only if the possibility of intercapillary diffusion is incorporated in the model. However, the sudden increase in capillary P_{O_2} as depicted can be found in any model that induces a heterogeneous capillary flow.

11.5 Oxygen diffusion from the ventricular cavity and thoracic space

Oxygen exchange may occur at the boundaries of the myocardium. Such a possibility should be especially considered at the endocardium. There is evidence [54] that with coronary occlusion, a thin layer at the subendocardium continues to consume oxygen, most probably due to oxygen diffusing from the ventricular cavity. Moreover, where the epicardial microcirculation is studied in an open thorax preparation, a layer with significant thickness is affected by the gas exchange between subepicardium and the medium with which the epicardium is in contact. It is therefore worthwhile to estimate the depth over which oxygen may diffuse into tissue from a flat surface. The solution to this diffusion problem is also worth knowing, because in many experimental preparations, tissue is submerged in a solution from which it receives its nutrients.

The mathematical problem is similar to that of the Krogh cylinder with maximal radius. It is assumed that oxygen only enters the tissue at the boundary. The oxygen pressure at this boundary is known and denoted as P_1. There is a region with thickness d_f in which oxygen is consumed at a constant rate independent of oxygen pressure. At a distance larger than d_f, oxygen pressure and oxygen consumption are zero.

The diffusion equation can be derived in a way similar to the oxygen diffusion in radial direction for the cylinder symmetric example, yielding

$$\frac{d^2 P(x)}{dx^2} = \frac{M}{\alpha D} \quad [11.19]$$

The general solution can be obtained by integration over x twice, yielding

$$P(x) = \frac{M}{2\alpha D} x^2 + K_1 x + K_2 \quad [11.20]$$

The boundary conditions are

$$\begin{cases} x = 0 & P = P_1 \\ x = d_f & \begin{cases} P = 0 \\ \dfrac{dP}{dx} = 0 \end{cases} \end{cases} \quad [11.21]$$

Substitution of the boundary conditions in Equation [11.20] yields expressions for the integration constants and d_f

$$K_1 = -\frac{M}{\alpha D}d_f \qquad [11.22]$$

$$K_2 = P_1 \qquad [11.23]$$

$$d_f = \sqrt{\frac{2\alpha D P_1}{M}} \qquad [11.24]$$

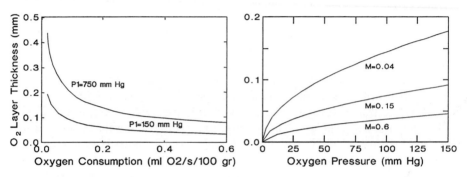

Figure 11.14: The thickness of a layer that can be supplied with oxygen from a flat surface. Left: Layer thickness as function of oxygen consumption at two different oxygen pressures. High values for oxygen pressure are chosen deliberately since such high values are often aimed at in experiments. Right: Layer thickness as a function of oxygen pressure at three levels of oxygen consumption (Units are ml $O^2 \cdot s^{-1} \cdot [100\ g]^{-1}$. These levels of oxygen consumption relate to the metabolism of the non-beating heart, the heart beating in control and at extreme work.

The Equations [11.22] to [11.24] completely define the oxygen pressure distribution within the oxygen consuming layer. This distribution obviously follows a parabolic function. The thickness of the layer that receives oxygen from the boundary layer is defined by Equation [11.24]. The dependency of this thickness on oxygen pressure at the boundary and oxygen consumption of the tissue is illustrated in Figure 11.14.

The thickness of the layer of influence can be much larger in practice, when oxygen is still being supplied by the capillaries, as this will reduce the effective oxygen consumption expressed by M in Equation [11.24].

11.6 Effect of oxygen consumption localized in the mitochondria

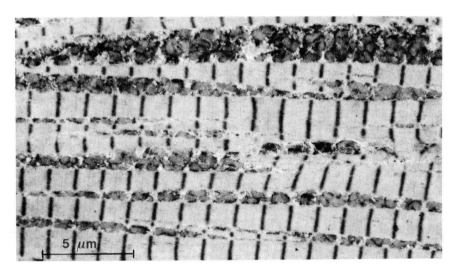

Figure 11.15: *Electron microscopic photograph of myocardial structure (human) elucidating the density and dimensions of mitochondria as well as the distance between them. The horizontal bands of granular structures consist of mitochondria. The distance between the dark vertical bands indicates the sarcomere length. (Courtesy of Dr. K.P. Dingemans of the Academic Medical Center, the University of Amsterdam.)*

In the theoretical analysis above, it was assumed that oxygen consumption was independent of the space coordinates. This, however, is not likely since oxygen consumption is concentrated in the mitochondria. An impression of mitochondrial density and dimensions is provided in Figure 11.15. By assuming a cylindrical structure of the mitochondria with a diameter of 1 μm and an intramitochondrial distance from center to center of about 4 μm, one arrives at a reasonable description of spatial structure.

In order to estimate the effect of localized oxygen consumption on the oxygen pressure distribution the following two models are compared as illustrated in Figure 11.16. The first model consists of a tissue cylinder with radius R_w. We assume that oxygen is consumed homogeneously over the cylinder. R_w equals half of the approximate intermitochondrial distance. The second model consists of a cylinder of tissue also with radius R_w but with a concentric inner cylinder representing the mitochondrium and hence with a radius R_m, equal to the approximate radius of the mitochondria. We assume that oxygen is exclusively consumed in the mitochondria and that the outer shell only serves as diffusion

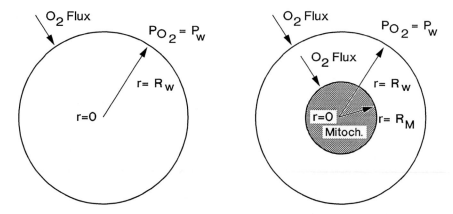

Figure 11.16: Models for evaluation of the effect of oxygen consumption restricted to the mitochondria on P_{O_2} distribution. Left: Tissue cylinder with radius R_w; P_{O_2} at the wall $= P_1$. Oxygen consumption is homogeneously distributed in the cylinder. Right: Same cylinder as on left, but now all oxygen consumption is within a smaller cylinder with radius R_m. The total oxygen consumptions of left and right cylinders are equal.

resistance to oxygen diffusing from the outer cylinder wall into the center. The oxygen consumption is located at the crista which are distributed over the mitochondria. One may, therefore, apply the first model of the homogeneously distributed oxygen consumption to the mitochondria after appropriate parameter selection.

11.6.1 Equations

For the first model the oxygen consumption is independent of radius. Oxygen consumption per unit mass is denoted M and equals the oxygen consumption of the tissue as can be estimated from, e.g., Fick's principle applied to the myocardium as a whole. For the second model, there are two regions: the outer shell with oxygen consumption zero and the inner cylinder with homogeneous oxygen consumption. Hence, the inner region is similar to the cylinder of model one but oxygen consumption per unit mass, M_m, will be larger. Since in the second model all oxygen consumption of the cylinder with radius R_w is concentrated in the cylinder R_m, one may write

$$M_m = \frac{\pi R_w^2}{\pi R_m^2} M \qquad [11.25]$$

Because the boundary conditions are different compared to the mathematics related to oxygen transfer out of a capillary it is useful to define the dimensionless

11.6 Effect of oxygen consumption localized in the mitochondria

variables differently as well. For both models it is convenient to make the independent variable r dimensionless with respect to R_w and the dependent variable $P(r)$ with respect to the oxygen pressure at $r = R_w$. This yields

$$r^* = \frac{r}{R_w} \qquad [11.26]$$

$$P^*(r^*) = \frac{P}{P_w} \qquad [11.27]$$

where:

R_w is the radius of the tissue cylinder,
P_w is the oxygen pressure at $r = R_w$.

Hence, the dimensionless oxygen pressure expresses the oxygen pressure as fraction of the pressure at $r = R_w$. Arbitrarily we define the dimensionless oxygen consumption for both models as

$$M^* = \frac{MR_w^2}{4\alpha D P_w} \qquad [11.28]$$

The boundary conditions for the two models at $r^* = 1$ are essentially the same since oxygen pressure and oxygen flux at the outer radius of both the tissue cylinders are equal. In dimensionless terms, the boundary conditions are

$$r^* = 1 \quad \begin{cases} P^* = 1 \\ \dfrac{dP^*}{dr^*} = 2M^* \end{cases} \qquad [11.29]$$

The following specific solutions can be derived, substituting the boundary conditions and the value of M^* in Equation [11.1].

First model; without mitochondrium:

$$P^*(r^*) = M^* r^{*2} + 1 - M^* \quad \text{with } M^* < 1 \qquad [11.30]$$

Second model; with mitochondrium:

$$P^*(r^*) = 2M^* \ln(r^*) + 1 \quad \text{with } r^* > e^{-1/(2M^*)} \qquad [11.31]$$

Note that Equation [11.31] describes the oxygen pressure distribution in the outer shell regardless of the radius of the mitochondrium as long as the condition with this equation is met. The conditions noted with the equations are required since otherwise the predicted oxygen pressure would be negative, which is impossible.

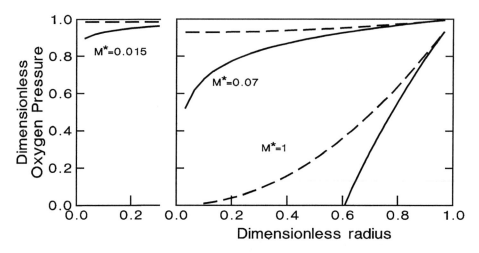

Figure 11.17: Solutions to the problem of oxygen diffusion from the wall of a tissue cylinder to the center. Broken curves: model with homogeneously distributed oxygen consumption, model 1. Solid curves: model with the outer shell and O_2 consumption concentrated in mitochondria, model 2. Horizontal axis: dimensionless radius in the tissue cylinder, which equals 1 at the outer wall. Vertical axis: dimensionless oxygen pressure being also one at the outer cylinder wall. Right: Distribution of oxygen pressure at a value $M^* = 1$ and $M^* = 0.07$. $M^* = 1$ corresponds to the limit for model 1. For $M^* > 1$ an anoxic core is predicted. $M = 0.07$ is a limit for model 2. All oxygen consumption may be concentrated closely around $r = 0$. For $M > 0.07$ the mitochondrium must have a finite diameter, otherwise the diffusion resistance of the outer shell would be too large. $M^* = 0.07$ corresponds to a heart using 4 times more oxygen than under control conditions and a tissue oxygen pressure of about 2 mm Hg. Left: Part of the solution for $M^* = 0.015$ which corresponds to a heart using 4 times more oxygen than at control and a tissue pressure of about 10 mm Hg.

11.6.2 Effect of mitochondrial oxygen consumption on oxygen pressure distribution

The oxygen distribution within the tissue cylinder as predicted for model 1 and the outer shell of model 2 for three different values of M^* is depicted in Figure 11.17. These values of M^* were chosen because of the following reasons.

$M^* = 1$ is a limit for the homogeneous model. For higher values of M^* the model predicts an anoxic core. For $M^* = 1$, the second model shows a rapid drop of oxygen pressure which becomes zero at approximately $r^* = 0.62$. This solution is only physically real if the radius of the mitochondrium were 0.62 times the radius of the tissue cylinder and all oxygen would be consumed at the outer surface of the mitochondrium at an oxygen pressure of zero. This is not realistic,

11.6 Effect of oxygen consumption localized in the mitochondria

apart from the last condition, since mitochondria may use oxygen at their maximal rate at a very low pressure. However, the radius of the mitochondrium is about 1 μm and about 25% of the radius of the tissue cylinder. Moreover, oxygen consumption is distributed within the mitochondria. The solutions at $M^* = 1$ of the two models illustrate that theoretically, in terms of oxygen uptake capacity, it would be better for oxygen consumption to be homogeneously distributed.

$M^* = 0.07$ is a limit of model 2. It describes a situation where all oxygen consumption is concentrated in a very small region around $r = 0$ and the region offering resistance to oxygen diffusion to the mitochondrium is maximal. This solution, in fact, illustrates that the concentration of oxygen consumption in mitochondria is not a major restriction under normal circumstances. $M^* = 0.07$ corresponds to an average tissue oxygen consumption of 0.6 ml $O_2 \cdot s^{-1} \cdot [100\ g]^{-1}$, being four times the control value, and an oxygen pressure at the outside of the tissue cylinder of 2 mm Hg.

$M^* = 0.015$ corresponds to a more realistic example, oxygen consumption being still four times above control, and oxygen pressure at the outside mitochondrial wall being 10 mm Hg. Note that in this instance the average oxygen pressure in the tissue cylinder will be close to that at the cylinder wall and not much different for either model. Small gradients of oxygen pressure around mitochondria with high oxygen consumption are also predicted when other geometries for mitochondria are assumed [5, 6].

When describing the distribution of oxygen pressure within the mitochondrium, assuming homogeneous distribution of oxygen consumption within it, one has to define its radius, R_m, and the boundary conditions at its outer wall. The boundary conditions should reflect the continuity of oxygen pressure and of oxygen flux at $r = R_m$. The first, $P(r = R_m)$ follows from the solution to the outer shell of model 2, the second from the fact that no oxygen is consumed in the outer shell. Hence, the total flow of oxygen at $r = R_m$ must equal that at $r = R_w$. We have seen from Figure 11.17 that for realistic values of oxygen consumption and tissue oxygen pressure ($M^* < 0.07$) the pressure drop from $r = R_w$ to $r^* = 0.25 \times R_w$ is small. For simplicity's sake we neglect this pressure drop. Hence, the solution for model 1 now also applies to the inner cylinder of model 2.

It is important to note that the values of M^* in Figure 11.17 correspond to the same operational conditions for both the first model and the mitochondrium. This is so because in the definition of M^*, Equation [11.28], MR_w^2 appears in the numerator. If the model applies to the mitochondrium, R_w should be replaced by R_m but M should be replaced by the oxygen consumption per unit weight of mitochondria, M_m. In order to have model 1 and model 2 describe the same tissue, MR_w^2 must equal MR_m^2 in order to keep the total oxygen consumption of the tissue the same (Equation [11.25]).

After having established that the dotted curves in Figure 11.17 also apply to the inner part of the mitochondrium we now may evaluate the oxygen pressure distribution within the mitochondrium. Let us first consider $M^* = 0.07$, a value applied to exercise and oxygen pressure of 2 mm Hg at $r = R_m$. The minimum oxygen pressure within the center of the mitochondrium will only be about 5% lower than at $r = R_m$. Oxygen consumption should be 14 times (1/0.07) higher, or P_{O_2} at $r = R_m$ 14 times lower before an anoxic core within the mitochondrium will result.

If one subdivides the tissue space in between capillaries into imaginary cylinders as in our model 2, it is plausible that the error made by the assumption of homogeneous distributed O_2 consumption is small close to the capillary wall but increases with distance from the capillary wall when oxygen pressure drops. As was discussed above, the error made in estimating the space averaged oxygen pressure over a cylinder increases with increasing M^*. M^* increases with decreasing oxygen pressure which in turn decreases with distance from the capillary. One should note that the homogeneous model overestimates the possibility for transfer of oxygen from the capillary because oxygen pressure within small tissue cylinders including a mitochondrium is overestimated by the homogeneous models.

11.6.3 Oxygen pressure near mitochondria

It has been found that especially in muscle with high metabolism mitochondria may be concentrated around the capillaries [23]. This may be interpreted as a compensation for higher diffusion distances. Such a compensatory mechanism is difficult to understand from the analysis of oxygen transfer in this chapter. Obviously, a location close to a capillary wall reduces the diffusion distance to a specific capillary, but it increases the diffusion distance to other capillaries on which it might depend when oxygen pressure in the capillary close by becomes too low. In order to test the hypothesis that mitochondria migrate to locations of higher oxygen pressure, one should look at a correlation between mitochondrial density and, e.g., capillary oxygen saturation. Such a study has, to our knowledge, not been performed yet. Recently, it was found that the concentration of mitochondria close to sarcolemma was also higher than interfibrillar mitochondria in myocytes of hypermetabolic rats. However, interfibrillar mitochondria exhibited a larger oxidative capacity [45]. Hence, for interpretation of effects of diffusion distances related to mitochondrial densities, only counting of mitochondria is not sufficient. The inhomogeneity of mitochondrial oxygen consumption should be taken into account too.

When mitochondria are suspended in a well-mixed solution, oxygen consumption is constant and high up to very low oxygen pressures; the oxygen pressure at which oxygen consumption of isolated skeletal muscle drops to half the maximal value is then 0.05 mm Hg [7], and that of isolated cells from adult rat ventricles is about 0.15 mm Hg [55]. The fact that mitochondrial oxygen consumption can be maximal at such a low pressure does not imply that oxygen pressure must be at such a level within a normal cell. This is confirmed by experiments of Katz et al. [22] in which it was shown that the difference between oxygen pressure inside and outside isolated myocytes in a well-mixed solution can be smaller than 2 mm Hg when the outside oxygen pressure is between 6 and 25 mm Hg. The rate by which mitochondria consume oxygen is probably not determined by oxygen pressure within the cell but by feedback from the ATP producing chain [1].

11.7 Intracellular oxygen transfer and resistance of the capillary wall to oxygen

11.7.1 Diffusion coefficient of oxygen in tissue

The interior of the myocardial cells is not just an aqueous solution but contains more or less solid structures. The limitation of aqueous space and its tortuosity makes oxygen diffusion per unit area of tissue slower than through a layer of pure water [4]. The diffusion coefficient applied for the calculation of dimensionless oxygen consumption was 1.5×10^{-5} cm$^2 \cdot$ s^{-1}, being close to that of water. The protein concentration of the interior of the cardiac cell is between 20 and 30 g%. The diffusion coefficient for oxygen in a protein solution of 30 g% is about 1.1×10^{-5} cm$^2 \cdot$ s^{-1}. However, lower diffusion coefficients for oxygen through tissue have been published as well. Jones [21] reported a range of 0.6×10^{-5} to 1.5×10^{-5} cm$^2 \cdot$ s^{-1} with an average of 1.1×10^{-5} cm$^2 \cdot$ s^{-1} for 8 studies. However, other arguments have been put forward by Jones which lead him to conclude the O$_2$ diffusion coefficient within cytoplasm would be about 5- to 10-fold lower than in water, meaning about 2.5- to 5-fold lower than for 30 g% protein solutions. Such a low diffusion coefficient for oxygen would imply, according to our calculations, that with a capillary oxygen pressure of 25 mm Hg the maximal radius for oxygenation in exercise would be reduced to less than half the intercapillary distance. Such a low diffusion coefficient would therefore be incompatible with exercise.

11.7.2 Facilitation of oxygen by myoglobin

Besides factors that hamper the diffusion of oxygen in the cell interior there are factors that will enhance the transfer of oxygen. Heart cells contain myoglobin which may facilitate oxygen diffusion. A second factor is intracellular convection which may be induced by fiber shortening and myocyte thickening. This factor of convection has not received a lot of attention yet. However, facilitated diffusion has been well studied, especially in model systems. A recent review has been published by Kreuzer and Hoofd [27].

A requirement for facilitated diffusion is a gradient in myoglobin oxygen saturation. The driving force for oxygen is then not only a gradient of oxygen concentration but also a gradient in oxyhemoglobin concentration. One-dimensional oxygen transfer including facilitated diffusion yields:

$$J_{O2} = \alpha D \frac{\Delta P}{\mathrm{d}x} + h_m D_m [M_b] \frac{\mathrm{d}S_m}{\mathrm{d}x} \qquad [11.32]$$

where:

J_{O2} is the total flux of oxygen (ml O_2 cm^{-2}),
h_m is the oxygen binding capacity of myoglobin (ml $O_2 \cdot$ g^{-1}),
S_m is the oxygen saturation of myoglobin (fraction),
D_m is the diffusion coefficient of myoglobin in the cytoplasm (cm$^2 \cdot$ s^{-1}),
$[M_b]$ is the myoglobin concentration (g%).

Since myoglobin is almost saturated at an oxygen pressure of 10 mm Hg, facilitation only occurs at low values of intracellular P_{O_2}.

An estimate of the maximal effect that can be expected from facilitated diffusion by myoglobin follows from the example where it is assumed that dissociation of MbO_2 and association of Mb with O_2 are so rapid that the reaction may be considered to be in equilibrium. One may then write

$$\begin{aligned} J_{O2} &= \alpha D \frac{\mathrm{d}[P_{O_2}]}{\mathrm{d}x} + h_m D_m \frac{\mathrm{d}S_m}{\mathrm{d}[P_{O_2}]} \frac{\mathrm{d}P_{O_2}}{\mathrm{d}x} \\ &= \left[\alpha D + h_m D_m [Mb] \frac{\mathrm{d}S_m}{\mathrm{d}[P_{O_2}]} \right] \frac{\mathrm{d}[P_{O_2}]}{\mathrm{d}x} \qquad [11.33] \\ &= \alpha D \left[1 + \frac{h_m D_m [Mb]}{\alpha D} \frac{\mathrm{d}S_m}{\mathrm{d}[P_{O_2}]} \right] \frac{\mathrm{d}[P_{O_2}]}{\mathrm{d}x} \end{aligned}$$

The second term between brackets can be considered as a facilitation factor and expresses in relative terms how much oxygen is transported by myoglobin in excess of that due to diffusion of oxygen alone. Myoglobin concentration in heart muscle has been estimated at 0.7 g% of wet weight [2, 31]. The diffusion coefficient for myoglobin in a solution of 20 g% is approximately 4×10^{-7} cm$^2 \cdot$ s^{-1} [25] whereas in muscle homogenate a lower value of 2.7×10^{-7} cm$^2 \cdot$ s^{-1} [35] has been reported. This latter value will be used in our further calculations. The oxygen binding capacity of 1 g% of myoglobin is of the same order as that for hemoglobin and amounts to 1.4 ml $O_2 \cdot$ g^{-1}. In contrast to hemoglobin which has an S-shaped saturation curve the saturation curve for myoglobin is hyperbolic. The P_{50} of myoglobin is about 5 mm Hg resulting in a maximal slope of 0.2 mm Hg^{-1} at $P_{O_2} = 0$. Substitution of these values and of αD into the facilitation factor results in a value of approximately 1. Hence on theoretical grounds oxygen transport may be twice that calculated on the basis of oxygen diffusion alone. However, one should note that this facilitation is less when reaction kinetics are incorporated into this prediction. Since dS_m/dP_{O_2} is decreasing with increasing P_{O_2}, the predicted facilitations at P_{O_2} of 5 and 10 mm Hg are 0.5 and 0.1 of the maximum at $P_{O_2} = 0$ respectivily.

11.7.3 Diffusion resistance of the capillary wall

Intracellular myoglobin gradients have been studied by Gayeski and Honig [11] with a cryospectrophotometer. In anesthetized dogs the gracilis muscle was surgically isolated and wrapped with a material that prevented O_2 exchange with the environment. The muscle was stimulated to contract isometrically. Flow through the muscle as well as arterial and venous oxygen saturation were measured, and oxygen consumption was computed applying the Fick principle. The muscle was quickly frozen in situ with a copper block cooled in liquid nitrogen ($-196\ ^0C$). The frozen muscle was fractured and myoglobin saturations measured in cellular cross sections approximately 200 μm beneath the surface. Measurements were done on muscle brought to what was thought to be maximal O_2-consumption which was about 0.25 ml $O_2 \cdot [100\ g]^{-1} \cdot s^{-1}$, a factor three to four times less than in the heart (e.g., Figure 9.17).

The results of Gayeski and Honig are striking. When recalculating the local oxygen pressure from the myoglobin oxygen saturation curve they found P_{O_2} to be about 3.2 mm Hg and a decrease in P_{O_2} of about 1.3 mm Hg over a distance of 40 μm. When analyzing these numbers in the dimensionless oxygen consumption one arrives at $M^* = 0.029$. The homogeneous model predicts for this example a maximal tissue radius of about 10 μm. This number is too small compared to the dimensions of the muscle cell. Over this distance the oxygen partial pressure should reduce to zero according to our model, but the calculated P_{O_2} drop from the experiment was only 30% over 40 μm. Gayeski and Honig explain the low intracellular oxygen pressure gradients in combination with high oxygen consumption on the basis of facilitated oxygen diffusion by myoglobin. This possibility has recently theoretically been studied [13, 14]. However, the degree of facilitation assumed in these studies exceeds substantially the degree that above was reasoned to be realistic.

Because of the low intracellular myoglobin saturation, corresponding with intracellular oxygen pressures lower than 4 mm Hg and assumed capillary oxygen pressures of 30 mm Hg or higher Gayeski and Honig concluded that the capillary walls would have a large resistance to oxygen diffusion.

When reading the paper of Gayeski and Honig, one is impressed by the care taken in experimentation. However, it seems difficult to fit their conclusions into more complete pictures of oxygen transfer to tissue. We reasoned above that facilitated diffusion by myoglobin could only explain a doubling of oxygen flux, whereas a factor of 4 to 10 is needed. Moreover, measurements of tissue oxygen pressure with surface electrodes on the heart reveal oxygen pressures of 10 mm Hg on average. Since the contact is predominantly with cell surfaces and capillary walls would have a large diffusion resistance to oxygen, the surface oxygen tension should reflect intracellular oxygen pressure. The low intracellular oxygen pressure in combination with a high resistance of the capillary for oxygen is also not compatible with the large variations in capillary oxygen pressures. Capillary oxygen pressures will be between arterial and venous values and hence may vary from 50 mm Hg to 10 mm Hg. Since oxygen flow through the capillary wall would be proportional to the oxygen pressure difference across the wall, and since intracellular oxygen pressure would be fixed around 3 mm Hg, the oxygen flux from the capillary to the tissue would vary over a factor 6. In order to explain a constant intracellular oxygen pressure, the resistance of the capillary wall to oxygen flow would have to decrease proportionally with capillary oxygen pressure and hence to vary by a factor of 6 as well.

Differences between extracellular oxygen pressure and oxygen pressure at the surface of mitochondria have been estimated by Katz et al. [22] with myocytes isolated from adult rat hearts suspended in a well-stirred iso-osmotic medium. The oxygen pressure at the mitochondrial surface was measured by the activity of monoamine oxidase, an enzyme located almost exclusively at the outer mitochondrial membrane, on the substrate phenylethylamine. The estimation of the oxygen pressure difference was at most 2 mm Hg. This result was also interpreted as indicating that the main resistance to oxygen diffusion must be located in the capillary wall. However, such a conclusion cannot be drawn directly from such an observation. A cell suspended in a well-stirred solution is in contact with oxygen all around whereas the same cell in tissue is only in contact with oxygen where it touches capillaries. This contact area and the gradients of oxygen pressure must be inversely proportional to each other. Moreover, the estimated maximal oxygen consumption per unit wet weight, assuming that 25% of the cell is protein, was 0.23 ml $O_2 \cdot s^{-1} \cdot [100 \text{ g}]^{-1}$ which is low compared to the earlier value for exercise in the dog of 0.6 ml $\cdot O_2^{-1} \cdot s^{-1} \cdot [100 \text{ g}]^{-1}$. Hence, for the dog myocyte, the difference between inside and outside oxygen pressure must again be a factor three times higher than that measured by Katz et al..

A way to evaluate the experimental data of Katz et al. [22] with reference to inside and outside oxygen pressure differences of in situ myocytes can be done by the models developed in this chapter. The experiment of Katz et al. would be described by model 1 of Figure 11.16 with homogeneously distributed oxygen consumption. The solution to this model, Equation [11.31], predicts the oxygen pressure in the center of a tissue cylinder. Assuming maximal O_2 consumption in their experiments and the radius of the tissue cylinder equal to half of the intercapillary distance of 10 μm, this results in a relative pressure drop of 13%. With an outside oxygen pressure of 10 mm Hg this corresponds to a maximal pressure difference of 1.3 mm Hg, the average oxygen pressure drop being lower.

This value corresponds nicely with the experimental value found by Katz et al.. The difference of the experiment with an in situ cell can then be evaluated by assuming a Krogh cylinder with a radius of 10 μm but now supplied by oxygen from a capillary in the center with a radius of 2.5 μm. The solution to this problem is provided by Equation [11.14]. For the same oxygen consumption we arrive then at a relative pressure difference between capillary wall and tissue cylinder wall of 0.35, being about three times larger than the calculated difference when the tissue was oxygenated from outside. Hence, in translating the in vitro results of Katz et al. to the in situ dog myocyte at exercise, a factor of three must be taken into account for both the difference in oxygen contact area and higher level of oxygen consumption. Together, this makes a factor of nine and hence there must be the possibility for the dog heart during exercise to generate an oxygen pressure difference between inside and outside of about $9 \times 1.3 = 11.7$ mm Hg, which is close to the venous oxygen pressure to be deduced from the experiments on exercising dogs reported on by VonRestorff et al. [49]. Hence, this quantitative analysis leaves little room for a large oxygen resistance of the capillary wall.

From the reasoning above one has to reject the possibility of low intracellular oxygen pressure in all cells at exercise. We then are left with the problem that myoglobin saturations can be about 35%, corresponding to oxygen pressures in the order of a few mm Hg, whereas for several reasons one would expect a much higher near capillary intracellular oxygen pressure in general.

11.7.4 Myoglobin as an oxygen store

The potential storage capacity of myoglobin can be compared with that of hemoglobin. Expressed per gram the oxygen binding capacities of both substances is approximately equal and amounts 1.34 mm $O_2 \cdot g^{-1}$. Hundred gram of myocardium contains about 0.9 g myoglobin and, assuming 10 volume% of capillary blood with a hemoglobin concentration of 16 g%, 1.6 g of hemoglobin. At a capillary oxygen pressure of about 23 mm Hg capillary hemoglobin is saturated for 50% and hence the oxygen storage of myoglobin is quit similar to that of capillary hemoglobin: 1.2 ml O_2 and 1.07 ml O_2 for myoglobin and hemoglobin respectively. For a basal oxygen consumption of 0.2 ml $\cdot$ s^{-1} $\cdot$ [100 g]$^{-1}$ the total oxygen store equals the oxygen consumption of about 6 seconds. This predicted time [42] agrees well with experimental observations from near-infrared spectroscopy [38].

Some spectrophometric studies on the beating heart concluded that myoglobin oxygen saturation varied during the heart cycle [18]. However, a similar more recent study [33] demonstrated that these early studies were probably hampered by some artifacts. In the Tyrode perfused rat heart the myoglobin saturation in the subepicardium is constant during the heart cycle.

11.8 Summary

Because of strong limitations in studying oxygen transfer at the microcirculatory level, the field of oxygen transfer to tissue has always had a strong emphasis on theoretical analysis. Theories were developed from the study of oxygen transfer from a capillary to surrounding tissue. The strength and limitations of the Krogh cylinder analysis were discussed. The Krogh cylinder is valuable since it provides an estimate of how much tissue can be supplied by oxygen from a single capillary. However, because of the relatively short intercapillary distances, shunting of oxygen from capillaries with high P_{O_2} to capillaries with low P_{O_2} may occur. The effect of this shunting on the distribution of oxygen in a network was analyzed by applying solutions of the two-dimensional diffusion equation to a model of a slab of tissue perforated with hexagonally stacked capillary segments. The consequence of shunting can further be analyzed by composing a model of the capillary bed by the addition of these model slabs. This model predicts heterogeneous distribution of oxygen pressure over tissue units. However, the width of this distribution is only half of the histogram that results from the assumption of absence of oxygen shunting. The oxygen transfer from the left ventricular cavity to the subendocardium was analyzed as well. Without capillary blood flow in the subendocardium this layer of influence will only be in the order of 80 μm. The oxygen transfer to the mitochondria was analyzed as well. The conclusion of some studies that the major part of the resistance to oxygen transfer of red cells to the mitochondria is located in the capillary wall, was doubted. Such a high resistance would require that the resistance for oxygen diffusion would be strongly dependent on capillary oxygen pressure.

References

[1] BALABAN RS (1990) Regulation of oxidative phosphorylation in the mammalian cell. *Am. J. Physiol.* **258** (Cell Physiol. **27**): C377–C389.
[2] BLESSING MH (1967) Über den Myoglobin Gehalt des Herzmuskels den Menschen. *Archiv für Kreislaufforschung* **52**: 236–278.
[3] BOAG JW (1969) Oxygen diffusion and oxygen depletion problems in radiobiology. *Curr. Top. Radiat. Res.* **5**: 141–195.
[4] CAILLÉ JP, HINKE JAM (1974) The volume available to diffusion in the muscle fiber. *Can. J. Physiol. Pharmacol.* **52**: 814–828.
[5] CLARK A JR, CLARK PAA (1985) Local oxygen gradients near isolated mitochondria. *Biophys. J.* **48**: 931–938.
[6] CLARK A JR, CLARK PAA, CONNETT RJ, GAYESKI TEJ, HONIG CR (1987) How large is the drop in P_{O2} between cytosol and mitochondrion? *Am. J. Physiol.* **252** (*Cell Physiol.* **21**): C583–C587.

[7] COLE RP, SUKANEK PC, WITTENBERG JB, WITTENBERG BA (1982) Mitochondrial function in the presence of myoglobin. *J. Appl. Physiol.* **53**: 1116–1124.

[8] DULING, BR, BERNE RM (1970) Longitudinal gradients in peri-arteriolar oxygen tension. A possible mechanism for the participation of oxygen in local regulation of blood flow. *Circ. Res.* **27**: 669–678.

[9] GAMBLE WJ, LAFARGE CG, FYLER DC, WEISUL J, MONROE RG (1974) Regional coronary venous oxygen saturation and myocardial oxygen tension following abrupt changes in ventricular pressure in the isolated dog heart. *Circ. Res.* **34**: 672–681.

[10] GAYESKI TEJ (1981) *A cryogenic cryospectrophotometric method for measuring myoglobin saturation in subcellular volume; application to resting dog gracilis muscle.* Thesis, Dept. of Physiology University of Rochester. Rochester, NY., University microfilms international, Ann Arbor, Michigan, USA, nr. 8224720, 1986: 303.

[11] GAYESKI TEJ, HONIG CR (1986) O_2 gradients from sarcolemma to cell interior in the red muscle at maximal $\dot{V}O_2$. *Am. J. Physiol.* **251** (*Heart Circ. Physiol.* **20**): H789–H799.

[12] GROEBE K (1990) A versatile model of steady state O_2 supply to tissue. Application to skeletal muscle. *Biophys. J.* **57**: 485–498.

[13] GROEBE K, THEWS G (1990) Calculated intra- and extracellular P_{O_2} gradients in heavily working red muscle. *Am. J. Physiol.* **259** (*Heart Circ. Physiol.* **28**): H84–H92.

[14] GROEBE K, THEWS G (1990) Role of geometry and anisotropic diffusion for modelling P_{O2} profiles in working red muscle. *Resp. Physiol.* **79**: 255–278.

[15] GRUNEWALD WA, LUBBERS DW (1975) Determination of intracapillary HbO_2 saturation with a cryo-microphotometric method, applied to the rabbit myocardium. *Pflügers Arch.* **353**: 255–273.

[16] GRUNEWALD WA (1970) Diffusion error and specific consumption of the Pt electrode during P_{O_2} measurements in the steady state. *Pflügers Arch.* **320**: 24–44.

[17] GRUNEWALD WA, SOWA W (1977) Capillary structures and O_2 supply to the tissue. An analysis with a digital diffusion model as applied to the skeletal muscle. *Rev. Physiol. Biochem. Pharmacol.* **77**: 149–209.

[18] HASSINEN IE, HILTUNEN H, TAKELA TES (1981) Reflectance spectrophotometric monitoring of the isolated heart as a method of measuring the oxidation-reduction of cytochrome and oxygenation of myoglobin. *Cardiovasc. Res.* **15**: 86–91.

[19] HILL AV (1928/1929) The diffusion of oxygen and lactic acid through tissues. *Proc. Roy. Soc. B* **104**: 39–96.

[20] HOLTZ J, GRUNEWALD WA, MANZ R, VONRESTORFF W, BASSENGE E (1977) Intracapillary hemoglobin oxygen saturation and oxygen consumption

in different layers of the left ventricular myocardium. *Plügers Arch.* **370**: 253–258.

[21] JONES DP (1986) Intracellular diffusion gradients of O_2 and ATP. *Am. J. Physiol.* **250** (*Cell Physiol.* **19**): C663–C675.

[22] KATZ IR, WITTENBERG JB, WITTENBERG BA (1984) Monoamine oxidase, an intracellular probe of oxygen pressure in isolated cardiac myocytes. *J. Biol. Chem.* **259**: 7504–7509.

[23] KAYAR SR, CLAASSEN H, HOPPELER H, WEIBEL ER (1986) Mitochondrial distribution in relation to changes in muscle metabolism in rat soleus. *Respir. Physiol.* **64**: 1–11.

[24] KREUZER F, YAHR WZ (1960) Influence of red cell membrane on diffusion of oxygen. *J. Appl. Physiol.* **15**: 1117–1122.

[25] KREUZER F (1970) Facilitated diffusion of oxygen and its possible significance; a review. *Resp. Physiol.* **9**: 1–30.

[26] KREUZER F, HOOFD LJC (1984) Facilitated diffusion of oxygen: possible significance in blood and muscle. *Adv. Exp. Med. Biol.* **169**: 3–21.

[27] KREUZER F, HOOFD LJC (1987) Facilitated diffusion of oxygen and carbon dioxide. In: *Handbook of Physiology. The respiratory system IV, Gas exchange.* Eds: FAHRI LE AND TENNEY SM. Am. Physiol. Soc., Bethesda, **3** chapter 6: 89–111.

[28] KROGH A (1919) The supply of oxygen to the tissue and the regulation of the capillary circulation. *J. Physiol. Lond.* **52**: 457–474.

[29] KROGH A (1919) The number and the distribution of capillaries in muscles with the calculation of the oxygen pressure head necessary for supplying the tissue. *J. Physiol. Lond.* **52**: 409–415.

[30] KROGH A (1930) *The anatomy and physiology of capillaries.* Yale University Press, New Haven. Mrs Hepsa Ely Silliman Memorial Lectures.

[31] LENIGER-FOLLERT E, LÜBBERS DW (1973) Determination of local myoglobin concentration in the Guinea pig heart. *Pflügers Arch.* **341**: 271–280.

[32] LOSSË BS, SCHUCHHARDT S, NIEDERLE N (1975) The oxygen pressure histogram in the left ventricular myocardium of the dog. *Pflügers Arch.* **356**: 121–132.

[33] MAKINO N, KANAIDE H, YOSHIMURA R, NAKAMURA M (1983) Myoglobin oxygenation remains constant during the cardiac cycle. *Am. J. Physiol.* **245** (*Heart Circ. Physiol.* **14**): H237–H243.

[34] MILLIKAN GA (1937) Experiments in muscle haemoglobin in vivo; the instantaneous measurement of muscle metabolism. *Proc. Roy. Soc. B*: 123–218.

[35] MOLL W (1968) The diffusion coefficient of myoglobin in muscle homogenate. *Pflügers Arch.* **299**: 247–251.

[36] MOLL W, NIENABER D, BÜLOW H (1969) Measurements of facilitated diffusion of oxygen in red blood cells at 37^0C. *Plügers Arch.* **305**: 269–278.

[37] NAKAMURA T, WAKAO Y, MUTO M, TAKAHASHI M (1990) Studies on

the changes in myocardial oxygen tension. *Nippon Juigaku Zasshi (Jap. J. Veterin. Sci.)* **52**: 79–84.
[38] PARSONS WJ, REMBERT JC, BAUMAN RP, GREENFIELD JR JC, PAINTA-DOSI CA (1990) Dynamic mechanisms of cardiac oxygenation during brief ischemia and reperfusion. *Am. J. Physiol.* **259** (*Heart Circ. Physiol.* **28**): H1477–H1485.
[39] POPEL AS (1980) Mathematical modeling of convective and diffusive transport in the microcirculation. In: *Mathematics of microcirculation phenomena*. Eds: GROSS JF, POPEL AS. Raven Press, New York.
[40] POPEL AS (1982) Oxygen diffusive shunts under conditions of heterogeneous oxygen delivery. *J. Theor. Biol.* **96**: 533–541.
[41] POPEL AS (1989) Theory of oxygen transport to tissue. *Crit. Rev. Biomed. Eng.* **17**: 257–321.
[42] RUITER JH, SPAAN JAE, LAIRD JD (1977) Transient oxygen uptake during myocardial reactive hyperemia in the dog. *Am. J. Physiol.* **232** (*Heart Circ. Physiol.* **1**): H437–H440.
[43] SARELIUS IH (1986) Cell flow path influences transit time through striated muscle capillaries. *Am. J. Physiol.* **250** (*Heart Circ. Physiol.* **19**): H899–H907.
[44] SEGAL A (1981) *AFEP user manual*. Delft University of Technology, The Netherlands.
[45] SILLAU AH, ERNST V, REYES N (1990) Oxidative capacity distribution in the cardiac myocytes of hypermetabolic rats. *Resp. Physiol.* **79**: 279–292.
[46] SILVER IA (1965) Some observations on the cerebral cortex with an ultramicromembrane-covered oxygen electrode. *Med. Electron. Biol. Eng.* **3**: 377.
[47] SPAAN JAE, KREUZER F, HOOFD L (1980) A theoretical analysis of nonsteady-state oxygen transfer in layers of hemoglobin solution. *Pflügers Arch.* **384**: 231–239.
[48] SPAAN JAE, KREUZER F, VANWELY FK (1980) Diffusion coefficients of oxygen and hemoglobin as obtained simultaneously from photometric determination of the oxygenation of layers of hemoglobin solutions. *Pflügers Arch.* **384**: 241–251.
[49] VONRESTORFF W, HOLTZ J, BASSENGE E (1977) Exercise induced augmentation of myocardial oxygen extraction in spite of normal coronary dilatory capacity in dogs. *Pflügers Arch.* **372**: 181–185.
[50] WEISS HR, SINHA AK (1978) Regional oxygen saturation of small arteries and veins in the canine myocardium. *Circ. Res.* **42**: 119–126.
[51] WHALEN WJ (1971) Intracellular $\dot{P}O_2$ in heart skeletal muscle. *Physiologist* **14**: 69–82.
[52] WHALEN WJ, RILEY J, NAIR P (1967) A microelectrode for measuring intracellular $\dot{P}O_2$. *J. Appl. Physiol.* **23**: 798–801.
[53] WIERINGA PA (1985) *The influence of the coronary capillary on the dis-*

tribution and control of local blood flow. PhD Thesis. Delft University of Technology, The Netherlands (ISBN 90-9001042).

[54] WILENSKY RL, TRANUM-JENSEN J, CORONEL R, WILDE AAM, FIOLET JWT, JANSE MJ (1986) The subendocardial border zone during acute ischemia of the rabbit heart: an electrophysiological, metabolic and morphological correlation. *Circulation* **74**: 1137–1146.

[55] WITTENBERG BA, ROBINSON TF (1981) Oxygen requirements, morphology, cell coat and membrane permeability of calcium-tolerant myocytes from hearts of adult rats. *Cell Tissue Res.* **216**: 231–251.

Chapter 12

Limitation of coronary flow reserve by a stenosis

Jos AE Spaan and Jan Verburg

12.1 Introduction

IN THE PREVIOUS CHAPTERS the control of coronary flow as well as the effect of heart contraction on coronary flow were analyzed under more or less normal perfusion conditions. It is clear that under normal circumstances, coronary flow is much lower than maximum which allows the coronary control vessels to be able to adapt the flow to an increased level of metabolism. The extent to which coronary flow can increase above control is generally referred to as coronary reserve. This reserve is obviously reduced by a coronary stenosis since this imposes additional resistance in large arteries which will reduce the effective perfusion pressure of the downstream coronary circulation. In several studies, the ratio between peak velocity and control velocity in a coronary artery is used as a measure of the capacity of the coronary system to adapt to an increased cardiac metabolism.

It is confusing in the literature that the term of flow reserve is used for the possible maximal increase of flow above control as well as for the ratio between control and maximal flow. It seems reasonable to restrict the notion reserve to the former: the difference between maximal and control flow. This is because a reserve of flow has the same physical dimension as flow but a ratio of flows is dimensionless. In this chapter, the term 'flow reserve' is used for the difference between maximal and basal flow, and 'flow ratio' for the ratio between maximal and basal flow.

Following the pioneering studies of Gould *et al.* [11, 12], there have been attempts to use the possible increase in coronary flow due to vasodilation induced by coronary vasodilators or 20 s occlusion as a measure of the severity of a coronary stenosis. Early studies were discussed by Marcus [25]. The ratio between maximal coronary flow and control flow showed little correlation with the percent stenoses when measured in humans. More recent studies, however, showed a better correlation which was attributed to better standardized conditions and selection of patients [40].

Some of the factors leading to a poor correlation in human studies are quite obviously due to a poorly defined baseline flow from which the flow increase is measured, as well as the fact that the flow at maximal vasodilation is affected by heart rate and the presence of diffuse disease which could lead to erroneous conclusions about the degree to which the vessel was obstructed [17, 18, 23, 32].

Also the flow at maximal vasodilation is determined by arterial pressure [9, 27] as follows from the pressure–flow relations discussed in Chapters 6 and 7. Only recently have attempts been made to normalize the coronary flow ratio so as to compensate for functional alterations in heart function and to quantify the impeding effect of the stenosis per se [13]. A complete picture of the reduction of coronary reserve is complicated because of the interaction between the different processes involved. The heart needs to contract to generate pressure to perfuse the coronary vessels although to minimize coronary resistance ensuing from heart contraction, the heart would do better at rest.

However, although coronary reserve may be troublesome in terms of quantifying these factors, it is a useful concept to discuss the limits of the operational range of the coronary control system. Hence, first the concept of coronary flow reserve will be discussed, after which the physics of the pressure drop across a coronary stenosis will be described. In conclusion, the interaction between coronary flow reserve, heart rate and the hemodynamic hindrance due to stenosis will be analyzed by a simple model.

12.2 Coronary flow reserve

In the following we will refer to coronary flow reserve as the amount of flow that the coronary bed can accommodate above control and hence the difference between maximal and control flow. A distinction should be made between physiological reserve and pharmacological reserve, the former being induced by a physiological stimulus such as a coronary occlusion and the latter by a drug, e.g., adenosine or papaverine. It has been shown [4, 14] that the pharmacological reserve may exceed the physiological one by a factor of two. The physiological reserve as determined by a reactive hyperemia resulting from an occlusion of long enough duration was depicted by Figure 1.9.

A second way to illustrate coronary reserve and its dependency on several

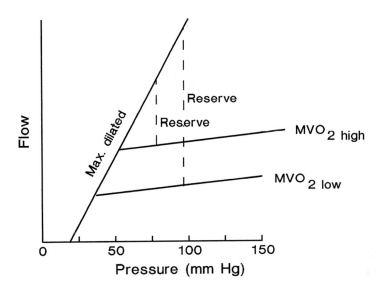

Figure 12.1: Dependency of coronary reserve on arterial pressure and oxygen consumption, MVO_2. Pressure-flow relations with autoregulation intact at two different levels of oxygen consumption and with obliteration of arteriolar smooth muscle tone by means of coronary arterial occlusion. Coronary reserve at a certain arterial pressure is the difference between the autoregulation and peak reactive hyperemic pressure–flow relations.

factors is the pressure–flow diagram of the coronary circulation. These pressure–flow lines were discussed in Chapters 1, 5, 6 and 7 and are schematically presented in Figure 12.1. The steepest curve represents the dependency of peak reactive hyperemic flow on arterial pressure (e.g., [9]). Because of the ischemic stimulus, arteriolar smooth muscle is relaxed and this curve represents the pressure–flow relation without control of the coronary circulation. The flatter curves illustrate autoregulation of the coronary bed at two different levels of constant oxygen consumption. These curves show the tendency of the local coronary control system to maintain coronary flow relatively independent of perfusion pressure, but adapted to the oxygen needs of the heart. In Chapter 9 we noted that these autoregulation curves shift in parallel with a change in oxygen consumption.

Figure 12.1 illustrates two factors that influence coronary reserve: arterial pressure and oxygen consumption. However, there are also other factors. The pressure–flow relation obtained under maximal vasodilatory stimulus is not unique but depends on heart rate and can be made steeper by the administration of drugs. With a coronary stenosis the perfusion pressure of the distal coronary bed drops as flow increases through the stenosis. The matter is even more complicated when the distribution of coronary flow and reserve over the myocardial wall is considered [17, 18]. It is well-known that the subendocardium is more vulnerable than the subepicardium to ischemia. This probably has to do with the compression effect of the contracting myocardium on the blood vessels which, as discussed in earlier chapters, is more pronounced in the inner layers of the heart muscle. Moreover, in recent years it has become clear that the reserve can be very heterogenous, even in a layer of constant depth within the myocardial wall [1, 6].

12.3 Coronary stenosis and flow reserve

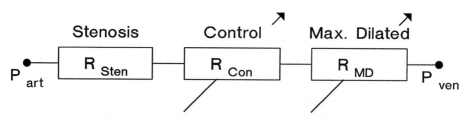

Figure 12.2: Model of the coronary resistance including a stenosis. R_{sten} represents the stenosis resistance. The local control resistance, R_{con}, is responsible for the compensatory change in perfusion pressure and for adjusting flow to an increase of oxygen demand. The minimal resistance R_{MD} is also variable due to compression of the coronary microcirculation by cardiac contraction. The pressure loss by the stenosis will be compensated for by decreasing arteriolar resistance, when possible, and reduce the ability for further metabolic flow adaptation.

In the presence of a stenosis the indication of coronary reserve in Figure 12.1 is not very realistic because if flow is increased at constant mean systemic pressure, the pressure drop over the stenosis will increase. As a result, the perfusion pressure of the coronary bed distal to the stenosis will decrease. The incorporation of this pressure drop over the stenosis in the analysis can be done by the model illustrated in Figure 12.2. The coronary circulation including the stenosis is thought to consist of three resistances in series: the stenosis resistance, R_{sten}, a variable resistance, R_{con} which is responsible for the local control mechanism, and a third resistance representing the resistance of the coronary bed when it is fully dilated, R_{MD}.

The variable resistance R_{con} describes the ability of the coronary circulation to adapt to changes in perfusion pressure and changes in metabolism. At maximal vasodilation the value of this resistance is zero. In the presence of a stenosis the resistance will decrease in order to compensate for the pressure drop over the stenosis. The third resistance, R_{MD}, reflects the resistance of the coronary bed

12.3 Coronary stenosis and flow reserve

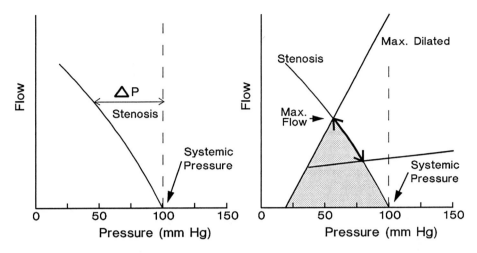

Figure 12.3: Schematic illustration of the effect of coronary stenosis on coronary reserve. Left: Illustrates the nonlinear pressure–flow relation of a stenosis. ΔP represents the pressure drop over the stenosis as a function of flow. Right: The pressure–flow relation of the stenosis is superimposed on the pressure–flow diagram applying to the coronary bed as discussed in relation to Figure 12.1. The only combinations of pressure and flow possible are within the shaded area delineated by the pressure–flow relation at maximal vasodilation and the one pertaining to the stenosis. Although the distal pressure at the control autoregulation curve is only reduced to about 80 mm Hg the maximal flow can only be twice control because of the progressive pressure drop with increasing flow through the stenosis.

at maximal vasodilation and without the coronary stenosis. This resistance can be deduced from the pressure–flow relation at maximal vasodilation as has been discussed in Chapters 6 and 7. It was shown that this resistance is also nonlinear and, moreover, not constant since it is influenced by several factors, such as heart rate. However, for the sake of simplicity the resistance at maximal vasodilation in Figure 12.2 will initially be assumed to be constant.

To illustrate its influence on flow reserve, an arbitrary pressure–flow relation of a stenosis is presented in Figure 12.3, left panel. The curvilinearity of this relation points to the flow dependency of a stenosis resistance. The relation shown does not pass through the origin since it is intended to express the pressure drop in relation to the systemic pressure, arbitrarily set at 100 mm Hg. The pressure drop over the stenosis follows from the horizontal distance between the pressure–flow relation and the line described by $P = $ systemic pressure. The reducing effect of a stenosis on coronary reserve is illustrated in the right panel of Figure 12.3. This panel combines the pressure–flow relation of the coronary stenosis with the relation holding for the coronary circulation without stenosis. The autoregulation curve depicted applies for the control oxygen consumption. The maximal coronary flow value is limited by the pressure–flow relation for the coronary bed at maximal vasodilation on the one hand and the pressure–flow relation for the stenosis on the other hand. The shaded area in the figure is where any combination of pressure and flow may occur which is bounded by these two pressure–flow relations. The figure clearly shows that when the flow demand by the myocardial metabolism is increased, resulting in further vasodilation, this increase in flow will reduce the effective perfusion pressure of the coronary bed. The stenosis resistance will cause this pressure reduction to be more than proportional.

The importance of the reduction in effective perfusion pressure by increasing coronary flow can hardly be overestimated. Note that in the control condition, where the pressure–flow relation of the stenosis crosses the autoregulation curve, the effective perfusion pressure is only reduced by 20 mm Hg. According to Figure 12.3 coronary flow would be able to increase by more than a factor of three if effective perfusion pressure could be maintained at that same pressure. However, because of the flow dependent pressure drop, this increase is limited to a factor of two. It should also be realized that factors which increase oxygen demand of the myocardium, e.g., heart rate and systolic left ventricular pressure, also augment the resistance at maximal vasodilation.

12.4 Prediction of pressure drop over a coronary stenosis

There are two fluid dynamic mechanisms that are responsible for the undesired pressure drop over a coronary stenosis. The first is due to frictional or viscous losses, the effect of which can be estimated by Poiseuille's law. The second has to do with the convective acceleration of blood where the resulting pressure drop can be estimated by the law of Bernoulli.

12.4.1 Pressure drop by viscous losses

Blood is a viscous medium, meaning that a shear stress is needed to have neighboring layers of blood moving at different rates. Since fluid sticks to the wall of a conduit, fluid velocity will be zero at the wall and maximal in the center of the conduit. For so-called Newtonian fluids shear stress is proportional to shear rate, the constant of proportionality being the viscosity. Shear rate equals per definition the gradient of velocity in the space coordinates. Blood is a suspension of cells within plasma and therefore behaves in a non-Newtonian manner. However, for conduits with a diameter larger than 0.4 mm it may be treated as a Newtonian fluid.

12.4 Prediction of pressure drop over a coronary stenosis

For cylindrical conduits the relation between pressure drop and flow as determined by viscous effects is described by Poiseuille's law

$$\Delta P = \frac{8\mu L Q}{\pi R^4}, \qquad [12.1]$$

where:

- μ is viscosity,
- L is the length of the tube considered,
- R is the tube radius,
- Q is flow through the tube.

The limitation of the law of Poiseuille as formulated in equation [12.1] is that it applies to a cylindrical tube with a fully developed parabolic flow profile. However, real stenoses are seldom cylindrical. Moreover, in general, stenoses are relatively short and hence unable to fully develop a parabolic flow profile. The limitations of these assumptions will be discussed later in this chapter. Equation [12.1] describes the pressure drop as a linear function of flow and length. However, the radius is the most important parameter since this appears in the formula to the power of four.

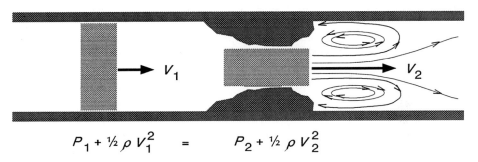

Figure 12.4: *Illustration of the convective acceleration of blood in a stenotic region. Because flow is constant over the length of the tube, the velocity in the constriction must be greater than in front or behind it. Velocity is inversely proportional to cross-sectional area as described by Equation [12.2]. The kinetic energy of the mass, represented by the filled box in the narrowing, is larger then that of the same mass in the unrestricted vessel. This increase in kinetic energy is at the expense of pressure, being a potential energy per unit volume. Therefore $P_2 < P_1$. Because of eddies, the pressure recovers incompletely distal to the stenosis. Energy is lost by heat production in this area.*

12.4.2 Pressure loss by convective acceleration

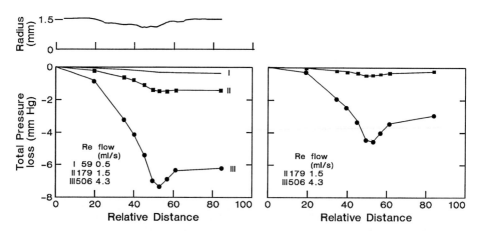

Figure 12.5: *Pressure drop along a replica of a stenosis of the left human circumflex artery as recalculated from Back [2]. Left top: The radius of the replica as function of axial position. Left bottom: Total pressure loss in the stenosis as a function of axial position for three different Reynolds numbers. The actual flow values are also given in the figure. In the prestenotic region the pressure gradient is small and is completely due to frictional losses. The fall in pressure because of the stenosis is due to both frictional losses within the stenosis and acceleration of blood. Right: The dynamic pressure loss calculated from the left bottom panel by assuming that the pressure loss at Reynolds number = 59 is completely due to frictional losses. From that relationship, the pressure drop component related to viscous losses is estimated for the higher Reynolds numbers and subtracted from the total pressure drop measured at these higher Reynolds numbers. Note that the dynamic pressure loss is only partly recovered.*

The second mechanism is the pressure drop due to convective acceleration. This acceleration is necessary since the lumen in the stenosis is smaller than in the prestenotic region while the same amount of blood has to pass per unit time. The relation between area and velocity is elucidated in Figure 12.4. Flow equals the product of average velocity in the cross-sectional area and of the cross-sectional area. Consequently, the relation between blood velocities in the prestenotic and stenotic area follows from the simple relation

$$v_1 A_1 = v_2 A_2 = Q \qquad [12.2]$$

where:

v_1 and v_2 are the velocities in the prestenotic and stenotic region,
A_1 and A_2 are the areas in the prestenotic and stenotic regions.

12.4 Prediction of pressure drop over a coronary stenosis

Equation [12.2] is known as the continuity equation and has been applied to determine coronary stenosis severity by relating a velocity increase measured by a Doppler tip velocity catheter to area reduction [21] in analogy to the estimation of valve area reduction [33].

The acceleration of fluid implies an increase in kinetic energy density which reduces potential energy density. The latter is equal to the pressure. The notion of energy density is used here since the energy terms refer to energy per unit volume of blood. The energy balance for a unit volume of blood is then equal to the energy balance of a point mass in solid mechanics. The conservation of energy yields

$$P + \frac{1}{2}\rho v^2 = \text{constant} \qquad [12.3]$$

where ρ is the fluid density and v the local velocity.

Equation [12.3] is known as Bernoulli's law.

The pressure drop between the prestenotic region and stenotic region is calculated from Equations [12.2] and [12.3]:

$$\begin{aligned} P_1 - P_2 &= \frac{1}{2}\rho[v_2^2 - v_1^2] \\ &= \frac{1}{2}\rho Q^2 \frac{[1 - \frac{A_2^2}{A_1^2}]}{A_2^2} \end{aligned} \qquad [12.4]$$

In theory, this pressure loss is reversible, because when blood flows out of the narrowing it decelerates and the kinetic energy could once again be converted into potential energy or pressure. This in contrast to the viscous pressure loss which cannot be recovered because energy is lost by heat production. Experimentally, however, it has been found that recovery of kinetic energy into pressure is negligible. This deviation from the prediction of the Bernoulli equation is caused by flow patterns proximal and distal to the constriction, which deviate from the parabolic Poiseuille flow and thereby cause extra viscous losses. Even in an ideal experimental preparation, where the conversion from the constriction to the wider tube is made very smoothly and gradually, pressure does not fully recover. Hence, for practical purposes in coronary pathology, it may be assumed that the dynamic pressure term is lost and therefore the pressure drop over the stenosis exceeds that predicted by Poiseuille's law.

Note that the dynamic pressure drop is inversely proportional to the cross-sectional area of the stenosis, and thus inversely proportional to the radius of the stenosis to the power of four. This dependency is the same just as for the frictional loss predicted by the law of Poiseuille. The dynamic pressure drop is, however, proportional to the square of the flow in contrast to viscous pressure loss, which is proportional to flow.

The pressure loss for a mild stenosis has been analyzed both theoretically and experimentally by Back et al. [2] and Mates et al. [26]. Both studies report the pressure drop relative to the dynamic pressure in the prestenotic region as a function of the axial position in the stenosis with the Reynolds number as parameter. The experiments of Back et al. were performed on a replica of a segment of the left circumflex human coronary artery with a mild stenosis. In order to facilitate the interpretation of their results, these were recalculated in terms of absolute pressure drop from the prestenotic reference point. The results of these recalculations are depicted in Figure 12.5. The left top panel illustrates the variation of cross-sectional area of the replica of the stenosis. The left bottom panel shows the total pressure drop as a function of the axial position in the stenosis for three different values of the Reynolds number corresponding in this specific experiment to three different flow values. As is clear from this panel there is some pressure recovery at the higher flow rates. Most certainly there is a better recovery of dynamic pressure at the lower Reynolds number which, however, is not noticeable in the axial pressure distribution because of the magnitude of the dynamic pressure relative to the pressure drop due to viscosity. A better illustration of the behavior of dynamic pressure as function of axial position is depicted in the right panel. Here, the dynamic pressure component has been calculated assuming that the total pressure drop at a small Reynolds number is completely due to viscous losses. Hence, the viscous pressure drop at higher flow values can be calculated simply by multiplying the viscous drop at low flow by the proportional increase in flow. Therefore, the dynamic pressure drop at higher flow rates can be calculated by subtraction of the viscous pressure loss from the total pressure drop.

As is shown in the right panel of Figure 12.5 the dynamic pressure drop component becomes relatively more important at higher flow values and only a partial recovery of dynamic pressure into static pressure is achieved.

12.4.3 Dependence of pressure drop over stenosis on stenosis diameter

As is clear from the formulas describing the pressure drop due to friction and due to dynamic pressure losses, the diameter of the stenosis is the most important parameter. In order to gain some insight into the sensitivity of the pressure drop on stenosis diameter, we will consider an imaginary cylindrical stenosis of variable diameter but with a fixed length of 10 mm. Four different levels of flow were used for the calculations ranging between 100 ml $\cdot$ min^{-1} and 500 ml $\cdot$ min^{-1}. Considering that under normal physiological conditions the coronary flow is about 100 ml $\cdot$ min^{-1} $\cdot$ [100 g]$^{-1}$ tissue, this range applies to the perfusion area of a large coronary branch in the human heart. Moreover, it covers the flow range from control to strenuous exercise. In the calculation the viscosity of blood, μ,

12.4 Prediction of pressure drop over a coronary stenosis

was taken as 3×10^{-3} Pa s (3 cP). The two components of pressure drop were calculated as a function of stenosis diameter. The sum of the two components forms the total pressure drop over the stenosis.

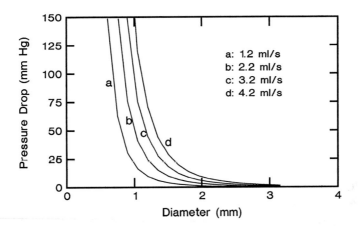

Figure 12.6: *Theoretical pressure drop as a function of diameter over a stenosis with length of 10 mm for four different levels of flow. Viscosity was assumed to be 3×10^{-3} Pa s. The pressure drop on the vertical axis is the sum of viscous and dynamic pressure losses. Assuming 50 mm Hg to be a critical pressure drop, the critical stenosis diameter is between 0.8 and 1.3 mm.*

The calculated total pressure drop as a function of diameter is illustrated in Figure 12.6. The diameter of a normal coronary artery carrying a flow of 60 to 350 ml · min^{-1} is 3 to 4 mm. A vessel segment with a length of 10 mm will therefore hardly generate any pressure drop. With a diameter of 2 mm the maximum pressure loss is still only about 10 mm Hg. This is negligible since from the study of autoregulation it is known that the myocardium can be adequately perfused under basal metabolic conditions with a perfusion pressure of 50 mm Hg. In conscious dogs at rest, adequate blood supply is still provided down to 40 mm Hg [5]. Arbitrarily assuming a threshold of only 50 mm Hg as the critical pressure below which there will be a shortage of blood supply to the heart, the theoretical curves indicate that a stenosis will only cause serious trouble if the stenosis diameter is less than 0.8 to 1.3 mm, depending on the flow value required.

The relative importance of the two pressure components is illustrated in Figure 12.7, where the ratio of the components is drawn as a function of the flow. Note that this pressure drop ratio is not dependent on the stenosis diameter. Obviously the relationship between this ratio and flow depends on the parameters of stenosis length and blood viscosity. If we assume that 60 ml · min^{-1} approximately equals the lowest value of coronary flow for a heart to function normally, we observe that both pressure drop components are about equal. However, at

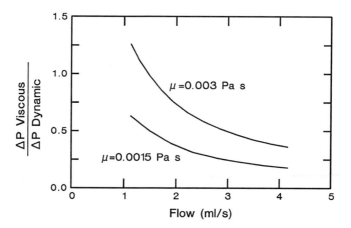

Figure 12.7: The ratio between the pressure drop due to viscous losses and dynamic losses at two different values of viscosity. Note that the ratio is independent of stenosis diameter. At flow rates about basal coronary flow the relative importance of both mechanisms is about equal at normal blood viscosity. At the higher flow rates the dynamic pressure component becomes dominant. Note that at the same heart rate, the ratio decreases in proportion to viscosity, because frictional losses decrease but dynamic loss is unaltered.

higher flow rates the pressure drop due to dynamic losses becomes dominant.

The same holds for the effect of stenosis length. For a shorter stenosis, the pressure drop predicted by the viscous term will become smaller, whereas the dynamic pressure term will remain constant and hence become relatively more important. Note that the importance of dynamic pressure loss increases with decreasing viscosity since it reduces the viscous pressure drop but has no effect on the dynamic losses.

The concept of dynamic pressure loss is not only useful in coronary pathology. It is routinely applied to estimate the pressure drop across stenotic mitral [20] and aortic valves [8].

12.5 Absolute versus relative definition of a stenosis

Illustration of the use of an impaired coronary flow ratio as measure for stenosis severity is provided in Figure 12.8. This figure is based on data of Wilson *et al.* [40]. In the right panel the flow ratio is plotted versus the ratio between minimum stenosis diameter and diameter proximal to the stenosis. In the right panel the minimum cross-sectional area is plotted on the horizontal axis. The data

12.5 Absolute versus relative definition of a stenosis

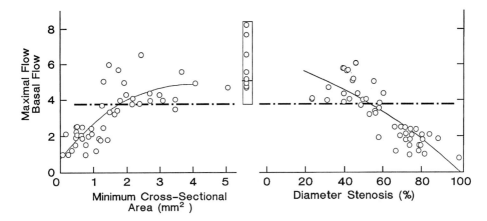

Figure 12.8: *Maximal flow ratio expressed as function of percent diameter reduction (right panel) and minimum cross-sectional area (left panel). The data points in the boxes are from subjects without coronary stenosis. The horizontal dash-dotted line indicates the underbound for the normal subjects. For further explanation: see text. (Redrawn from Wilson et al. [40].)*

were obtained from 50 patients selected who had one discrete lesion in the vessel under study and no more than two coronary vessels with obstructive lesions. Two hemodynamic conditions determining control and peak flow, i.e., heart rate and arterial pressure, were rather constant and approximately 65 beats $\cdot$ min^{-1} and 86 mm Hg respectively. Coronary blood velocity was measured with a catheter tip ultrasound Doppler instrument. Maximal vasodilation was obtained by intracoronary infusion of papaverine. The figure includes data from 13 patients with coronary arteries without stenosis. In the panels a horizontal line is added at the level coinciding with the lower values found in normal coronary arteries. The right panel indicates that coronary flow ratio is seriously impaired only at a vessel diameter below 1.5 mm. This stenosis diameter corresponds well with the theoretical range indicated in Figure 12.6.

The correlations between flow ratio and stenosis parameters are fairly good: 0.82 for the stenosis diameter and 0.79 for the minimum cross-sectional area. These correlations are much better than reported earlier [25] and are due to the patient selection.

In clinical practice, it is customary to report the severity of a coronary stenosis in terms of percentage of stenosis. This percentage is either the reduction in lumen diameter or cross-sectional area. On theoretical grounds one would not advise the use of such a ratio to quantify the hemodynamic importance of the stenosis. The unrestricted vessel has a very low resistance over a length comparable to the length of a stenosis and dynamic pressure drop is almost negligible. Moreover, although there is a correlation between diameter of vessels and the amount of tissue perfused [24], there might be a considerable scatter in such a correlation in disease. Consequently, the hemodynamic properties of the undisturbed vessel form a very insensitive standard for the hemodynamic events in stenotic area. This point may be clarified by the following example. Assume two conditions in which the same amount of myocardium is perfused by a major coronary vessel with a lumen of 3 or 4 mm and a stenosis of 10 mm length with a lumen of 1 mm. In absolute terms, the expected pressure drop over the stenosis is the same in both arteries while the stenosis severities are 66% and 75% respectively when expressed in diameter ratios.

A decision on the best choice of stenosis parameter, absolute cross-sectional area or percent stenoses, cannot be made on the basis of Figure 12.8. The range of diameters proximal to the stenosis was fairly small, being 7.5 ± 0.4 (SEM) mm^2. Hence, the variation in proximal diameters is too small to distinguish between the two parameters. It should be noted that a different set of data from the same center [15] showed no correlation between flow ratio and percent stenoses. However, normal and abnormal flow ratios could be distinguished when plotted versus absolute minimal stenosis cross-sectional area [25]. The range of diameters proximal to the stenosis was twice as large as in the data set shown in Figure 12.8. Moreover, the data were obtained from patients undergoing heart surgery. More data under a variety of conditions are needed to allow a rational choice of stenosis parameter indicating physiological significance.

12.6 Effect of stenosis geometry and flow pulsatility on pressure drop

In the two sections above, the pressure drop over either a very mild stenosis or a stenosis with a neat cylindrical geometry was considered. Such an analysis is very useful for assessing the relative importance of several parameters. In reality, however, a stenosis is only clinically significant if the lumen diameter is smaller than 2 mm and is considered serious at half of this diameter. Moreover, in most patients severe stenoses are not cylindrical.

As discussed above, for short stenoses the most important factor is the pressure loss due to the lack of dynamic pressure recovery. However, for longer stenoses, especially if the minimal area is not severely reduced, the frictional loss should not be neglected. Hence, it is worthwhile to consider the effect of stenosis geometry on this.

An idea of the importance of the deviation from cylindrical shape for frictional pressure loss can be obtained by calculating the pressure drop over a tube with elliptical cross section. If a constant cross-sectional area is maintained, the

12.6 Effect of stenosis geometry and flow pulsatility on pressure drop

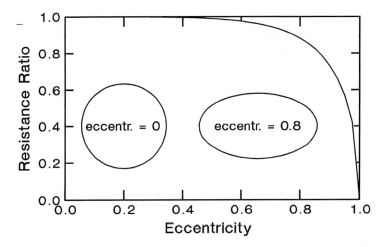

Figure 12.9: Effect of asymmetry of a vessel with an elliptic cross-sectional area. On the horizontal axis, the ratio between short and long axis of the ellipse is plotted. On the vertical axis, the ratio between pressure drop of the elliptic vessel and a circular channel, both with the same cross-sectional area and flow, are shown.

asymmetry can be expressed by the ratio between the shorter and the longer axis. The ratio between the resistance of the eccentric vessel and the cylindrical vessel as function of eccentricity is illustrated in Figure 12.9. The effect of asymmetry on the pressure drop follows from the calculated resistance per unit length. As is clear from this figure, it is not until a high degree of asymmetry is reached that the pressure drop deviates from the prediction for the symmetrical cylinder with the same cross-sectional area.

Seeley and Young [30] investigated the effect of a smooth but irregular cross section of the constriction on the pressure drop experimentally. They found for high Reynolds numbers, that the deviation from a regular model with the same area reduction was smaller than 1%, and for low Reynolds numbers the deviation was never larger than 16%. These findings are in fair agreement with our theoretical analysis. At a high Reynolds number, the dynamic pressure loss is dominant and the increase in fluid velocity is more related to the magnitude of the area than to the shape, whereas at lower Reynolds numbers the viscous effects become more important but have an effect only with strong deviations from cylinder symmetry.

The eccentric position of the stenosis lumen has been studied experimentally in hydraulic models by Seeley and Young et al. [30] and Mates et al. [26]. The differences with the concentric model are very small and can be neglected for practical purposes.

The total pressure drop ΔP due to friction over a stenosis with length L and cross-sectional area $A(x)$ as function of axial position x can be estimated by

$$\Delta P = 8\pi\mu Q \int_{-L/2}^{+L/2} \frac{1}{A^2(x)}\,\mathrm{d}x. \qquad [12.5]$$

where Q is flow through the stenosis. This integral expresses the weighted average of the cross-sectional area over the stenosis length.

Up to now, we have not taken the possible effect of flow pulsatility into account. The pulsatile character of the flow introduces an extra inertial factor since the fluid in the vessel goes through a period of acceleration and deceleration. The inertia of a tube with a length L and radius r is: $\rho L/[\pi r^2]$. It is clear that a constriction in a tube increases this term. The effect of flow pulsatility has been studied by several authors [26, 28, 29, 41]. It was shown that for severe stenoses, the problem can be regarded in the same way as for steady flow. Moreover, it was discovered that instead of having a magnifying effect on the pressure drop, when severe constrictions were studied, the pulsatility had an attenuating effect. The pressure drop over the stenosis was 10% lower due to the fact that the development of turbulence and flow separation were delayed. In contrast, there is some extra pressure drop due to pulsatility with milder stenoses. However, since the pressure drop over such a stenosis can be ignored, the effect of pulsatility in that instance has very little practical value. An added argument for neglecting the pulsatility effect of flow on pressure drop is the reduction of the pulsatility of coronary flow in an artery with a coronary stenosis [31].

12.7 Theoretical optimization of coronary reserve

12.7.1 Effect of heart rate

Obviously, without stenosis, coronary reserve is determined by the same parameters that determine the two quantities by which it is defined: actual coronary flow and the maximal coronary flow under the given set of operational conditions. The analysis of the determinants of reserve is complicated, since they affect both control and maximal flow. Coronary flow, if regulation is still active, is mainly determined by oxygen consumption, which in turn depends on mechanical factors such as heart rate and systolic left ventricular pressure. The same factors affect the maximal possible coronary flow by squeezing the myocardial microvessels. The interaction is further complicated since the maximal coronary flow especially depends on average systemic arterial pressure, which in turn is dependent on the mechanical function of the left ventricle with its interaction with the system circulation. Consequently, a full analysis of the present problem would require a coronary circulation model coupled to a model of the circulation as a whole. In itself, such a model would be very useful especially for studying the effects of pharmacological interactions directed at the management of systemic blood pressure and or heart rate. However, no such an overall analysis is attempted. The influence of mechanical factors on the coronary circulation will be discussed independently of how these are determined by the systemic circulation.

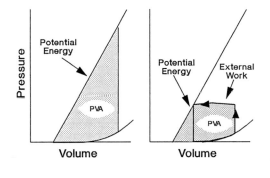

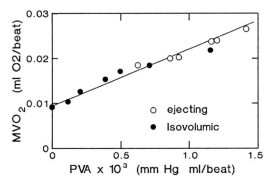

Figure 12.10: Dependence of oxygen consumption, MVO_2, on energy due to a single heart, PVA, beat according to the concept of Suga et al. [34]. Top panels: Total energy needed for a heart beat is determined by the potential energy built up by the myocardium and the external work. This energy depends on the pressure–volume area (PVA) independent of how it is established. Top left illustrates an isovolumic beat and top right an ejecting beat. Bottom panel: A typical result obtained by Suga, in support of his concept. The open circles represent ejecting ventricles and the closed circles are from isovolumic contractions.

A concept of how oxygen consumption is related to mechanical work has been established by Suga and coworkers. In this concept, the myocardium uses a certain amount of oxygen for each contraction, which is determined by a pressure–volume area as illustrated in the top panels of Figure 12.10 This area is delineated by the diastolic pressure–volume and end-systolic pressure–volume relations. The area illustrates the sum of potential energy and external work and it is assumed that this total determines the oxygen consumption independent of the ratio between potential energy and external work. In a subsequent paper [36] a good correlation between the pressure–volume area and oxygen consumption was demonstrated. These results obtained in isolated hearts were confirmed by an in vivo study using anesthetized dogs [38]. A correlation between pressure–

volume area and oxygen consumption, found in an isolated heart preparation, is demonstrated in the bottom panel of Figure 12.10. Hence, in the concept of Suga et al., the oxygen consumption for the beating heart can simply be related to the mechanical performance of individual beats. From these beats, the end-diastolic volume and the systolic pressure must be known, both of which are determined by the interplay of ventricle and systemic circulation. Obviously, these determinants will vary depending on heart function and alterations in systemic circulation. However, it is clear that heart rate is the main determinant of myocardial oxygen consumption. The effects of the other determinants will be neglected at first. Hence it will be assumed that oxygen consumption is linearly related to heart rate. More recently, Suga et al. [35] established that an increase in contractility can shift the PVA–MVO$_2$ relationship parallel to higher values of MVO$_2$.

The assumed linear relation between oxygen consumption and heart rate is defined by two coordinates: MVO$_2$ = 0.01 ml O$_2$ · s^{-1} [100 g]$^{-1}$ at heart rate zero, and MVO$_2$ = 0.15 ml O$_2$ · s^{-1} · [100 g]$^{-1}$ at HR = 100 · min^{-1}. As was shown in Chapter 9, coronary flow can be related to oxygen consumption and arterial pressure by the following equation:

$$\mathrm{CBF} = 0.0034 P_p + 1.4 \frac{\mathrm{MVO}_2}{1.34 \mathrm{Hb}} - 0.167 \qquad [12.6]$$

where:

    CBF   is coronary blood flow
    P_p is perfusion pressure
    MVO$_2$ is the oxygen consumption

    $\frac{\mathrm{MVO}_2}{1.34\,\mathrm{Hb}}$ is MVO$_{2,n}$ is normalized oxygen consumption

    Hb   is the hemoglobin concentration in g · [100 ml]$^{-1}$
    1.34   is the oxygen binding capacity of 1 g of hemoglobin.

The constants are from Vergroesen et al. [37] and were obtained from a study on dogs. We will refer to this equation as the coronary flow demand. It is graphically represented in Figure 12.11.

The second relation needed to evaluate the effect of mechanical parameters on coronary reserve is the dependency of maximal possible coronary flow on heart rate, systolic pressure and perfusion pressure. Again, heart rate is the main determinant and the modulating effects of systolic pressure and contractility on the maximal coronary flow will be neglected. We will further assume a constant coronary arterial pressure of 100 mm Hg such that the results in Figure 7.5 can be applied. These results will be approximated by a linear relation between maximal coronary flow and HR. This relationship is determined by the maximal

12.7 Theoretical optimization of coronary reserve

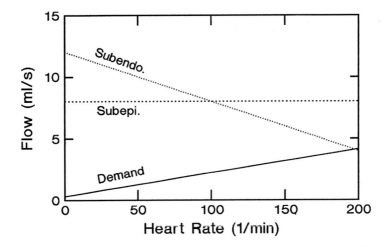

Figure 12.11: *Schematic representation of maximal flow through subendocardium and subepicardium as a function of heart rate, compared with flow demand as function of heart rate. It is assumed that coronary arterial pressure is kept at 100 mm Hg. Flow demand was calculated by Equation [12.6]. Note that as a result of choice of parameter values in the present example demand equals maximal flow in the subendocardium at a heart rate of 200 beats/min.*

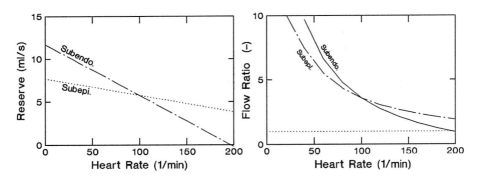

Figure 12.12: *Flow reserve (left panel) and ratio between maximum and control flow (right panel) as a function of heart rate as calculated from Figure 12.11. Note that the indices are more sensitive to HR at the subendocardium than at the subepicardium. Shortage of flow occurs when reserve approaches zero and flow ratio approaches unity.*

possible flow at $HR = 100 \cdot min^{-1}$ and the slope of the relationship. For the subepicardium, this slope is assumed to be zero and for the subendocardium this is chosen such that at $HR = 0$, the flow is 50% above and at $HR = 200$, 50%

below the reference value at HR = 100. Coronary flow is distributed relatively evenly over the myocardial wall at this heart rate, as was discussed in Chapter 1.

The reference flow for maximal vasodilation is chosen such that at HR = 100, the ratio between maximal flow and flow with autoregulation intact equals four. The results of this reasoning for the maximal flow as a function of heart rate for both the subepicardium and subendocardium are also depicted in Figure 12.11.

The dependency of coronary flow reserve and flow ratio as a function of heart rate can readily be calculated from the results presented in Figure 12.11 and are depicted in Figure 12.12. The shapes of these relationships are not surprising. Reserve depends linearly on heart rate. For the subepicardium the slope is only determined by the slope of the HR–demand relation whereas at the subendocardium the slope is additionally determined by the dependency of maximal flow on heart rate. The latter has, based on the assumed numbers, a larger effect than the former. The flow ratio curves exhibit a hyperbolic relation with heart rate because demand increases with heart rate and is in the denominator of the ratio. It appears that at heart rates higher than 100 beats · min^{-1} the flow ratio is less sensitive to heart rate than is reserve. However, the analysis illustrates that because of the hyperbolic relation it becomes very important to know the effect of heart rate on flow ratio in practical circumstances, this ratio is used to indicate the compensatory capacity of the coronary bed during disease.

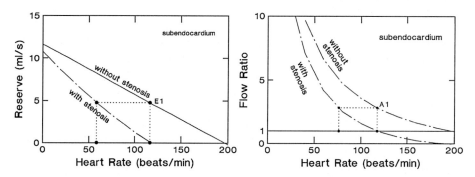

Figure 12.13: *Effect of stenosis on coronary reserve and the maximal/basal flow ratio for the subendocardial layer. It is assumed that the resistances induced by the stenoses are independent of flow. The resistance value equaled $2 \times R_{min}$, where R_{min} equals the resistance at maximal vasodilation and HR = 100 min^{-1}. Obviously, heart rate has an important effect on the two indices. In the example given the threshold for ischemia is about 120 beats min^{-1}. At a lower heart rate, 59 and 76 min^{-1} respectively, the indices would indicate a reserve in flow or ratio equaling the condition at 120 min^{-1} without stenosis. This is illustrated by the dotted lines.*

12.7.2 Reserve and flow ratio in the presence of a stenosis

The notions of reserve and flow ratio (ratio between maximal and basal flow) are meant to quantify the capacity of the coronary bed to accommodate an increase in flow demand when vessels are obstructed. We now will calculate the effects of a stenosis on the effect of heart rate on these variables. In order to calculate the effect of a stenosis on coronary flow reduction, the dependency of flow on two variables must be known: heart rate and perfusion pressure. The effect of HR on maximal flow at a coronary pressure of 100 mm Hg was defined above. The effect of coronary pressure was incorporated by assuming that at a given heart rate, maximal flow would decrease linearly from its value at 100 mm Hg to zero at a constant pressure intercept of 10 mm Hg.

The calculated effect of stenosis on coronary reserve and flow ratio is presented in Figure 12.13 for a value of stenosis resistance equal to twice the resistance of the coronary circulation at maximal vasodilation and a heart rate of $100 \cdot \text{min}^{-1}$. As is obvious from Figure 12.13, the effect of stenosis is especially clear at higher heart rates. The effect will even be stronger when the nonlinear behavior of the stenosis resistance is considered, because it implies an increasing resistance value at higher flow demands.

Both flow ratio and reserve at constant heart rate are diminished by the coronary stenosis. However, because of the effect of heart rate on the indices, its application here to indicate the severity of the stenosis should be done with care. This is illustrated in Figure 12.13. For the chosen conditions, both indices indicate an absence of further flow adaptation at a heart rate of 120 beats $\cdot \text{min}^{-1}$ with stenosis present. Without stenosis, each index would have a certain value at this heart rate, indicated by E1 and A1 for reserve and ratio respectively. In the presence of the stenosis, the same values will be predicted at heart rates of 59 and 76 beats $\cdot \text{min}^{-1}$ for reserve and flow ratio respectively. This simple calculation shows that heart rate should be defined in interpreting the indices. Since there is a larger difference in heart rate needed for making this error with flow reserve than with maximal/basal flow ratio the notion of reserve is less likely to produce a falsely positive result than is the flow ratio.

12.7.3 Hemodilution in the presence of a stenosis

In the presence of a stenosis the question of hemodilution becomes an important one. Hemodilution reduces blood viscosity, but also decreases the oxygen carrying capacity of the blood. These two factors may compensate for each other partly [3] in the sense that at the same driving pressure and constant vascular resistance, the oxygen flow into the organ will diminish less than the decrease in oxygen binding capacity of the blood. Hence, under normal circumstances and constant oxygen consumption, reserve will be less altered by hemodilution than is expected on the basis of a lower hematocrit since not only will flow demand increase, but so will maximal allowable flow. However, this relationship changes with a coronary stenosis. As was discussed above, an important fraction of the pressure drop over the stenosis is caused by loss of dynamic energy which is proportional to the blood velocity to the power two. In order to provide the same oxygen flow with hemodilution, the blood flow, and with it velocity, has to increase. The increase in velocity results in a more than proportional increase in dynamic pressure loss and therefore a more than proportional reduction in maximal allowable flow through the vascular system. Obviously, this effect is stronger when the contribution of the dynamic pressure loss to the total pressure loss (viscous plus dynamic) is larger. Since normal velocity will be lower in the more distal coronary branches, it is likely that the extra risk induced by hemodilution will be larger with stenosis in the larger branches.

12.8 Reflections on the clinical use of coronary flow reserve

In this chapter we attempted to elucidate the theoretical basis for the interpretation of coronary reserve measurements and the quantification of the hemodynamic severity of a coronary stenosis. Coronary flow measurements in human are scarce and until recently were limited to the coronary sinus [10, 22]. This latter method is not suitable for determining reserve restriction by a major vessel stenosis, because the blood collected in the coronary sinus will have originated from other vessels. With the introduction of Doppler tip coronary catheters, the coronary arterial blood velocity signal has become available [7, 16]. In the clinical application of this catheter, we were confronted with the problem of the introduction of some resistance introduced by the guiding catheter at the coronary ostium. The interpretation of a coronary arterial flow signal obviously requires an accurate measurement of the coronary arterial pressure signal concomitant with the flow measurement. A problem not solved by the measurement of coronary arterial flow by either method is the difference between subendocardial and subepicardial perfusion. As has been underlined, the subendocardium is the most susceptible to ischemia.

It has been shown in this chapter, on theoretical grounds, that coronary flow reserve or the ratio between maximal and basal flow is highly dependent on the working condition of the heart. The problem with measuring coronary reserve in the clinical setting is that this mostly is done under resting conditions providing an optimistic estimate for either reserve or flow ratio. As has been pointed out, coronary reserve may even be larger in the subendocardium than in the subepicardium in resting conditions which might lead to an underestimate of the severity of the impairment of flow. Since reserve decreases more rapidly in the subendocardium than in the subepicardium with increasing cardiac work, the subendocardium will be more vulnerable despite a possible higher subendocardial reserve measured at rest. This illustrates that flow reserve measured at rest is in itself not a proper index to estimate vulnerability of the myocardium. What is needed is the definition of an index that quantifies the remaining ability of the heart to adapt to an increase in cardiac work above a working point corresponding with a person's normal daily level of activity.

In an animal study Gould et al. [13] addressed the problem of dependency of flow ratio on physiological variables, specifically systemic pressure. Experiments were done in anesthetized dogs with an adjustable stenosis on the left circumflex artery. These authors indeed showed that the standard deviation of maximal/basal flow ratio could amount to around 40% if systemic pressure varied between 70 and 150 mm Hg. This is a rather wide range of systemic pressure, but the study shows the potential of systemic pressure as an error source in the estimation of flow ratio. Heart rate variability was much less than pressure variability and hence was not really addressed.

McGinn et al. [27] investigated the effect of heart rate, mean arterial pressure and preload on coronary blood velocity in man with regulation intact and after vasodilation with papaverine. The influences of these factors were most clear on resting coronary flow. As to be expected mean arterial pressure also affected maximal flow. However, from experimental studies one would expect a decrease of coronary flow with heart rate. It should be noted that in this study the heart rate was changed by pacing and and only moderately, from 76 to 100 beats per minute and that contractility was not determined. Since flow was measured in a large coronary artery alteration in subendocardial flow might have been present but not noticed.

Gould et al. [13] suggested a relative change of flow ratio as index. This relative change is the flow ratio in the presence of the stenosis divided by the flow ratio without stenosis. Both ratios have to be obtained under the same physiological conditions. Standard deviation could be reduced by a factor of 10 by this normalization. The normalization could be done by these authors because flow ratio was obtained in the same artery with and without stenosis. In patients the flow ratio without stenosis would have to be determined from an unobstructed vessel within the same heart; this would require the catheterization of a healthy vessel. The normalization can however also be obtained from alternative perfusion measurements. A nice illustration applying positron emission tomography was presented by Gould et al. [13]. Activity distribution over the myocardium was measured under rest and after vasodilation with intravenously administered dipyridamole. Flow ratio distribution was then calculated. The highest flow ratio was designated as normal and used to normalize the flow ratio distribution over the heart. As was also shown by the authors, even with positron emission tomography it might be difficult to find a 'normal' area without diffuse reduction of coronary flow reserve.

When reading clinical literature, the concept of supply and demand ratio is generally accepted. Management of patients is directed to maximize the factors beneficial to blood supply and to minimize the factors that dominate oxygen consumption. However, to these factors the impeding effect of cardiac contraction on coronary flow should be added. Heart rate increases this impediment. Since heart rate is a major determinant of oxygen demand one should, in management of the cardiovascular system under critical conditions, try to minimize heart rate. However, based on the analysis in this chapter, minimizing heart rate is even more important because of its impediment on flow. As illustrated in Figure 12.11, the maximal coronary flow in the subendocardium decreases faster with heart rate than demand increases.

Heart rate can obviously not be lowered to the extent that the lowered systemic pressure can endanger coronary flow. However, systemic blood pressure is not expected to prove an important determinant of flow reserve or ratio between maximal and control flow. Systolic pressure has some effect on the resistance of intramyocardial vessels, but much less than heart rate. Moreover, a decrease in pressure would result in a lower flow demand than the situation where pressure was constant, because of a reduction in oxygen consumption per beat. These two effects are compensatory in their effect on the indices.

In the concept of Suga [34], the oxygen consumption per heart beat is determined by the systolic left ventricular pressure and end-diastolic volume. This is a different way of stating that the heart works most efficiently with a large ejection fraction. At a given systemic pressure, the ejection fraction can be increased by increasing contractility or increasing end-diastolic volume. According to Suga, the effect of an increase in contractility to increase the ejection fraction costs less oxygen than an increase in end-diastolic volume. However, although it has been established that contractility is an important determinant of phasic coronary arterial flow, a quantitative relation between contractility and extravascular resistance has not yet been well-established.

The theoretical analysis of the pressure drop over a coronary stenosis closely agrees with the conclusions of some clinical studies, that the smallest absolute diameter of a coronary stenosis is a much better measure of the severity of a coronary stenosis than the often used ratio between stenosis diameter and the diameter of the vessel without stenosis. One should appreciate that the choice for an absolute measure is also supported by the observations that often the non-stenotic parts of the vessels are also affected by diffuse diseases and hence their diameters are not suited to be a standard. It should be noted that the clinical measurements of the pressure drop over a stenosis cannot be used to validate the analysis of a pressure drop over a stenosis. In these types of measurements the pressure drop is measured by means of a catheter through the lumen of the stenosis which strongly affects the cross-sectional area available for flow.

To simplify matters, several very relevant aspects related to the pathophysiology of coronary stenoses have been left out of the analysis in this chapter and which are recently reviewed by others [19, 39, 42]. Obviously, the net effect of a stenosis in a main branch can only be judged taking into account the possible collateral flow from other branches. This, undoubtedly, is an additional cause for the large scatter in clinical data. It also explains why sometimes a very severe stenosis of over 90% does not cause an infarct.

A major point to be considered is the heterogeneity of coronary reserve [1, 6], which can vary 6- to 20-fold. However, there will be no strong alterations in the picture outlined above if heterogeneity is taken into account. The analysis should then be applied to the areas with the lowest reserve.

In the literature up to now it seems that one either emphasizes the assessment of stenosis severity from a reserve measurement or reserve from a geometrical definition of a stenosis. There are, however, good reasons to uncouple these problems. The nature, extent and distribution of coronary narrowing are as important as the disease process itself. The question related to myocardial perfusion should be approached independently and preferably by methods that give information on perfusion distribution. Moreover, emphasis should be placed on definition of the working range of coronary perfusion and especially the maximal perfusion possible.

12.9 Summary

The coronary bed is normally capable of sustaining a flow through it four to six times larger than under resting conditions. Due to local control mechanisms flow is adapted to the needs of the heart. In the presence of a stenosis the control system is used to compensate for the pressure loss over the stenosis whereby the range over which flow normally can vary is reduced. There are two ways to quantify this reduction effect of the stenosis:

1. coronary reserve, being the difference between maximal flow and control flow and,

2. the ratio between control flow and maximal flow.

The pressure drop induced by the stenosis is caused by two physical principles. The first principle states that pressure is reduced because of viscous losses. Theory predicts that this pressure loss is proportional to the length of the stenosis and blood viscosity but inversely proportional to the square of an average cross-sectional area of the stenosis.

The second principle states that pressure is reduced because of the increase in kinetic energy of the blood when it is accelerated due to vessel narrowing. In theory this pressure reduction is reversible, but because of eddies at the outlet of the stenosis this is not so. In theory, this so-called dynamic pressure loss is independent of blood viscosity and stenosis length. The two pressure losses, viscous and dynamic, are additive. Similarly to the viscous losses, the dynamic pressure loss is proportional to the inverse of the square of the cross-sectional area. However, the viscous pressure loss is proportional to flow through the stenosis but the dynamic pressure loss is proportional to the flow to the power two. This latter property ensures that, especially with short stenoses, the dynamic pressure loss is dominant.

In predicting the reducing effect of a stenosis on coronary flow reserve one should take into account the fact that the pressure loss by the stenosis is increased with flow. This is best illustrated by a model analysis. An additional effect that should be taken into account is the increase in flow impediment from contraction of the heart. An increasing heart rate reduces coronary flow reserve by an increase in flow demand but even more importantly by increasing the extravascular component of coronary resistance. This is especially true for the subendocardium where the impeding effect of heart contraction on coronary flow is much more pronounced than at the subepicardium where this effect is almost absent.

References

[1] AUSTIN RE JR, ALDEA GS, COGGINS DL, FLYNN AE, HOFFMAN JIE (1990) Profound spatial heterogeneity of coronary reserve. Discordance between patterns of resting and maximal myocardial blood flow. *Circ. Res.* **67**: 319–331.

[2] BACK LH, RADBILL JR, CHO YI, CRAWFORD DW (1986) Measurement and prediction of flow through a replica segment of a mildly atherosclerotic coronary artery of man. *J. Biomech.* **19**: 1–17.

[3] BAER RW, VLAHAKES GJ, UHLIG PN, HOFFMAN JIE (1987) Maximum myocardial oxygen transport during anemia and polycythemia in dogs. *Am. J. Physiol.* **252** (*Heart Circ. Physiol.* **21**): H1086–H1095.

[4] CANTY JM JR, KLOCKE FJ (1985) Reduced regional myocardial perfusion in the presence of pharmacologic vasodilator reserve. *Circulation* **71**: 370–377.

[5] CANTY JM JR (1988) Coronary pressure-function and steady state pressure-flow relations during autoregulation in the unanesthetized dog. *Circ. Res.* **63**: 821–836.

[6] COGGINS DL, FLYNN AE, AUSTIN RE JR, ALDEA GS, MUEHRCKE D, GOTO M, HOFFMAN JIE (1990) Nonuniform loss of regional flow reserve during myocardial ischemia in dogs. *Circ. Res.* **67**: 253–264.

[7] COLE JS, HARTLEY CJ (1977) The pulsed Doppler coronary artery catheter. Preliminary report of a new technique for measuring rapid changes in coronary artery flow velocity in man. *Circulation* **56**: 18–25.

[8] CURRIE PJ, SEWARD JB, READER GS, VLIETSTRA RE, BRESNAHAN DR, BRESNAHAN JF, SMITH HC, HAGLER DJ, TAJIK A (1985) Continuous wave Doppler echocardiographic assessment of severity of calcific aortic stenosis: a simultaneous Doppler-catheter study in 100 adult patients. *Circulation* **71**: 1162-1169.
[9] DOLE WP, MONTVILLE WJ, BISHOP VS (1981) Dependency of myocardial reactive hyperemia on coronary artery pressure in the dog. *Am. J. Physiol.* **240** (*Heart Circ. Physiol.* **9**): H709-H715.
[10] GANZ W, TAMURA K, MARCUS HS, DONOSO R, YOSHIDA S, SWAN HJC (1971) Measurement of coronary sinus blood flow by continuous thermodilution in man. *Circulation* **44**: 181-195.
[11] GOULD KL, LIPSCOMB K, HAMILTON GW (1974) Physiologic basis for assessing critical coronary stenosis. Instantaneous flow response and regional distribution during coronary hyperemia as measures of coronary flow reserve. *Am. J. Cardiol.* **33**: 87-94.
[12] GOULD KL (1978) Pressure-flow characteristics of coronary stenoses in unsedated dogs at rest and during coronary vasodilation. *Circ. Res.* **43**: 242-253.
[13] GOULD KL, KIRKEEIDE RL, BUCHI M (1990) Coronary flow reserve as a physiologic measure of stenosis severity. *J. Am. Coll. Cardiol.* **15**: 459-474.
[14] GRATTAN MT, HANLEY FL, STEVENS ML, HOFFMAN JIE (1986) Transmural coronary flow reserve patterns in dogs. *Am. J. Physiol.* **250** (*Heart Circ. Physiol.* **19**): H276-H283.
[15] HARRISON DG, WHITE CW, HIRATZKA LF, DOTY DB, MILLER MR, EASTHAM CL, MARCUS ML (1981) Can the significance of a coronary stenosis be predicted by quantitative coronary angiography? Abstract. *Circulation* **64** *Suppl.* IV: 160.
[16] HARTLEY CJ, COLE JS (1974) A single-crystal ultrasonic catheter-tip velocity probe. *Med. Instrum.* **8**: 241-243.
[17] HOFFMAN JIE (1984) Maximal coronary flow and the concept of coronary vascular reserve. *Circulation* **70**: 153-159.
[18] HOFFMAN JIE (1987) A critical view of coronary reserve. *Circulation* **75** *Suppl.* I: 6-11.
[19] HOFFMAN JIE (1989) Coronary flow reserve. *Ann. of Cardiol. Surg.* **1989**: 90-96.
[20] HOLEN J, SIMONSEN S (1979) Determination of pressure gradient in mitral stenosis with Doppler echocardiography. *Br. Heart J.* **41**: 529-534.
[21] JOHNSON EL, YOCK PG, HARGRAVE VK, SREBRO JP, MANUBENS SM, SEITZ W, PORTS TA (1989) Assessment of severity of coronary stenoses using a Doppler catheter. Validation of a method based on the continuity equation. *Circulation* **80**: 625-635.
[22] KLOCKE FJ (1976) Coronary blood flow in man. *Prog. Cardiovasc. Dis.* **19**: 117-166.

[23] KLOCKE FJ (1987) Measurements of coronary flow reserve: defining pathophysiology versus making decisions about patient care. *Circulation* **76**: 1183–1189.
[24] KOIWA Y, BAHN RC, RITMAN EL (1986) Regional myocardial volume perfused by the coronary artery branch: estimation in vivo. *Circulation* **1**: 157–163.
[25] MARCUS ML (1983) *The coronary circulation in health and in disease.* McGraw-Hill, New York: 242–269.
[26] MATES RE, GUPTA RL, BELL AC, KLOCKE FJ (1978) Fluid dynamics of coronary artery stenosis. *Circ. Res.* **42**: 152–162.i
[27] MCGINN AL, WHITE CW, WILSON RF (1990) Interstudy variability of coronary flow reserve. Influence of heart rate, arterial pressure, and ventricular preload. *Circulation* **81**: 1319–1330.
[28] NEWMAN DL, WESTERHOF N, SIPKEMA P (1979) Modeling of aortic stenosis *J. Biomech.* **12**: 229–235.
[29] REUL H, SCHOENMACKERS J, STARKE W (1972) Loss of pressure, energy and performance at simulated stenoses in pulsatile quasiphysiological flow *Med. Biol. Eng.* **10**: 711–718.
[30] SEELEY BD, YOUNG DF (1976) Effect of geometry on pressure losses across models of arterial stenoses *J. Biomech.* **9**: 439–448.
[31] SPAAN JAE, BREULS NPW, LAIRD JD (1981) Diastolic-systolic coronary flow differences are caused by intramyocardial pump action in the anesthetized dog. *Circ. Res.* **49**: 584–593.
[32] SPAAN JAE, BRUINSMA P, LAIRD JD (1983) Coronary flow mechanics of the hypertrophied heart. In: *Cardiac left ventricular hypertrophy.* Eds. TERKEURS HEJD, SCHIPPERHEIJN JJ. Martinus Nijhoff, Dordrecht, The Netherlands: 171–191.
[33] SKJAERPE T, HEGRENAES L, HATLE L (1985) Non-invasive estimation of valve area in patients with aortic stenosis by Doppler ultrasound and two-dimensional echocardiography. *Circulation* **72**: 810–819.
[34] SUGA H (1979) External mechanical work from relaxing ventricle. *Am. J. Physiol.* **236** (*Heart Circ. Physiol.* **5**): H494–H497.
[35] SUGA H, GOTO Y. FUTAKI S, YAKU H, KAWAGUCHI O (1990) Ventricular elastance and oxygen consumption. *Proceedings First World Congress of Biomechanics.* **II**: 61.
[36] SUGA H, HAYASHI T, SHIRAHATA M (1981) Ventricular systolic pressure-volume area as predictor of cardiac oxygen consumption. *Am. J. Physiol.* **240** (*Heart Circ. Phsysiol.* **9**): H39–H44.
[37] VERGROESEN I, NOBLE MIM, WIERINGA PA, SPAAN JAE (1987) Quantification of O_2 consumption and arterial pressure as independent determinants of coronary flow. *Am. J. Physiol.* **252** (*Heart Circ. Physiol.* **21**): H545–H553.

[38] VINTEN-JOHANSEN J, DUNCAN HW, FINKENBERG JG, HUME MC, ROBERTSON JM, BARNARD RJ, BUCKBERG GD (1982) Prediction of myocardial O_2 requirements by indirect indices. *Am. J. Physiol.* **243** (*Heart Circ. Physiol.* **12**): H862–H868.
[39] WILSON RF (1990) An artery has many masters. *Circulation* **81**: 1147–1150.
[40] WILSON RF, MARCUS ML, WHITE CW (1987) Prediction of the physiologic significance of coronary arterial lesions by quantitative lesion geometry in patients with limited coronary artery disease. *Circulation* **75**: 723–732.
[41] YOUNG DF, TSAI FY (1973) Flow characteristics in models of arterial stenoses - II. Unsteady Flow. *J. Biomechanics* **6**: 547–559.
[42] ZIJLSTRA F, VANOMMEREN J, REIBER JH, SERRUYS PW (1987) Does the quantitative assessment of coronary artery dimensions predict the physiologic significance of a coronary stenosis? *Circulation* **75**: 1154–1161.

Appendix A

Equivalent schematic for calculation of pressure distribution

FIGURE 2.11 ILLUSTRATES that in order to calculate the pressures at branch points of a symmetrical branching tree this system can be simplified to a series of resistances, each of which are equal to the parallel equivalent of the resistances at that same order. This equivalent schematic seems obvious, but is surprisingly difficult to prove. A simple way is the following. Because of symmetry the pressure at branch points distal of segments of a certain order should be equal. Hence, the substitution of the branching network by a series of resistance formed an obvious solution. Now it remains to be proved that each resistance is the parallel equivalent of the segments of the respective order. Let us look at the pressure drop over resistance R_i, $P_{i+1} - P_i$. We can write:

$$P_{i+1} - P_i = R_i Q \qquad [A.1]$$

where:

R_i is resistance in the equivalent schematic,
Q is flow through the system.

Let q_i be the flow through segment i, with resistance r_i. Hence in the branching tree:

$$P_{i+1} - P_i = r_i q_i = r_i \cdot \frac{Q}{N_i} \qquad [A.2]$$

The most right part of Equation [A.2] holds because the flows through all N_i segments are equal. Since $P_{i+1} - P_i$ calculated by Equation [A.1] and Equation [A.2] should be equal, it follows that:

$$R_i = \frac{r_i}{N_i} \qquad [\text{A.3}]$$

which would be correct if all resistances r_i were directly connected in a parallel fashion.

It is clear that the above derivation only works if the tree is indeed symmetrical. As soon as the pressures proximal and distal to segments of a certain order are not equal, the parallel equivalence no longer holds. The precise distribution of resistance over all orders must therefore be known then in order to calculate approximate pressure distribution from a simplified series schematic.

Appendix B

Nonlinear pump model

IN THIS APPENDIX a description of the mathematical methods used with the nonlinear pump model as presented by Bruinsma et al. [1] will be given.

In the model the vascular wall is divided into eight concentric layers. Each layer consists of three compartments: an arteriolar, capillary and venular compartment in series. Each compartment consists of a transmural pressure dependent compliance in between two transmural pressure dependent resistances. The blood volume depends on the transmural pressure according to a nonlinear relation (Figure 6.8).

For every compartment the resistance, R, is defined according to the law of Poiseuille for tubes with constant length:

$$R = \frac{K}{V^2} \qquad [\text{B.1}]$$

where:

V is the volume of a compartment, and
K a constant specific for each compartment.

The vascular transmural pressure is the difference between intravascular pressure, P_b, and hydrostatic pressure in the surrounding tissue, P_{im}

$$P_{\text{tr}} = P_b - P_{\text{im}} \qquad [\text{B.2}]$$

The compliance C of a compartment is defined by

$$C = \frac{dV}{dP_{\text{tr}}} \qquad [\text{B.3}]$$

The compliance is equal to the slope of the transmural pressure-volume relation (Figure 6.8).

The flows into and out of a compartment, Q_{in} and Q_{out}, are determined by the distribution of hydrostatic pressures:

$$\begin{cases} Q_{in} = \dfrac{P_p - P_b}{R} \\ \\ Q_{out} = \dfrac{P_b - P_d}{R} \end{cases} \quad [B.4]$$

in which P_p, P_d, and P_b are the hydrostatic pressures at the proximal end, at the distal end, and within the compartment respectively.

The volume of a compartment is related to inflow and outflow according to

$$\frac{dV}{dt} = Q_{in} - Q_{out} \quad [B.5]$$

The numerical solution method applied to our equations requires a mathematical formulation of the pressure-volume relations (Figure 6.8). The characteristics of the pressure-volume relations are a rest volume at $P_{tr} = 0$, possible total collapse, and decreasing dV/dP_{tr} with increasing P_{tr}. These are met by the following equation:

$$P_{tr} = ae^{cV} + b\ln(cV) - p_0 \quad [B.6]$$

The first term dominates at high and the second term at low volume values. The coefficients a, b and p_0 influence the shape of the curve, whereas the constant c acts as a scaling factor for the volume axis. The constants a, b and p_0 for the different compartments were estimated such that the pressure distensibility curve agreed over a range of positive transmural pressure [2]. The curves are shown in Figure 6.8. The values for a, b and c are given in Table B.1, $p_0 = 5$ mmHg. The reference condition is the nonbeating heart with zero tissue pressure in all layers. The reference condition is defined by the data in Table B.1 as well.

In the reference situation it is assumed that the pressure distribution from arteries to veins is the same for all layers. This distribution was taken to be 50, 35, 15, 7.5 and 5 mmHg for the arterial, arteriolar, capillary, venular and venous pressures respectively.

In the reference situation total coronary flow was assumed to be 4 ml · s^{-1} · [100 g]$^{-1}$ LV. However, the flow distribution from endocardium to epicardium is not uniform in the arrested heart (Figure 1.10). An endo/epi flow ratio of 1.56 was assumed. The flow values in the intermediate layers were determined by linear interpolation.

A total coronary blood volume of 9.4 ml · [100 g]$^{-1}$ LV was assumed. Using the ration for the three compartmental volumes, as given by Spaan (1985) one arrives at a distribution of volume of 1.8, 4.0 and 3.6 ml · [100 g]$^{-1}$ LV for the arteriolar, capillary and venular compartments respectively. The coronary volume is not uniformly distributed from subendocardium to subepicardium. We assumed an endo/epi ratio of 1.14 [3] for all three compartments in the reference condition.

Table B.1: *Value variables and parameters in the reference condition.*

	Pressure mm Hg	Volume ml/100 g	Flow ml/s/100 g	a mm Hg	b mm Hg	c ml/s
Arteriolar	35	1.8	4	0.01	4.13	4.5
Capillary	15	4.0	4	0.17	7.57	1.0
Venular	7.5	3.6	4	0.14	5.89	1.0
Endo/epi ratio	1	1.14	1.56	1	1	1/1.14

The volume, pressure and flow distribution through each layer are now defined. This allows us to calculate all the resistances in the reference condition (Equation [B.4] and Equation [B.5]) and the constant K (Equation [B.1]) and parameter c (Equation [B.6]) for each compartment.

Each layer is now described by three coupled first order nonlinear differential equation of the form ($i = 1,2,3$):

$$\frac{dV_i}{dt} = \frac{P_{p,i} - 2P_{b,i} + P_{d,i}}{R_i} \qquad [B.7]$$

where index i refers to the arteriolar, capillary and venular compartment respectively. $P_{p,1} = P_a$, coronary arterial pressure and $P_{d,3} = P_v$, coronary venous pressure.

If P_a, P_v and P_{im} are defined as a function of time then the solution can be obtained by numerical integration. The solutions for the layers are different mainly because P_{im} differs from layer to layer. It was assumed that intramyocardial pressure was equal to left ventricular pressure at the endocardium and decreased linearly to zero at the epicardium.

References

[1] BRUINSMA P, ARTS T, DANKELMAN J, SPAAN JAE (1988) Model of the coronary circulation based on pressure dependence of coronary resistance and compliance. *Basic Res. Cardiol.* **83**: 510–524.

[2] SPAAN JAE (1985) Coronary diastolic pressure-flow relation and zero flow pressure explained on the basis of intramyocardial compliance. *Circ. Res.* **56**: 293–309.

[3] WEISS HR, WINBURY MM (1974) Nitroglycerin and chromonar on small-vessel blood content of the ventricular walls. *Am. J. Physiol.* **226**: 838–843.

Appendix C

Calculation of oxygen consumption with changing flow

IN THIS APPENDIX, the dynamic change of oxygen consumption will be derived from arterial and venous flow signals and from the arterial-venous oxygen difference as is proposed by Vergroesen and Spaan [3]. The model schematically given in Figure 9.5 will be used for the calculation.

The mass balance of oxygen in capillary space equals:

$$FO_2 = CAF\ O_{2a} - CCF\ O_{2c} + \frac{d[V_c O_{2c}]}{dt} \qquad [C.1]$$

where:

- FO_2 is the oxygen leaving the capillary space and entering the tissue space,
- CAF, CCF are the flows entering and leaving the capillary space,
- O_{2a}, O_{2c} are the arterial and capillary oxygen contents,
- V_c is the volume of the capillary blood space.

The last term of Equation [C.1] can be rewritten:

$$\frac{d(V_c O_{2c})}{dt} = O_{2c} \frac{dV_c}{dt} + V_c \frac{dO_{2c}}{dt} \qquad [C.2]$$

where dV_c/dt is the change of capillary volume which can be calculated by

$$\frac{dV_c}{dt} = CAF - CCF \qquad [C.3]$$

Combining Equations [C.1], [C.2] and [C.3] yields:

$$FO_2 = CAF[O_{2a} - O_{2c}] + V_c \frac{dO_{2c}}{dt} \qquad [C.4]$$

Assuming that the capillary compartment is well-mixed, the capillary oxygen content can be calculated from the venous oxygen content as follows:

$$O_{2c} = O_{2v} + \left[\frac{V_v}{CCF}\right] \frac{dO_{2v}}{dt} \qquad [C.5]$$

Combining Equations [C.4] and [C.5] yields:

$$\begin{aligned} FO_2 &= CAF\left[O_{2a} - O_{2v} - \left[\frac{V_v}{CCF}\right] \frac{dO_{2v}}{dt}\right] \\ &+ \left[V_c + V_c \frac{[CCF - CVF]}{CCF} - \frac{V_c \cdot V_v}{CCF^2} \cdot \frac{dCCF}{dt}\right] \frac{dO_{2v}}{dt} \\ &- \frac{V_c \cdot V_v}{CCF} \frac{d^2 O_{2v}}{dt^2} \end{aligned} \qquad [C.6]$$

where CCF−CVF equals dV_v/dt.

The oxygen flux can now be calculated from arterial and venous signals by Equation [C.6] if the values for the volumes of the different compartments and CCF are known. An estimate of the volume values is given by Spaan(Chapter 9 [50]). By assuming that the distribution of the volumes over the compartments does not change, the change in the volumes of these compartments can be calculated from the arterial and venous flow signals (Chapter 9 [2]).

The capillary flow, CCF, can not be measured. However, by assuming that the distribution of volumes over the compartments does not change, CCF can be calculated by:

$$CCF = CAF - \frac{V_c(0)}{[V_c(0) + V_v(0)]}[CAF - CVF] \qquad [C.7]$$

where $V_c(0)$ and $V_v(0)$ are the volumes of the capillary and venous compartment in the reference condition (steady state).

For the calculation of the oxygen flux change during a long diastole, Equation [C.6] can be simplified. After 3–4 s of diastole CAF can be assumed to be equal to CVF and consequently equal to CCF. Furthermore, total volume undergoes no further change and thus it can be assumed that $dCCF/dt = 0$. Hence after 3 s the second term of the right hand side reduces to $[V_c + V_v]dO_{2v}/dt$. In the first 3 s of diastole, when CCF is not known, dO_{2v}/dt is close enough to zero to allow the second term to be completely disregarded. The last term is important during the first 3 s of diastole. In this period CCF was assumed to be equal to CVF. The resulting error is similar to the errors induced by the assumption of volume distribution.

Equation [C.6] then becomes:

$$FO_2 = CAF[O_{2a} - O_{2v}] - [V_c + V_v]\frac{dO_{2v}}{dt} - \frac{V_c \cdot V_v}{CCF}\frac{d^2O_{2v}}{dt^2} \qquad [C.8]$$

The relation between oxygen consumption and the oxygen flux from blood to tissue (FO_2) is given by Equation [9.6]:

$$MVO_2 = FO_2 - d(V_t O_{2t}) \qquad [C.9]$$

where:

V_t is the tissue volume and,
O_{2t} is the oxygen content in tissue.

The solubility of oxygen in tissue is about 28.09^{-6} ml $O_2 \cdot g^{-1}$ tissue $\cdot$ mm Hg^{-1}. Assuming that 85% tissue consists of extravascular tissue yields an oxygen storage change of 2.4 μl O_2 per mm Hg per 100 g. The same value can be calculated for the capillary blood per 100 g LV by linearization of the oxygen saturation curve around the P_{50} value. This gives a value of 16.5 $\mu l \cdot$ mm Hg^{-1}. Assuming that the oxygen pressure in tissue and blood are in equilibrium, the variation of oxygen storage in tissue is only 15% of that in blood. The effect of oxygen storage in tissue can then be accounted for by increasing the volume of the capillary compartment by 15%. The last term of Equation [C.9] can then be neglected. In this calculation it is assumed that tissue P_{O_2} is at such a level that myoglobin is saturated with oxygen. Combining Equations [C.8] and [C.9] yields:

$$MVO_2 = CAF[O_{2a} - O_{2v}] - [V_c + V_v]\frac{dO_{2v}}{dt} - \frac{V_c \cdot V_v}{CCF}\frac{d^2O_{2v}}{dt^2} \qquad [C.10]$$

References

[1] SPAAN JAE (1985) Coronary diastolic pressure-flow relation and zero flow pressure explained on the basis of intramyocardial compliance. *Circ. Res.* **56**: 293–309.

[2] VERGROESEN I, NOBLE MIM, SPAAN JAE (1987) Intramyocardial blood volume change in first moments of cardiac arrest in anesthetized goats. *Am. J. Physiol.* **253** (*Heart Circ. Physiol.* **22**): H307–H316.

[3] VERGROESEN I, SPAAN JAE (1988) Rate of decrease of myocardial O_2 consumption due to cardiac arrest in anesthetized goats. *Pflügers Arch.* **413**: 160–166.

Appendix D

The Krogh model

D.1 Definition of the problem

THE PROBLEM DISCUSSED HERE is that of a single capillary with radius R_c surrounded by a cylinder of tissue with radius R_k. A mass balance is formulated for a cylindrical shell of tissue having an inner radius of r and outer radius of $r + \Delta r$. It is not hard to see that the mass balance for this shell can be written as:

$$\underbrace{2\pi r J(r)}_{A} - \underbrace{2\pi (r + \Delta r) J(r + \Delta r)}_{B} = \underbrace{2\pi r \Delta r M}_{C} \qquad [\text{D.1}]$$

where:

    r is radial coordinate,
    Δr is distance between the concentric cylinders,
    $J(r)$ is flux of oxygen through a cylinder wall at radius r,
    M is oxygen consumption.

In Equation [D.1] the terms A and B represent the amount of oxygen diffusing through the inner and outer cylindrical surfaces of the shell respectively. These amounts are formed by the product of the flux (rate per unit area) and the surface area per unit length. Term C represents the amount of oxygen that is consumed in the concentric space per unit length. Dividing all terms by $2\pi r \Delta r$ and taking the limit for $\Delta r \to 0$ yields:

$$\frac{dJ(r)}{dr} + \frac{J(r)}{r} = -M \qquad [\text{D.2}]$$

The radial oxygen flux is related to the radial gradient in oxygen pressure by:

$$J(r) = -\frac{D dC(r)}{dr} = -\alpha D \frac{dP(r)}{dr} \qquad \text{[D.3]}$$

where:

$C(r)$ is oxygen concentration,
α is the solubility for oxygen in the tissue,
D is diffusion coefficient.

Oxygen pressure and oxygen concentration are related by the law of Henry, $C = \alpha P$.

The use of the partial gas pressure instead of the concentration is advantageous since it is constant across boundaries between media with different solubilities, whereas the oxygen concentration shows stepwise changes across such a boundary. Hence, in the following, the oxygen partial pressure will be used as the dependent variable.

Substitution of Equation [D.3] into Equation [D.2] and some rewriting results in the one-dimensional diffusion equation for cylindrical coordinates:

$$\frac{d}{r dr}\left(r\frac{dP(r)}{dr}\right) = \frac{M}{\alpha D} \qquad \text{[D.4]}$$

This equation can be solved by integrating twice which yields

$$P(r) = +\frac{M}{4\alpha D}r^2 + A_1 \ln(r) + A_2 \qquad \text{[D.5]}$$

where:

$\ln(r)$ is the natural logarithm of radius r,
A_1, A_2 are integration constants to be determined from the boundary conditions.

Derivation of the integration constants, as well as the representation of the results of the diffusion equation, is made easier by the introduction of dimensionless variables and parameters. This is done by means of the following relations.

$$r^* = \frac{r}{R_c} \qquad \text{[D.6]}$$

is the relative radius within the tissue with reference to the capillary radius, R_c.

$$P^*(r^*) = \frac{P}{P_c} \qquad \text{[D.7]}$$

is the oxygen pressure as fraction of the pressure at $r = R_c$ being P_c.

$$M^* = \frac{M R_c^2}{4\alpha D P_c} \qquad \text{[D.8]}$$

D.3 Simplified equation for maximal Krogh radius

is the ratio between oxygen consumption per unit mass and maximal flux at $r = R_c$.

The general solution can then be reduced to

$$P^*(r^*) = M^* r^{*2} + K_1 \ln(r^*) + K_2 \qquad [D.9]$$

where K_1, and K_2 are constants to be determined by boundary conditions.

D.2 Simplified equation for maximal Krogh radius

In Chapter 11 an implicit equation was derived for the relation between maximal Krogh radius and dimensionless oxygen consumption. Also a simplified equation was presented:

$$R_f^* = 1.242 M^{*-0.35} \qquad [D.10]$$

The relative error made by this equation is documented in Figure D.1.

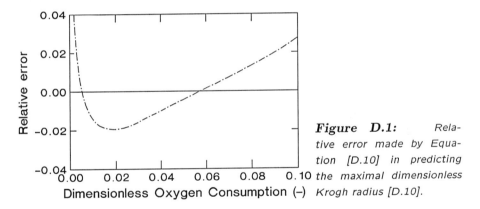

Figure D.1: Relative error made by Equation [D.10] in predicting the maximal dimensionless Krogh radius [D.10].

D.3 Derivations of the Krogh model

In order to derive the mathematical equations a thin slice of the Krogh cylinder, tissue and capillary with thickness Δz and perpendicular to the axis of the capillary will be considered. One may equate the oxygen flow over that distance to the amount of oxygen consumed per unit time by the tissue within the slice. The latter can be expressed by

$$VO_2 = \pi(R_K^2 - R_c^2) M \Delta z \qquad [D.11]$$

where:

> VO_2 is the amount of oxygen consumed in the slice per unit time,
> R_K is the radius of Krogh cylinder,
> R_c is the capillary radius.

The reduction in oxygen flow within the capillary over distance Δz can be related to the drop in capillary P_{O_2} by

$$VO_2 = Qh\beta\Delta P \qquad [D.12]$$

where:

> Q is the magnitude of capillary flow, being independent of z,
> h is the oxygen binding capacity of blood in ml $O_2 \cdot$ ml^{-1} blood,
> β is the slope of the oxygen saturation curve of the capillary blood,
> ΔP is the drop in oxygen pressure of the capillary blood over Δz.

Substitution of the first expression for the second, dividing both sides of the resulting expression by Δz with $\Delta z \to 0$ results in the simple first order differential equation:

$$\frac{dP}{dz} = -\frac{M\pi(R_t^2 - R_c^2)}{Qh\beta} \qquad [D.13]$$

If the Krogh radius is larger than that oxygen can diffuse maximally allowed, the radius of the tissue cylinder R_K becomes a function of the capillary oxygen pressure. In that case, integration becomes more complex. We will disregard this possibility. Integration of Equation [D.13] and applying the boundary condition at the capillary inlet where oxygen pressure equals inlet pressure, P_i yields:

$$P(z) = P_i - \frac{M\pi(R_t^2 - R_c^2)}{Qh\beta} z \qquad [D.14]$$

The oxygen pressure in the tissue as function of radius r and at given z can be calculated by the Krogh equation, Equation 11.3. As is to be expected, the gradient in capillary oxygen pressure in the axial direction depends on the ratio between the oxygen consumption per unit length and the oxygen flow through the capillary.

Author index

Ashikawa, K, 74
Allela, A, 12
Areskog, NH, 265
Armour, JA, 92
Arts, MGJ, 46, 47, 48, 49, 137, 140
Arts, T, 8, 11
Ashikawa, K, 74, 75, 186
Aukland, K, 261, 264, 276, 284
Austin, RE Jr, 24, 27, 336
Aversano, T, 184, 185
Avolio, AP, 23
Azuma, T, 185, 200
Bache, RJ, 22, 25, 168, 169, 247
Back, LH, 340, 342
Baer, RW, 353
Balaban, RS, 323
Barcroft, J, 12
Bardenheuer, H, 245
Bassingthwaighte, JB, 26, 27, 28, 60, 69, 70, 71, 79, 87
Bayliss, WM, 23
Becker, BF, 50, 55
Bellamy, RF, 15, 155, 180, 186
Belloni, FL, 18, 223, 225
Berne, RM, 22, 243, 244
Beyar, R, 92
Bishop, VS, 182, 183, 185
Blessing, MH, 324
Bolwig, TG, 267
Borg, TK, 73
Broten, TP, 237, 252
Brown, RE, 38
Bruinsma, P, 140, 187, 365

Burattini, R, 140
Burrows, ME, 199
Buss, DD, 70
Caille, JP, 323
Canty, JM Jr, 20, 92, 115, 116, 118, 119, 121, 179, 184, 334, 343
Carew, TE, 186
Caro, CG, 96
Chadwick, RS, 177
Chien, G, 56
Chilian, WM, 49, 50, 56, 92, 183, 186
Chvapil, M, 264
Ciuffo, AA, 87
Coffman, JD, 20
Coggins, DL, 336, 357
Cole, RP, 322, 354
Conley, KE, 70
Crone, C, 276
Curry, FE, 266, 284
Damon, DH, 74, 82
Dankelman, J, 20, 140, 179, 224, 226, 232, 234, 236, 239
Daut, J, 23
Davis, MJ, 49, 51
Demoment, G, 100
Desjardins, C, 76
Dobrin, PB, 213
Dole, WP, 20, 22, 181, 182, 183, 185, 247, 253, 334, 335
Domenech, RJ, 25
Douglas, JE, 49
Downey, HF, 13, 20, 25, 135

Downey, JM, 8, 26, 137, 138, 164, 165
Drake-Holland, AJ, 232, 252
Dreisbach, RH, 243
Driscol, DE, 19, 20
Duling, BR, 74, 76, 79, 236, 237, 309
Eckenhoff, JE, 13
Edlund, A, 245
Eichling, JO, 267
Eikens, E, 242
Eliassen, E, 276
Elzinga, G, 231
Eng, C, 48, 121, 181, 182, 183, 184
Eriksson, E, 79
Fåhraeus, R, 77
Fam, WM, 57
Feigl, EO, 5, 22
Feldstein, ML, 265
Fenton, BM, 75
Fleisch, A, 23
Flynn, AE, 169
Franzen, D, 29
Fronek, K, 60
Fulton, WFM, 40
Fung, YC, 72
Furchgott, RF, 23
Gamble, WJ, 294
Ganz, W, 354
Gayeski, TEJ, 293, 325
Gellai, M, 232
Gerdes, AM, 70, 82
Gerlach, E, 232, 243
Gibbs, CL, 231
Giezeman, MJMM, 212
Goldberger, AL, 28, 61
Goldsmith, HL, 77
Gorczynski, RJ, 236, 237
Goto, M, 155
Gould, KL, 334, 355
Grande, PO, 242
Granger, HJ, 244, 247
Grattan, MT, 20, 334

Grayson, J, 88
Greensmith, JE, 194, 195
Gregg, DE, 8, 12, 14, 38, 132, 221
Gross, L, 87
Grunewald, WA, 292, 293, 294
Gundry, SR, 87
Guyton, AC, 276
Han, Y, 274
Hanley, FL, 22, 166, 167, 247, 253
Harasawa, Y, 111
Harris, TR, 265
Harrison, DG, 346
Hartley, CJ, 354
Hassinen, IE, 327
Hausdorff, F, 61
Heineman, FW, 8, 137, 164
Henquell, L, 70
Heslinga, G, 24
Hevesy, G, 267
Hill, AV, 293
Hiramatsu, O, 6, 10
Hof, RA, 89
Hoffman, JIE, 11, 73, 137, 186, 334, 336, 357
Holtz, J, 23, 294
Ignarro, LJ, 23
Intaglietta, M, 199
Ito, Y, 185
Johansson, B, 198
Johnson, PC, 196
Jones, DP, 323
Kajiya, F, 8, 10, 175, 177
Kanatsuka, H, 185
Katz, SA, 5, 322, 326
Kayar, SR, 322
Kedem, O, 268
Kendall, MG, 60
Kerber, RE, 27
King, RB, 28
Kirk, ES, 8, 135, 137, 138, 165
Kitamura, K, 248
Klassen, GA, 92, 174

Author Index

Klitzman, B, 79
Klocke, FJ, 16, 165, 181, 186, 334, 354
Koch, AR, 253
Koiwa, Y, 346
Krams, R, 5, 8, 26, 110, 120, 151, 152, 154, 174, 179
Kreuzer, F, 292, 323, 324
Krogh, A, 74, 292, 298
Kroll, K, 22, 245, 247, 253
Kuo, L, 23, 197, 198, 205, 214, 251, 252
Laine, GA, 268, 269, 270
Laird, JD, 253
Lansman, JB, 220
Lee, J, 111, 140, 178, 179
Leniger-Follert, E, 324
Levy, BI, 73, 155
Lew, HS, 75
Lie, M, 23
Ljung, L, 100
Lossë, BS, 294
Lowensohn, RE, 6, 7
Magder, S, 185
Makino, N, 327
Mandelbrot, B, 61
Marcus, ML, 27, 28, 92, 334, 345, 346
Martini, J, 70, 82, 83
Marzilli, M, 8, 172, 173
Mates, RE, 184, 342, 347, 348
McDonald, N, 44
McGillivary, KM, 253
McGinn, AL, 334, 355
McHale, PA, 196, 242
Meer, JJ van de, 8
Meininger, GA, 49, 51, 253
Messina, LM, 186
Michel, CCH, 262, 265, 267, 276, 284
Miller, AJ, 261, 265
Millikan, GA, 294
Mohrman, DE, 14, 253

Moll, W, 292, 324
Munch, DF, 155
Murphy, RA, 213
Murray, CD, 44
Nagata, Y, 205
Nakamura, T, 295
Nellis, SH, 49
Newman, DL, 348
O'Keefe, DD, 70, 82
Oka, S, 200
Okun, EM, 70
Olsson, RA, 245, 246, 247
Osol, G, 199
Pelosi, G, 49
Perl, W, 276
Permutt, S, 135
Pogatsa, G, 261
Polimeni, PI, 264
Popel, AS, 60, 292
Porter, WT, 5, 8, 10, 92
Potter, RF, 70
Raff, WK, 132
Rakusan, K, 69
Ratajczyk-Pakalska, E, 88
Reneman, RS, 8
Reul, H, 348
Rhodin, JAG, 194, 204
Roberts, JT, 70
Rose, CP, 83, 276
Rouleau, J, 24, 107
Rubio, R, 244, 247
Ruiter, JH, 20, 21
Sabiston, DC, 5, 132
Sadick, N, 243
Sagawa, K, 100
Saint-Felix, D, 100
Saito, D, 247
Salisbury, PF, 261
Sarelius, IH, 75, 314
Scaramucci, J, 5
Schaper, W, 40
Scharf, SM, 89, 90

Schoenmackers, J, 40
Schrader, J, 245, 247
Schwartz, GG, 227, 243
Seeley, BD, 347
Seely, S, 104
Segal, A, 305
Sestier, FJ, 28
Shapiro, HM, 49, 51
Shepherd, AP, 228
Sillau, AH, 322
Silver, IA, 293
Smaje, LH, 72
Smiseth, OA, 94
Sowa, W, 292
Spaan, JAE, 5, 9, 10, 11, 16, 17, 59, 96, 106, 108, 110, 111, 176, 181, 186, 228, 230, 278, 292, 334, 348, 366, 369
Starling, EH, 267
Steenbergen, C, 28
Steinhausen, M, 70, 74, 82
Suga, H, 151, 153, 349, 350, 356
Sun, Y, 140
Suwa, N, 44
Taira, A, 263
Tangelder, GJ, 185
Taylor, MG, 117
Tillmanns, H, 49, 70, 73, 74
Tomanek, RJ, 40, 41, 69, 70, 72
Tomonaga, G, 92, 183, 184
Tsujioka, K, 177
Tyml, K, 74
Uchida, E, 196
Uhlig, PN, 95
VanBavel, E, 22, 42, 43, 45, 59, 196, 197, 198, 199, 242, 245, 246
VanBeek, JHGM, 61, 62, 228, 231
VanDijk, AM, 201
VanHuis, GA, 117, 118
VanWezel, HB, 249
VanWinkle, DM, 26, 173
Vargas, FF, 271, 272, 277

Vergroesen, I, 12, 13, 110, 174, 175, 228, 231, 232, 233, 237, 244, 248, 250, 275, 350, 369
Vetterlein, F, 77, 82
Vinten-Johansen, J, 349
VonRestorff, W, 22, 248, 250, 251, 327
Wüsten, B, 25, 39, 49, 142
Watanabe, J, 185
Wearn, JT, 70
Weiss, HR, 294, 295, 367
Westerhof, N, 5, 110, 119, 120, 121, 140, 152, 187
Whalen, WJ, 293, 294
Wieringa, PA, 46, 48, 49, 79, 80, 81, 292, 305, 309, 310, 311
Wiggers, CJ, 10, 11, 92
Wilensky, RL, 315
Wilson, RF, 334, 344, 345, 357
Wittenberg, BA, 322
Wong, AYK, 92
Wright, AJA, 82
Wyatt, D, 111, 112, 113
Yamakawa, T, 74
Yanagisawa, M, 22
Yen, RT, 75
Yipintsoi, T, 27
Young, DF, 348
Yudilevich, DL, 267
Zamir, M, 44
Zijlstra, F, 357
Zweifach, BW, 49, 204

Subject Index

α-receptors, 253
α-tone, 253
β-lipoprotein, 270
PS product, 83
Acetylcholine, 196
Actin filaments, 194
ADA, 22, 247
Adenosine
    hypothesis, 22 ,244 ,247, 253
    pool, 244
    mass balance, 245
    washout, 253
Adventitia, 194
Afterload, 151
Anatomical
    capillary length, 79
    recruitment, 82
Anesthetized dog, 94
Anesthetized goat, 222
Anoxic vasodilation, 23
Anterior veins, 88
Aortic valve, 6
Arrested heart, 167, 168, 279
Arterial
    density, 46
    network, 28
    occlusion, 10, 242
    volume, 193
Arteriolar
    P_{O_2}, 301, 309, 311
    compartment, 149, 167
    density, 47
    mechanics, 200

    resistance, 110, 234
    smooth muscle, 335
    tone 185
    wall, 220
Arterioles, 23, 40, 51, 56, 74, 193, 252, 314
ATP, 23
Atrial contraction, 6
Autoregulation, 13, 51, 180, 205, 219, 222, 226, 232, 235
    curve, 23, 107, 335, 338
    plateau, 206
Backpressure, 139, 160
Backflow, 9, 284
Barium contraction, 73, 155
Batson, 40
Beat Coronary Index, BCI, 18, 239
Blackbox, 105
Boundary layer, 316
Branching, 111
    network, 37
    nodes, 62
    pattern, 40, 43, 265
Brownian motion, 291
Capacitive flow, 141, 149, 184
Capillaries hexagonally stacked, 79
Capillary, 261
    anastomoses, 79
    bed, 37, 75. 279
    blood velocities, 74, 78, 303
    co- and counter flow, 81
    compartment, 149, 156
    cross-sectional area, 70

density, 70, 77, 83
diameter, 73
distensibility, 73
endothelium, 276
filtration coefficient, 276
growth, 82
hexagons, 310
interconnections, 83
lattice, 305
membrane, 284
network, 76, 81
pressure, 51
recruitment, 82
surface area, 267
transmural pressure, 262
wall, 262
Cardiac
arrest, 170
contraction, 117
cycle, 74
lymph, 264, 268
metabolism, 291
work, 220
Casts, 40
Characteristic time, 151
Collagen struts, 73
Collagen, 194, 264
Collapse, 95, 135, 149, 183
Collapse pressure, 181, 185
Collateral(s), 39
flow, 111, 357
load line, 113
resistance, 114
Collecting vein, 311
Colloid osmotic pressure, 267
Compartmentalization, 140
Complex system, 99
Compliance, 118, 210, 263
of microcirculation, 271
of interstitial space, 271, 276
per unit length, 210
Compression, 19, 30

Connective fibers, 194
Connective structures, 263
Constant pressure perfusion, 153, 174, 222, 225, 235
Constant flow perfusion, 222, 225, 235, 241
Contractility, 9, 94, 151, 172, 356
Control
engineering, 21, 224
of blood flow, 291, 333
Convection, 268
Convective acceleration, 338
Convective flux of proteins, 270
Coronary
peripheral pressure, 10
arterial pressure, 106, 354
arterial occlusion, 122, 174
arterial tree, 37
arterioles, 199
conductance, 245
flow 5, 100, 230, 243, 261, 354
flow control, 107, 193
index, 241, 242
input impedance, 118
microcirculation, 106
reserve, 21, 333, 334, 352, 354
resistance, 232, 273, 334, 336
sinus, 88, 89, 269, 286
stenosis, 336, 353
tone, 14, 239
venous system, 87, 94
venous flow, 10
venous pressure, 166, 269
venous oxygen saturation, 22, 27
CR model, 119
Cremaster muscle, 79, 253
Cryomicrophotometric method, 294
Cumulative pressure drop, 57
Cumulative volume, 53
Cytoplasm, 266
Daughter

diameter, 43
branches, 41
segments, 59
Diastole, 14
Diastolic
    aortic pressure, 243
    capillary blood pressure, 282
    resistance index, 18
    flow, 139
    flow fraction, 160
    perfusion, 170
    pressure–flow lines, 181
    pressure–volume relation, 155
    time fraction, 147, 169, 240
Dichotomous branching tree, 38, 46
Diffusion, 268, 291
    equation, 315
Diffusional shunting, 310
Diffusive flux, 270
Dilated coronary bed, 111
Diode, 138
Dipyridamole, 50
Directional effect in the dynamic response of autoregulation, 223, 225, 241
Discharge hematocrit, 76
Distensibility, 72, 120, 174, 204, 210
Distribution
    of compliances, 279
    of flow, 24, 131
Dog, 70
Dynamic(s)
    distensibility, 213
    of coronary flow adjustment, 17
    of coronary flow control, 222, 238
    pressure, 341, 342,
    pressure losses, 344
Edema, 261
Ejection fraction, 356
Elastance, 110, 152, 158, 159, 225, 242, 262

Elastance model, 158, 164, 168
Elastic tubes, 103, 121
Elastic lamina, 194
Elasticity, 210
Elastin, 194
Electrical engineering, 115, 120
Electrical analog, 135
Electronic circuits, 81
Elliptical cross section, 346
End-segments, 59
End-diastolic resistance index, 15
End-diastolic resistance, 132
End diastolic volume, 356
Endo/epi ratio, 25, 169, 174
Endocardium, 24, 242
Endomurally, 40
Endothelial, 23, 193, 253, 266
Endothelin, 22
Epicardial
    arteries, 131
    capillary red cell velocities, 74
    lymph, 274
    veins, 96, 131, 177
Epicardium, 24, 242
Equivalent circuit, 105
Error signal, 21
Exponential, 107
External work, 152, 349
Extravascular
    resistance, 132, 134, 163, 225
    resistance model, 160
    space, 234
Fåhraeus-Lindquist effect, 55
Facilitated oxygen transport, 292
Feedback, 21, ,223 235
Fenestrae, 266
Fiber shortening, 110
Fibonacci series, 61
Fick equation, 228
Filament orientation, 194
Filtration coefficient, 267
Flow

adaptation to metabolism, 219
adjustment, 226, 235, 242
control, 220
induced relaxation, 23, 241, 252
pulsatility, 346, 348
reserve (see coronary reserve)
Fluid dynamic, 103
Fluorescence of NADH, 28
Fourier analysis, 115
Fractal models, 28, 62
Frequency domain, 103
Functional
    hyperemia, 219
    recruitment, 82
    segment length, 54
GAG, 264
Gamma camera, 271
Gas exchange, 315
Gel, 264
Goat, 94
Great cardiac vein, 88
Gregg effect, 13, 221
Growth function, 43
Hamster, 74, 79
Harmonics, 103, 117
Heart
    block, 243
    contraction, 126
    function, 350
    muscle, 193
    rate, 164, 242, 272, 282, 350
    weight, 271
Hematocrit, 75, 272
Hemodilution, 353
Hemodynamic importance of a stenosis, 344
Hemoglobin saturation, 294
Heterogeneity, 20, 24, 357
Heterogeneous distribution of myocardial perfusion, 61
Heterogeneous capillary flow, 82, 309

Hexamethonium, 13
His bundle, 115
Histograms, 311
Human, 70
Hydrated GAG's, 264
Hydraulic diameter, 194
Hydraulic conductivity, 267
Hydrodynamics, 115
Hydrostatic pressure, 262
Hyperemia, 219
Hypermetabolic rats, 322
Hypertension, 249
Hypertrophy, 264
Impedance of perfusion system, 174
Impulse response, 117
In vivo heart, 70
Incompressibility, 107
Inertia, 348
Input impedance, 100, 104, 115, 117, 126
Input compliance, 179, 184
Interaction of control mechanisms, 253
Intercapillary
    distance, 82, 292
    shunting, 310, 313
Intercellular fluid, 291
Interendothelial clefts, 276
Internal resistance, 105, 107
Interstitial
    adenosine, 22, 244
    fluid, 284, 291
    oncotic pressure, 23
    pressure, 262, 269, 275, 276
    proteins, 284
    water, 272
Interstitium, 261, 286
Intramural veins, 87
Intramyocardial
    blood pressure, 10
    blood volume, 10, 153, 174, 187
    compliance, 174, 183, 239, 267

pump model, 8, 151, 164, 170
   vessels, 9, 14
Ischemia, 40
Isoproterenol, 172
Isovolumetric conditions, 153
Kedem-Katchalsky, 268
Kinetic energy density, 341
Krogh, 292
   cylinder300, 315
   problem, 298
   radius, 300
LAD, 39, 94, 113, 172
Langendorff preparation, 46, 276
Large coronary arterial branches, 39, 46, 52
Large artery structure, 54
Law of Bernoulli, 338
LCX, 39
Left
   anterior descending, 39
   circumflex artery, 39
   main coronary artery, 106
   ventricular pressure, 132, 138, 151, 175, 262, 274, 348
Lidocaine, 172
Linear
   analysis, 111
   control system, 224
   intramyocardial pump model, 132, 179, 239, 278, 282, 287
Linearity, 101
Linearized oxygen saturation curve, 309
Lipophilic substances, 266
Load line analysis, 105, 111, 185
Local control of coronary flow, 12, 30, 219
Long diastoles, 115
Lumped, 140
Lung, 135
Lymph, 262
   capillaries, 264, 265

flow, 262, 268, 275
obstruction, 274
pressure, 274
Main capillaries, 70, 79
Mass density, 120
Mathematical models, 104
Maximal vasodilation, 222
Maximal vasoconstriction, 222
Maximal coronary flow 338
Mean resistance, 134
Mechanical work, 349
Mechanics of arteriolar wall, 193
Media, 194
Membranes, 266
Mesentery, 60, 199, 262
Metabolic flow adjustment, 13
Metabolism, 244, 333
Metabolites, 261
Microvascular pressure, 160
Microcirculation, 19, 74, 79, 107, 112, 261
Microsphere distribution, 135, 172, 174
Microspheres, 50, 88, 112
Microvascular resistance, 170
Microvessels, 64, 348
Mitochondria, 252, 317
   density of, 317
   oxygen consumption of, 229
Models, 277
   CR model, 119
   elastance model, 158, 164, 168
   extravascular resistance model, 132, 134, 163, 225
   fractal models, 28, 62
   intramyocardial pump models, 8, 151, 164, 170
   linear intramyocardial pump model, 132, 179, 239, 278, 282, 287
   mathematical models, 104
   nonlinear models, 132

nonlinear intramyocardial pump model, 140, 155, 160, 164, 239, 278, 281
nonsymmetrical tree model, 51
physical models, 104
predictive models, 131
RCR models, 119
relational models, 104
waterfall model, 95, 135, 137, 151, 160, 163, 225, 239, 285, 287
Morphology of arteriolar wall, 194
Mother branches, 41
Muscle fibers, 25
Myocardial wall, 186, 262
Myocytes, 73, 82, 263
Myogenic, 220, 252
mechanism, 193, 219
optimal strength of, 208
response, 23, 195, 242, 253
tone, 23, 196
working range, 207
Myoglobin, 292
Myosin filaments, 194
Necrotic areas, 48
Negative feedback, 220
Neighboring capillaries, 292
Nifedepine, 249
Nitroprusside, 249
Noise signals, 100
Nonsymmetrical model, 51
Nonlinear, 15, 223
intramyocardial pump model, 140, 155, 160, 164, 239, 278, 281
models, 132
response, 123
system, 103, 223
venous pressure–flow relations, 90
Normalized pressure–flow relations, 224

Normoxic, 30
Obstructed arterioles, 47
Osmotic transients, 271, 273
Osmotic pressure, 267, 271, 273
Oxygen
balance, 230
buffers, 228, 292
consumption, 110, 236, 219, 220, 228, 247, 300, 308, 338, 349, 356
content, 228
demand, 244
dissociation curve, 301
dose–response curves, 236
extraction, 250
hypotheses of coronary flow control, 21, 215, 232, 244
pressure distribution, 309, 316
supply, 244
transfer to tissue, 82
transport, 291
uptake, 228
Parallel-perfused capillaries, 83
Pathophysiology, 357
Peak reactive hyperemic flow, 20
Perfusion system, 14
Perfusion pressure, 13, 221, 275
Pericardial pressure, 94
Pericardium, 93, 95
Perivascular P_{O_2}, 253
Permanent diastole, 147, 158
Permanent systole, 147, 281
Permeability, 82, 276
Pharmacological interventions, 349
Pharmacological reserve, 334
Phasic venous flow, 92
Phasic tissue pressure, 278
Physical models, 104
Plasma, 74
Plasma oncotic pressure, 275, 285
Poiseuille's law, 37, 194, 338, 339, 341

Subject Index

Positive feedback, 220
Post mortem heart, 70
Posterior, 88
Potassium channels, 23
Potential energy, 349
Prestenotic region, 341
Precapillary sphincters, 51, 83
Predictive models, 131
Preload, 151
Pressure–flow relations, 16, 100, 164, 181, 208, 335
Pressure distribution, 37, 49, 52, 55
Pressure source, 105
Pressure volume relationships, 142, 165, 193, 285
Pressure–cross-sectional area relations, 214
Pressure dependent resistances, 165
Propagation of asymmetry, 62
Proteins, 262, 265, 267
Protein concentration of the interstitium, 284
Proximal resistance vessels, 23
Pulsatile flow, 110, 159
Rabbit, 276
Radioactive microspheres, 60
Radioactivity, 273
Rat, 70
Ratio between maximal and control flow, 356
RC time constant, 146
RCR model, 119
Reactive hyperemic response, 20, 181, 197, 334
Red cells, 74, 271, 313
Reference point, 99
Reflection coefficients, 121, 267, 276
Relational models, 104
Relative pressure distribution, 55
Relative compliance, 210, 211
Repayment of flow, 242
Residence time, 265

Resistance
 control, 63
 index, 14
 of the lymph system, 265
 vessels, 23
Retrograde flow, 9, 111, 163, 183
Retrograde load line, 113
Rheological factors, 37, 82
Right ventricular wall, 38
Right coronary artery, 111
Right coronary arterial tree, 49
Right heart bypass, 166
Right atrial pressure, 181
Right ventricle, 294
Rigid tubes, 14
River structure, 63
Saline, 275
Segment length, 45
Sensitivity of resistance to pressure, 209
Short circuit, 110
Shortening, 25
Sine wave, 103
Sinus of Valsalva, 38
Skeletal muscle, 242
Small arteries, 38, 40, 48, 52, 54, 252
Smooth muscle
 cells, 38, 193, 241, 273
 tone, 220
Solute flux, 271
Solute, 267
Solvent, 267
Space averaged flow, 131
Spatial heterogeneity, 83
Spatial resolution, 294
Square wave, 132, 147, 278
Squeezing effect of systole, 170
Starling resistance, 87, 90
Starling hypothesis, 267
Static compliance, 210
Stenosis, 333, 334
 diameter, 342

geometry 346
length, 343
resistance, 107
Step functions, 17, 115
Stochastic processes, 28
Strahler ordering, 58, 265
Stresses, 107
Striated muscle, 74, 79, 193
Subendocardium, 6, 20, 30, 48, 63, 134, 137, 149, 262, 278, 284, 292, 336, 351
  compartments in, 146, 149
  compression of, 25
  resistance in, 138
Subepicardium, 8, 20, 49, 63, 134, 262, 284, 315, 336, 351
  arterioles in, 186
  flow in, 164, 168
Substrates, 261
Sucrose, 271
Superposition principle, 103, 106
Supply/demand ratio, 28, 250
Symmetrical dichotomous branching model, 47, 51, 62
Symmetrical dichotomous tree model, 47
Symmetry factor, 41
Sympathetic vasoconstriction, 253
Systemic arterial pressure, 168, 336, 337
Systemic circulation, 350
Systole, 73
Systolic
  arterial flow, 139
  inhibition, 6
  left ventricular pressure, 356
  pressure, 94, 278
  time fraction, 283
  tissue pressure, 160
  venous flow, 92
  volumes, 158
Systolic–diastolic interaction, 281, 287
Temporal heterogeneity, 83
Tension, 202
Tenuissimus, 60
Tetanic contraction, 185
Thebesian channels, 88, 96
Thermodilution, 249
Thermostat, 252
Tibialis, 74
Time
  averaged signals, 102
  averaged flow, 131, 139
  constants, 18, 234
  varying elastance concept, 94, 152, 164, 286
Tissue
  adenosine, 245
  oxygen tension, 22, 220, 310
  pressure, 139, 158, 175, 187, 261, 279
  pressure, 278, 282
  unit, 308
Total capillary volume, 70
Transcapillary pressure, 278, 281
Transfer function, 103, 104, 115
Transients in the coronary index, 239
Transmission line, 120
Transmural
  arteries, 73
  capillary pressure, 278
  pressure, 151, 187
  veins, 73, 88
Tube hematocrit, 76
Unbranched
  arterial segments, 40
  capillary segment, 83
Unstressed volume, 175
Vascular
  architecture, 26
  smooth muscle, 242
  volume, 142, 271, 273

Vasoconstriction, 20, 23, 107, 177, 194, 220, 223
Vasoconstrictor, 243
Vasodilation, 20, 211, 220, 253
Vasodilator, 219, 243
Vasodilatory response, 107
Vasomotion, 198
Vasomotor tone, 50, 116, 222
Venous
    anastomoses, 88, 90
    collateral resistance, 92
    compartment, 168
    compliance, 95
    outflow, 149, 175, 242
    oxygen pressure, 294
    pressure–flow relations, 90
    pressure, 221, 279
    resistance, 239, 279, 285
Ventricular cavity, 6, 172
Ventricular pressure, 164
Venular pressure, 157, 178
Venules, 74, 281, 314
Vesicles, 266
Vessel collapse, 106
Viscoelastic properties, 118, 126, 215
Viscosity, 55, 344
Viscous pressure drop, 344
Voltage source, 138
Volume distribution, 52
Volume changes, 230
Wall stress, 216
Washout of adenosine, 245
Water transfer, 265
Water balance, 51, 277, 284
Waterfall model, 95, 135, 137, 151, 160, 163, 225, 239, 285, 287
Waterfall element, 114, 178
Waterfall concept, 164
Windkessel, 120, 174, 183
Working point, 99, 102, 126
Working range, 253

Working condition, 354
Zero flow, 181

Developments in Cardiovascular Medicine

1. Ch.T. Lancée (ed.): *Echocardiology.* 1979   ISBN 90-247-2209-8
2. J. Baan, A.C. Arntzenius and E.L. Yellin (eds.): *Cardiac Dynamics.* 1980
                                                                                                   ISBN 90-247-2212-8
3. H.J.Th. Thalen and C.C. Meere (eds.): *Fundamentals of Cardiac Pacing.* 1979
                                                                                 ISBN 90-247-2245-4
4. H.E. Kulbertus and H.J.J. Wellens (eds.): *Sudden Death.* 1980   ISBN 90-247-2290-X
5. L.S. Dreifus and A.N. Brest (eds.): *Clinical Applications of Cardiovascular Drugs.* 1980   ISBN 90-247-2295-0
6. M.P. Spencer and J.M. Reid: *Cerebrovascular Evaluation with Doppler Ultrasound.* With contributions by E.C. Brockenbrough, R.S. Reneman, G.I. Thomas and D.L. Davis. 1981   ISBN 90-247-2384-1
7. D.P. Zipes, J.C. Bailey and V. Elharrar (eds.): *The Slow Inward Current and Cardiac Arrhythmias.* 1980   ISBN 90-247-2380-9
8. H. Kesteloot and J.V. Joossens (eds.): *Epidemiology of Arterial Blood Pressure.* 1980
                                                    ISBN 90-247-2386-8
9. F.J.Th. Wackers (ed.): *Thallium-201 and Technetium-99m-Pyrophosphate. Myocardial Imaging in the Coronary Care Unit.* 1980   ISBN 90-247-2396-5
10. A. Maseri, C. Marchesi, S. Chierchia and M.G. Trivella (eds.): *Coronary Care Units.* Proceedings of a European Seminar, held in Pisa, Italy (1978). 1981
                                                                   ISBN 90-247-2456-2
11. J. Morganroth, E.N. Moore, L.S. Dreifus and E.L. Michelson (eds.): *The Evaluation of New Antiarrhythmic Drugs.* Proceedings of the First Symposium on New Drugs and Devices, held in Philadelphia, Pa., U.S.A. (1980). 1981   ISBN 90-247-2474-0
12. P. Alboni: *Intraventricular Conduction Disturbances.* 1981   ISBN 90-247-2483-X
13. H. Rijsterborgh (ed.): *Echocardiology.* 1981   ISBN 90-247-2491-0
14. G.S. Wagner (ed.): *Myocardial Infarction.* Measurement and Intervention. 1982
                                                  ISBN 90-247-2513-5
15. R.S. Meltzer and J. Roelandt (eds.): *Contrast Echocardiography.* 1982
                                                  ISBN 90-247-2531-3
16. A. Amery, R. Fagard, P. Lijnen and J. Staessen (eds.): *Hypertensive Cardiovascular Disease.* Pathophysiology and Treatment. 1982   IBSN 90-247-2534-8
17. L.N. Bouman and H.J. Jongsma (eds.): *Cardiac Rate and Rhythm.* Physiological, Morphological and Developmental Aspects. 1982   ISBN 90-247-2626-3
18. J. Morganroth and E.N. Moore (eds.): *The Evaluation of Beta Blocker and Calcium Antagonist Drugs.* Proceedings of the 2nd Symposium on New Drugs and Devices, held in Philadelphia, Pa., U.S.A. (1981). 1982   ISBN 90-247-2642-5
19. M.B. Rosenbaum and M.V. Elizari (eds.): *Frontiers of Cardiac Electrophysiology.* 1983   ISBN 90-247-2663-8
20. J. Roelandt and P.G. Hugenholtz (eds.): *Long-term Ambulatory Electrocardiography.* 1982   ISBN 90-247-2664-6
21. A.A.J. Adgey (ed.): *Acute Phase of Ischemic Heart Disease and Myocardial Infarction.* 1982   ISBN 90-247-2675-1
22. P. Hanrath, W. Bleifeld and J. Souquet (eds.): *Cardiovascular Diagnosis by Ultrasound.* Transesophageal, Computerized, Contrast, Doppler Echocardiography. 1982   ISBN 90-247-2692-1

Developments in Cardiovascular Medicine

23. J. Roelandt (ed.): *The Practice of M-Mode and Two-dimensional Echocardiography.* 1983 ISBN 90-247-2745-6
24. J. Meyer, P. Schweizer and R. Erbel (eds.): *Advances in Noninvasive Cardiology.* Ultrasound, Computed Tomography, Radioisotopes, Digital Angiography. 1983 ISBN 0-89838-576-8
25. J. Morganroth and E.N. Moore (eds.): *Sudden Cardiac Death and Congestive Heart Failure.* Diagnosis and Treatment. Proceedings of the 3rd Symposium on New Drugs and Devices, held in Philadelphia, Pa., U.S.A. (1982). 1983 ISBN 0-89838-580-6
26. H.M. Perry Jr. (ed.): *Lifelong Management of Hypertension.* 1983 ISBN 0-89838-582-2
27. E.A. Jaffe (ed.): *Biology of Endothelial Cells.* 1984 ISBN 0-89838-587-3
28. B. Surawicz, C.P. Reddy and E.N. Prystowsky (eds.): *Tachycardias.* 1984 ISBN 0-89838-588-1
29. M.P. Spencer (ed.): *Cardiac Doppler Diagnosis.* Proceedings of a Symposium, held in Clearwater, Fla., U.S.A. (1983). 1983 ISBN 0-89838-591-1
30. H. Villarreal and M.P. Sambhi (eds.): *Topics in Pathophysiology of Hypertension.* 1984 ISBN 0-89838-595-4
31. F.H. Messerli (ed.): *Cardiovascular Disease in the Elderly.* 1984
    Revised edition, 1988: see below under Volume 76
32. M.L. Simoons and J.H.C. Reiber (eds.): *Nuclear Imaging in Clinical Cardiology.* 1984 ISBN 0-89838-599-7
33. H.E.D.J. ter Keurs and J.J. Schipperheyn (eds.): *Cardiac Left Ventricular Hypertrophy.* 1983 ISBN 0-89838-612-8
34. N. Sperelakis (ed.): *Physiology and Pathology of the Heart.* 1984
    Revised edition, 1988: see below under Volume 90
35. F.H. Messerli (ed.): *Kidney in Essential Hypertension.* Proceedings of a Course, held in New Orleans, La., U.S.A. (1983). 1984 ISBN 0-89838-616-0
36. M.P. Sambhi (ed.): *Fundamental Fault in Hypertension.* 1984 ISBN 0-89838-638-1
37. C. Marchesi (ed.): *Ambulatory Monitoring.* Cardiovascular System and Allied Applications. Proceedings of a Workshop, held in Pisa, Italy (1983). 1984 ISBN 0-89838-642-X
38. W. Kupper, R.N. MacAlpin and W. Bleifeld (eds.): *Coronary Tone in Ischemic Heart Disease.* 1984 ISBN 0-89838-646-2
39. N. Sperelakis and J.B. Caulfield (eds.): *Calcium Antagonists.* Mechanism of Action on Cardiac Muscle and Vascular Smooth Muscle. Proceedings of the 5th Annual Meeting of the American Section of the I.S.H.R., held in Hilton Head, S.C., U.S.A. (1983). 1984 ISBN 0-89838-655-1
40. Th. Godfraind, A.G. Herman and D. Wellens (eds.): *Calcium Entry Blockers in Cardiovascular and Cerebral Dysfunctions.* 1984 ISBN 0-89838-658-6
41. J. Morganroth and E.N. Moore (eds.): *Interventions in the Acute Phase of Myocardial Infarction.* Proceedings of the 4th Symposium on New Drugs and Devices, held in Philadelphia, Pa., U.S.A. (1983). 1984 ISBN 0-89838-659-4
42. F.L. Abel and W.H. Newman (eds.): *Functional Aspects of the Normal, Hypertrophied and Failing Heart.* Proceedings of the 5th Annual Meeting of the American Section of the I.S.H.R., held in Hilton Head, S.C., U.S.A. (1983) 1984 ISBN 0-89838-665-9

Developments in Cardiovascular Medicine

43. S. Sideman and R. Beyar (eds.): [3-D] *Simulation and Imaging of the Cardiac System. State of the Heart.* Proceedings of the International Henry Goldberg Workshop, held in Haifa, Israel (1984). 1985 ISBN 0-89838-687-X
44. E. van der Wall and K.I. Lie (eds.): *Recent Views on Hypertrophic Cardiomyopathy.* Proceedings of a Symposium, held in Groningen, The Netherlands (1984). 1985
ISBN 0-89838-694-2
45. R.E. Beamish, P.K. Singal and N.S. Dhalla (eds.), *Stress and Heart Disease.* Proceedings of a International Symposium, held in Winnipeg, Canada, 1984 (Vol. 1). 1985 ISBN 0-89838-709-4
46. R.E. Beamish, V. Panagia and N.S. Dhalla (eds.): *Pathogenesis of Stress-induced Heart Disease.* Proceedings of a International Symposium, held in Winnipeg, Canada, 1984 (Vol. 2). 1985 ISBN 0-89838-710-8
47. J. Morganroth and E.N. Moore (eds.): *Cardiac Arrhythmias.* New Therapeutic Drugs and Devices. Proceedings of the 5th Symposium on New Drugs and Devices, held in Philadelphia, Pa., U.S.A. (1984). 1985 ISBN 0-89838-716-7
48. P. Mathes (ed.): *Secondary Prevention in Coronary Artery Disease and Myocardial Infarction.* 1985 ISBN 0-89838-736-1
49. H.L. Stone and W.B. Weglicki (eds.): *Pathobiology of Cardiovascular Injury.* Proceedings of the 6th Annual Meeting of the American Section of the I.S.H.R., held in Oklahoma City, Okla., U.S.A. (1984). 1985 ISBN 0-89838-743-4
50. J. Meyer, R. Erbel and H.J. Rupprecht (eds.): *Improvement of Myocardial Perfusion.* Thrombolysis, Angioplasty, Bypass Surgery. Proceedings of a Symposium, held in Mainz, F.R.G. (1984). 1985 ISBN 0-89838-748-5
51. J.H.C. Reiber, P.W. Serruys and C.J. Slager (eds.): *Quantitative Coronary and Left Ventricular Cineangiography.* Methodology and Clinical Applications. 1986
ISBN 0-89838-760-4
52. R.H. Fagard and I.E. Bekaert (eds.): *Sports Cardiology.* Exercise in Health and Cardiovascular Disease. Proceedings from an International Conference, held in Knokke, Belgium (1985). 1986 ISBN 0-89838-782-5
53. J.H.C. Reiber and P.W. Serruys (eds.): *State of the Art in Quantitative Cornary Arteriography.* 1986 ISBN 0-89838-804-X
54. J. Roelandt (ed.): *Color Doppler Flow Imaging and Other Advances in Doppler Echocardiography.* 1986 ISBN 0-89838-806-6
55. E.E. van der Wall (ed.): *Noninvasive Imaging of Cardiac Metabolism.* Single Photon Scintigraphy, Positron Emission Tomography and Nuclear Magnetic Resonance. 1987
ISBN 0-89838-812-0
56. J. Liebman, R. Plonsey and Y. Rudy (eds.): *Pediatric and Fundamental Electrocardiography.* 1987 ISBN 0-89838-815-5
57. H.H. Hilger, V. Hombach and W.J. Rashkind (eds.), *Invasive Cardiovascular Therapy.* Proceedings of an International Symposium, held in Cologne, F.R.G. (1985). 1987 ISBN 0-89838-818-X
58. P.W. Serruys and G.T. Meester (eds.): *Coronary Angioplasty.* A Controlled Model for Ischemia. 1986 ISBN 0-89838-819-8
59. J.E. Tooke and L.H. Smaje (eds.): *Clinical Investigation of the Microcirculation.* Proceedings of an International Meeting, held in London, U.K. (1985). 1987
ISBN 0-89838-833-3

Developments in Cardiovascular Medicine

60. R.Th. van Dam and A. van Oosterom (eds.): *Electrocardiographic Body Surface Mapping*. Proceedings of the 3rd International Symposium on B.S.M., held in Nijmegen, The Netherlands (1985). 1986 ISBN 0-89838-834-1
61. M.P. Spencer (ed.): *Ultrasonic Diagnosis of Cerebrovascular Disease*. Doppler Techniques and Pulse Echo Imaging. 1987 ISBN 0-89838-836-8
62. M.J. Legato (ed.): *The Stressed Heart*. 1987 ISBN 0-89838-849-X
63. M.E. Safar (ed.): *Arterial and Venous Systems in Essential Hypertension*. With Assistance of G.M. London, A.Ch. Simon and Y.A. Weiss. 1987
 ISBN 0-89838-857-0
64. J. Roelandt (ed.): *Digital Techniques in Echocardiography*. 1987
 ISBN 0-89838-861-9
65. N.S. Dhalla, P.K. Singal and R.E. Beamish (eds.): *Pathology of Heart Disease*. Proceedings of the 8th Annual Meeting of the American Section of the I.S.H.R., held in Winnipeg, Canada, 1986 (Vol. 1). 1987 ISBN 0-89838-864-3
66. N.S. Dhalla, G.N. Pierce and R.E. Beamish (eds.): *Heart Function and Metabolism*. Proceedings of the 8th Annual Meeting of the American Section of the I.S.H.R., held in Winnipeg, Canada, 1986 (Vol. 2). 1987 ISBN 0-89838-865-1
67. N.S. Dhalla, I.R. Innes and R.E. Beamish (eds.): *Myocardial Ischemia*. Proceedings of a Satellite Symposium of the 30th International Physiological Congress, held in Winnipeg, Canada (1986). 1987 ISBN 0-89838-866-X
68. R.E. Beamish, V. Panagia and N.S. Dhalla (eds.): *Pharmacological Aspects of Heart Disease*. Proceedings of an International Symposium, held in Winnipeg, Canada (1986). 1987 ISBN 0-89838-867-8
69. H.E.D.J. ter Keurs and J.V. Tyberg (eds.): *Mechanics of the Circulation*. Proceedings of a Satellite Symposium of the 30th International Physiological Congress, held in Banff, Alberta, Canada (1986). 1987 ISBN 0-89838-870-8
70. S. Sideman and R. Beyar (eds.): *Activation, Metabolism and Perfusion of the Heart*. Simulation and Experimental Models. Proceedings of the 3rd Henry Goldberg Workshop, held in Piscataway, N.J., U.S.A. (1986). 1987 ISBN 0-89838-871-6
71. E. Aliot and R. Lazzara (eds.): *Ventricular Tachycardias*. From Mechanism to Therapy. 1987 ISBN 0-89838-881-3
72. A. Schneeweiss and G. Schettler: *Cardiovascular Drug Therapoy in the Elderly*. 1988
 ISBN 0-89838-883-X
73. J.V. Chapman and A. Sgalambro (eds.): *Basic Concepts in Doppler Echocardiography*. Methods of Clinical Applications based on a Multi-modality Doppler Approach. 1987 ISBN 0-89838-888-0
74. S. Chien, J. Dormandy, E. Ernst and A. Matrai (eds.): *Clinical Hemorheology*. Applications in Cardiovascular and Hematological Disease, Diabetes, Surgery and Gynecology. 1987 ISBN 0-89838-807-4
75. J. Morganroth and E.N. Moore (eds.): *Congestive Heart Failure*. Proceedings of the 7th Annual Symposium on New Drugs and Devices, held in Philadelphia, Pa., U.S.A. (1986). 1987 ISBN 0-89838-955-0
76. F.H. Messerli (ed.): *Cardiovascular Disease in the Elderly*. 2nd ed. 1988
 ISBN 0-89838-962-3
77. P.H. Heintzen and J.H. Bürsch (eds.): *Progress in Digital Angiocardiography*. 1988
 ISBN 0-89838-965-8

Developments in Cardiovascular Medicine

78. M.M. Scheinman (ed.): *Catheter Ablation of Cardiac Arrhythmias.* Basic Bioelectrical Effects and Clinical Indications. 1988   ISBN 0-89838-967-4
79. J.A.E. Spaan, A.V.G. Bruschke and A.C. Gittenberger-De Groot (eds.): *Coronary Circulation.* From Basic Mechanisms to Clinical Implications. 1987
ISBN 0-89838-978-X
80. C. Visser, G. Kan and R.S. Meltzer (eds.): *Echocardiography in Coronary Artery Disease.* 1988   ISBN 0-89838-979-8
81. A. Bayés de Luna, A. Betriu and G. Permanyer (eds.): *Therapeutics in Cardiology.* 1988   ISBN 0-89838-981-X
82. D.M. Mirvis (ed.): *Body Surface Electrocardiographic Mapping.* 1988
ISBN 0-89838-983-6
83. M.A. Konstam and J.M. Isner (eds.): *The Right Ventricle.* 1988   ISBN 0-89838-987-9
84. C.T. Kappagoda and P.V. Greenwood (eds.): *Long-term Management of Patients after Myocardial Infarction.* 1988   ISBN 0-89838-352-8
85. W.H. Gaasch and H.J. Levine (eds.): *Chronic Aortic Regurgitation.* 1988
ISBN 0-89838-364-1
86. P.K. Singal (ed.): *Oxygen Radicals in the Pathophysiology of Heart Disease.* 1988
ISBN 0-89838-375-7
87. J.H.C. Reiber and P.W. Serruys (eds.): *New Developments in Quantitative Coronary Arteriography.* 1988   ISBN 0-89838-377-3
88. J. Morganroth and E.N. Moore (eds.): *Silent Myocardial Ischemia.* Proceedings of the 8th Annual Symposium on New Drugs and Devices (1987). 1988
ISBN 0-89838-380-3
89. H.E.D.J. ter Keurs and M.I.M. Noble (eds.): *Starling's Law of the Heart Revisted.* 1988   ISBN 0-89838-382-X
90. N. Sperelakis (ed.): *Physiology and Pathophysiology of the Heart.* (Rev. ed.) 1988
ISBN 0-89838-388-9
91. J.W. de Jong (ed.): *Myocardial Energy Metabolism.* 1988   ISBN 0-89838-394-3
92. V. Hombach, H.H. Hilger and H.L. Kennedy (eds.): *Electrocardiography and Cardiac Drug Therapy.* Proceedings of an International Symposium, held in Cologne, F.R.G. (1987). 1988   ISBN 0-89838-395-1
93. H. Iwata, J.B. Lombardini and T. Segawa (eds.): *Taurine and the Heart.* 1988
ISBN 0-89838-396-X
94. M.R. Rosen and Y. Palti (eds.): *Lethal Arrhythmias Resulting from Myocardial Ischemia and Infarction.* Proceedings of the 2nd Rappaport Symposium, held in Haifa, Israel (1988). 1988   ISBN 0-89838-401-X
95. M. Iwase and I. Sotobata: *Clinical Echocardiography.* With a Foreword by M.P. Spencer. 1989   ISBN 0-7923-0004-1
96. I. Cikes (ed.): *Echocardiography in Cardiac Interventions.* 1989
ISBN 0-7923-0088-2
97. E. Rapaport (ed.): *Early Interventions in Acute Myocardial Infarction.* 1989
ISBN 0-7923-0175-7
98. M.E. Safar and F. Fouad-Tarazi (eds.): *The Heart in Hypertension.* A Tribute to Robert C. Tarazi (1925-1986). 1989   ISBN 0-7923-0197-8
99. S. Meerbaum and R. Meltzer (eds.): *Myocardial Contrast Two-dimensional Echocardiography.* 1989   ISBN 0-7923-0205-2

Developments in Cardiovascular Medicine

100. J. Morganroth and E.N. Moore (eds.): *Risk/Benefit Analysis for the Use and Approval of Thrombolytic, Antiarrhythmic, and Hypolipidemic Agents.* Proceedings of the 9th Annual Symposium on New Drugs and Devices (1988). 1989 ISBN 0-7923-0294-X
101. P.W. Serruys, R. Simon and K.J. Beatt (eds.): *PTCA - An Investigational Tool and a Non-operative Treatment of Acute Ischemia.* 1990 ISBN 0-7923-0346-6
102. I.S. Anand, P.I. Wahi and N.S. Dhalla (eds.): *Pathophysiology and Pharmacology of Heart Disease.* 1989 ISBN 0-7923-0367-9
103. G.S. Abela (ed.): *Lasers in Cardiovascular Medicine and Surgery.* Fundamentals and Technique. 1990 ISBN 0-7923-0440-3
104. H.M. Piper (ed.): *Pathophysiology of Severe Ischemic Myocardial Injury.* 1990 ISBN 0-7923-0459-4
105. S.M. Teague (ed.): *Stress Doppler Echocardiography.* 1990 ISBN 0-7923-0499-3
106. P.R. Saxena, D.I. Wallis, W. Wouters and P. Bevan (eds.): *Cardiovascular Pharmacology of 5-Hydroxytryptamine.* Prospective Therapeutic Applications. 1990 ISBN 0-7923-0502-7
107. A.P. Shepherd and P.Å. Öberg (eds.): *Laser-Doppler Blood Flowmetry.* 1990 ISBN 0-7923-0508-6
108. J. Soler-Soler, G. Permanyer-Miralda and J. Sagristà-Sauleda (eds.): *Pericardial Disease.* New Insights and Old Dilemmas. Preface by Ralph Shabetai. 1990 ISBN 0-7923-0510-8
109. J.P.M. Hamer: *Practical Echocardiography in the Adult.* With Doppler and Color-Doppler Flow Imaging. 1990 ISBN 0-7923-0670-8
110. A. Bayés de Luna, P. Brugada, J. Cosin Aguilar and F. Navarro Lopez (eds.): *Sudden Cardiac Death.* 1991 ISBN 0-7923-0716-X
111. E. Andries and R. Stroobandt (eds.): *Hemodynamics in Daily Practice.* 1991 ISBN 0-7923-0725-9
112. J. Morganroth and E.N. Moore (eds.): *Use and Approval of Antihypertensive Agents and Surrogate Endpoints for the Approval of Drugs affecting Antiarrhythmic Heart Failure and Hypolipidemia.* Proceedings of the 10th Annual Symposium on New Drugs and Devices (1989). 1990 ISBN 0-7923-0756-9
113. S. Iliceto, P. Rizzon and J.R.T.C. Roelandt (eds.): *Ultrasound in Coronary Artery Disease.* Present Role and Future Perspectives. 1990 ISBN 0-7923-0784-4
114. J.V. Chapman and G.R. Sutherland (eds.): *The Noninvasive Evaluation of Hemodynamics in Congenital Heart Disease.* Doppler Ultrasound Applications in the Adult and Pediatric Patient with Congenital Heart Disease. 1990 ISBN 0-7923-0836-0
115. G.T. Meester and F. Pinciroli (eds.): *Databases for Cardiology.* 1991 ISBN 0-7923-0886-7
116. B. Korecky and N.S. Dhalla (eds.): *Subcellular Basis of Contractile Failure.* 1990 ISBN 0-7923-0890-5
117. J.H.C. Reiber and P.W. Serruys (eds.): *Quantitative Coronary Arteriography.* 1991 ISBN 0-7923-0913-8
118. E. van der Wall and A. de Roos (eds.): *Magnetic Resonance Imaging in Coronary Artery Disease.* 1991 ISBN 0-7923-0940-5
119. V. Hombach, M. Kochs and A.J. Camm (eds.): *Interventional Techniques in Cardiovascular Medicine.* 1991 ISBN 0-7923-0956-1